Molecular Methods in
Antibiotics Discovery

Molecular Methods in Antibiotics Discovery

Editor

Charlotte A. Huber

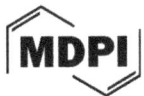

Basel • Beijing • Wuhan • Barcelona • Belgrade • Novi Sad • Cluj • Manchester

Editor
Charlotte A. Huber
Centre for Clinical Research
University of Queensland
Herston
Australia

Editorial Office
MDPI AG
Grosspeteranlage 5
4052 Basel, Switzerland

This is a reprint of articles from the Special Issue published online in the open access journal *Antibiotics* (ISSN 2079-6382) (available at: www.mdpi.com/journal/antibiotics/special_issues/Molecular_Methods).

For citation purposes, cite each article independently as indicated on the article page online and as indicated below:

Lastname, A.A.; Lastname, B.B. Article Title. *Journal Name* **Year**, *Volume Number*, Page Range.

ISBN 978-3-7258-2004-7 (Hbk)
ISBN 978-3-7258-2003-0 (PDF)
doi.org/10.3390/books978-3-7258-2003-0

© 2024 by the authors. Articles in this book are Open Access and distributed under the Creative Commons Attribution (CC BY) license. The book as a whole is distributed by MDPI under the terms and conditions of the Creative Commons Attribution-NonCommercial-NoDerivs (CC BY-NC-ND) license.

Contents

About the Editor vii

Preface ix

Charlotte A. Huber
Bacterial and Fungal Pathogens: New Weapons to Fight Them
Reprinted from: *Antibiotics* **2024**, *13*, 384, doi:10.3390/antibiotics13050384 1

Meltem Haktaniyan, Richa Sharma and Mark Bradley
Size-Controlled Ammonium-Based Homopolymers as Broad-Spectrum Antibacterials
Reprinted from: *Antibiotics* **2023**, *12*, 1320, doi:10.3390/antibiotics12081320 4

Lewis T. Ibbotson, Kirsten E. Christensen, Miroslav Genov, Alexander Pretsch, Dagmar Pretsch and Mark G. Moloney
Tricyclic Fused Lactams by Mukaiyama Cyclisation of Phthalimides and Evaluation of their Biological Activity
Reprinted from: *Antibiotics* **2023**, *12*, 9, doi:10.3390/antibiotics12010009 25

Leandro P. Bezerra, Cleverson D. T. Freitas, Ayrles F. B. Silva, Jackson L. Amaral, Nilton A. S. Neto, Rafael G. G. Silva, et al.
Synergistic Antifungal Activity of Synthetic Peptides and Antifungal Drugs against *Candida albicans* and *C. parapsilosis* Biofilms
Reprinted from: *Antibiotics* **2022**, *11*, 553, doi:10.3390/antibiotics11050553 39

Robert Penchovsky, Antoniya V. Georgieva, Vanya Dyakova, Martina Traykovska and Nikolet Pavlova
Antisense and Functional Nucleic Acids in Rational Drug Development
Reprinted from: *Antibiotics* **2024**, *13*, 221, doi:10.3390/antibiotics13030221 55

Juan Andrades-Lagos, Javier Campanini-Salinas, América Pedreros-Riquelme, Jaime Mella, Duane Choquesillo-Lazarte, P. P. Zamora, Hernán Pessoa-Mahana, et al.
Design, Synthesis, and Structure–Activity Relationship Studies of New Quinone Derivatives as Antibacterial Agents
Reprinted from: *Antibiotics* **2023**, *12*, 1065, doi:10.3390/antibiotics12061065 77

Ramasamy Kavitha, Mohammad Auwal Sa'ad, Shivkanya Fuloria, Neeraj Kumar Fuloria, Manickam Ravichandran and Pattabhiraman Lalitha
Synthesis, Characterization, Cytotoxicity Analysis and Evaluation of Novel Heterocyclic Derivatives of Benzamidine against Periodontal Disease Triggering Bacteria
Reprinted from: *Antibiotics* **2023**, *12*, 306, doi:10.3390/antibiotics12020306 103

Povilas Kavaliauskas, Birutė Grybaitė, Rita Vaickelionienė, Birutė Sapijanskaitė-Banevič, Kazimieras Anusevičius, Agnė Kriaučiūnaitė, et al.
Synthesis and Development of *N*-2,5-Dimethylphenylthioureido Acid Derivatives as Scaffolds for New Antimicrobial Candidates Targeting Multidrug-Resistant Gram-Positive Pathogens
Reprinted from: *Antibiotics* **2023**, *12*, 220, doi:10.3390/antibiotics12020220 117

Hansa Raj KC, David F. Gilmore and Mohammad A. Alam
Development of 4-[4-(Anilinomethyl)-3-phenyl-pyrazol-1-yl] Benzoic Acid Derivatives as Potent Anti-Staphylococci and Anti-Enterococci Agents
Reprinted from: *Antibiotics* **2022**, *11*, 939, doi:10.3390/antibiotics11070939 144

Atiah H. Almalki, Walid Hamdy Hassan, Amany Belal, Ahmed Farghali, Romissaa M. Saleh, Abeer Enaiet Allah, et al.
Exploring the Antimicrobial Activity of Sodium Titanate Nanotube Biomaterials in Combating Bone Infections: An In Vitro and In Vivo Study
Reprinted from: *Antibiotics* 2023, 12, 799, doi:10.3390/antibiotics12050799 160

Fayez Althobaiti, Ola A. Abu Ali, Islam Kamal, Mohammad Y. Alfaifi, Ali A. Shati, Eman Fayad, et al.
New Ionic Liquid Microemulsion-Mediated Synthesis of Silver Nanoparticles for Skin Bacterial Infection Treatments
Reprinted from: *Antibiotics* 2023, 12, 247, doi:10.3390/antibiotics12020247 182

Alessio Nocentini, Clemente Capasso and Claudiu T. Supuran
Carbonic Anhydrase Inhibitors as Novel Antibacterials in the Era of Antibiotic Resistance: Where Are We Now?
Reprinted from: *Antibiotics* 2023, 12, 142, doi:10.3390/antibiotics12010142 200

About the Editor

Charlotte A. Huber

Dr Charlotte Preston-Huber studied Pharmacy at the Swiss Federal Institute of Technology in Zurich, Switzerland, and completed her PhD in Microbiology at the Swiss Tropical and Public Health Institute in Basel, Switzerland.

Dr Preston-Huber was a Postdoctoral Research Fellow at the University of Queensland Centre for Clinical Research (Herston, Australia, Infection and Immunity Group), where she also received two annual grants by the Swiss National Science Foundation. Title: "Monitoring of structural alterations and intracellular concentrations of ß-lactam and aminoglycoside antibiotics using mass spectrometry as a rapid method to detect antibiotic resistance".

Her other activities include being a Ship Pharmacist on the Mercy Ship Anastasis, a Member of the Board of Mercy Ships Switzerland, and she is currently a Member of the Advisory Board of the Africa Capacity Building Council.

Preface

I want to thank my friend, Professor Ruth Ruprecht, for critically reviewing the draft of the Editorial and advising me regarding its content.

The introduction of antibiotics into clinical practice in the 20th century has revolutionised modern medicine, extending the average human lifespan by more than two decades. The discovery of penicillin in 1928 was the beginning of the golden age of antibiotic discovery, which peaked in the 1950s. However, today, only a few new antibiotics are in the clinical trial pipeline.

Antibiotics are mostly derived from natural sources, and antibiotic resistance has been known to exist since prehistoric times. Extensive use of antibiotics has resulted in a strong selective pressure and, consequently, the advancement of resistant bacterial strains, leading to the current antibiotic resistance crisis. New antibiotic compounds are urgently needed.

Financial incentives for the development of new antibiotics are limited, as antibiotics are usually inexpensive and only used for a short time. Additionally, new antibiotics are often reserved as a last resort, potentially limiting their use even further. This highlights the need for publicly funded academic laboratories to take on the task of antibiotic discovery.

This Special Issue welcomed manuscripts that describe new compounds with antibiotic activity.

Charlotte A. Huber
Editor

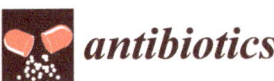

Editorial

Bacterial and Fungal Pathogens: New Weapons to Fight Them

Charlotte A. Huber

Centre for Clinical Research, The University of Queensland, Herston, Brisbane, QLD 4029, Australia; ca.prestonhuber@gmail.com

In high-income countries, degenerative diseases are the primary cause of death. In the past, however, most people worldwide were killed by infections and did not live long enough to die from degenerative diseases. Life expectancy was much lower, and in many cases, infant mortality exceeded ten percent.

One highly virulent pathogen was *Yersinia pestis*, the causative agent of the plague. It is considered to have killed between one- and two-thirds of Europe's population in one of its pandemics (1347–1352). Centuries later, but still in the pre-antibiotic era, the plague was held at bay by human intervention. Nowadays, the plague is treatable with antibiotics and is no longer such a menace [1].

The introduction of antibiotics has revolutionised modern medicine. In addition to the treatment of infectious diseases, antibiotics are used for prevention during medical procedures, such as cancer treatment and surgery. However, bacteria have been around for billions of years and have developed methods to evade compounds that are toxic to them. Extensive use of antibiotics has resulted in selection pressure in favour of resistant strains, causing the prevalence of antibiotic resistance to rise steadily. As a result, we run the risk of approaching a post-antibiotic era, and some pandrug-resistant bacterial strains are already untreatable.

Decades ago, the emergence of resistance was met with the introduction of new antibiotics into clinical practice. More recently, a lack of success and rising costs have resulted in large pharmaceutical companies discontinuing antibiotic discovery and development. As a result, few candidates are in the clinical trial pipeline while resistance continues to evolve and disseminate. Deaths associated with antibiotic resistance have exceeded one million, and, unless the situation improves, millions more are expected to die from previously easily treatable infections. New weapons to combat bacterial infections are imperative [2].

This Special Issue sought contributions on molecular methods in antibiotic discovery. Eleven papers were published, describing novel compounds, formulations, or repurposed drugs (https://www.mdpi.com/journal/antibiotics/special_issues/Molecular_Methods; accessed on 30 March 2024).

Most papers describe novel compounds, including homopolymers (contribution 1), cyclic imides (contribution 2), antimicrobial peptides (contribution 3), nucleic acids (contribution 4), and derivatives of quinone (contribution 5), benzamidine (contribution 6), thiazole (contribution 7), and pyrazole (contribution 8). Two papers describe novel galenic formulations of titanate (contribution 9) or silver nanoparticles (contribution 10), respectively. One contribution describes repurposed drugs (contribution 11).

Fungi, being eukaryotes, are distinctly different from bacteria. However, drug resistance has also become a concern for fungal infections, particularly in the immunocompromised. Resistance to antimicrobials is prevalent among several microbial kingdoms. Although systemic treatment of fungal infections has relied on only four classes of antifungals, fungi have been neglected when aiming to address the threat of antimicrobial resistance [3]. Furthermore, fungi are able to build interkingdom biofilms with bacteria, potentially worsening the outcome. While most of the contributions to this Special Issue

Citation: Huber, C.A. Bacterial and Fungal Pathogens: New Weapons to Fight Them. *Antibiotics* **2024**, *13*, 384. https://doi.org/10.3390/antibiotics13050384

Received: 4 April 2024
Accepted: 22 April 2024
Published: 24 April 2024

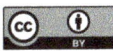

Copyright: © 2024 by the author. Licensee MDPI, Basel, Switzerland. This article is an open access article distributed under the terms and conditions of the Creative Commons Attribution (CC BY) license (https://creativecommons.org/licenses/by/4.0/).

describe compounds with antibacterial activity, two papers describe antimicrobial candidates that have both antibacterial and antifungal properties (contributions 7 and 9), and one paper describes compounds with antifungal activity (contribution 3).

Biofilms protect microorganisms from external influences, such as host immune responses and pharmaceuticals. This further exacerbates the problem of antimicrobial resistance. Three papers contributing to this Special Issue describe compounds (contributions 3 and 8) or formulations (contribution 10) with antibiofilm activity.

In vitro toxicity testing using cell lines was performed in many cases. Although describing a novel antibacterial mechanism of action, one contribution to this Special Issue describes repurposed drugs. Having undergone extensive safety testing, including in humans, repurposed drugs can undergo clinical trials relatively quickly and inexpensively (contribution 11).

Antimicrobials in preclinical research are innovative and diverse. However, less than 50 antibiotic candidates were in the clinical trial pipeline in December 2020. At the same time, the number of candidates for cancer treatment was estimated to be in excess of 1300. Not only did large pharmaceutical companies discontinue the development of new antibiotics, but smaller companies that took over suffered great financial loss or even insolvency. Paradoxically, this happened upon successful introduction of their product into clinical practice. New antibiotics are often inexpensive, and being used as last-line options, they have low sales volumes. A satisfactory return on investment cannot be guaranteed, even if a product successfully reaches the market. Therefore, antibiotic candidates are abandoned because of a lack of funding in preclinical and early clinical research stages (referred to as the "valleys of death"). What complicates the issue even further is that many experts in antibiotic development have retired, and there is little financial incentive for young scientists to enter the field.

Meanwhile, the development of novel antifungals faces similar issues. The clinical trials necessary for market approval are time-consuming and may cost hundreds of millions of US dollars. In the case of antifungals, too, it is a challenge to reach a market big enough to make a development project financially viable [3].

It has become clear that classic financing models give little incentive for the pharmaceutical industry to develop new antimicrobials. However, some funding strategies have been suggested, such as grants for basic antimicrobial drug discovery and preclinical research, and market entry rewards.

Finding new weapons to fight bacterial and fungal pathogens is of great urgency and importance to the public. However, free-market principles may not get us there, and we may instead depend on foundations and well-invested taxpayers' money [2–4].

Conflicts of Interest: The author declares no conflicts of interest.

List of Contributions:

1. Haktaniyan, M.; Sharma, R.; Bradley, M. Size-Controlled Ammonium-Based Homopolymers as Broad-Spectrum Antibacterials. *Antibiotics* **2023**, *12*, 1320. https://doi.org/10.3390/antibiotics12081320.
2. Ibbotson, L.T.; Christensen, K.E.; Genov, M.; Pretsch, A.; Pretsch, D.; Moloney, M.G. Tricyclic Fused Lactams by Mukaiyama Cyclisation of Phthalimides and Evaluation of their Biological Activity. *Antibiotics* **2023**, *12*, 9. https://doi.org/10.3390/antibiotics12010009.
3. Bezerra, L.P.; Freitas, C.D.T.; Silva, A.F.B.; Amaral, J.L.; Neto, N.A.S.; Silva, R.G.G.; Parra, A.L.C.; Goldman, G.H.; Oliveira, J.T.A.; Mesquita, F.P.; et al. Synergistic Antifungal Activity of Synthetic Peptides and Antifungal Drugs against *Candida albicans* and *C. parapsilosis* Biofilms. *Antibiotics* **2022**, *11*, 553. https://doi.org/10.3390/antibiotics11050553.
4. Penchovsky, R.; Georgieva, A.V.; Dyakova, V.; Traykovska, M.; Pavlova, N. Antisense and Functional Nucleic Acids in Rational Drug Development. *Antibiotics* **2024**, *13*, 221. https://doi.org/10.3390/antibiotics13030221.

5. Andrades-Lagos, J.; Campanini-Salinas, J.; Pedreros-Riquelme, A.; Mella, J.; Choquesillo-Lazarte, D.; Zamora, P.P.; Pessoa-Mahana, H.; Burbulis, I.; Vásquez-Velásquez, D. Design, Synthesis, and Structure–Activity Relationship Studies of New Quinone Derivatives as Antibacterial Agents. *Antibiotics* **2023**, *12*, 1065. https://doi.org/10.3390/antibiotics12061065.
6. Kavitha, R.; Sa'ad, M.A.; Fuloria, S.; Fuloria, N.K.; Ravichandran, M.; Lalitha, P. Synthesis, Characterization, Cytotoxicity Analysis and Evaluation of Novel Heterocyclic Derivatives of Benzamidine against Periodontal Disease Triggering Bacteria. *Antibiotics* **2023**, *12*, 306. https://doi.org/10.3390/antibiotics12020306.
7. Kavaliauskas, P.; Grybaitė, B.; Vaickelionienė, R.; Sapijanskaitė-Banevič, B.; Anusevičius, K.; Kriaučiūnaitė, A.; Smailienė, G.; Petraitis, V.; Petraitienė, R.; Naing, E.; et al. Synthesis and Development of N-2,5-Dimethylphenylthioureido Acid Derivatives as Scaffolds for New Antimicrobial Candidates Targeting Multidrug-Resistant Gram-Positive Pathogens. *Antibiotics* **2023**, *12*, 220. https://doi.org/10.3390/antibiotics12020220.
8. Raj KC, H.; Gilmore, D.F.; Alam, M.A. Development of 4-[4-(Anilinomethyl)-3-phenyl-pyrazol-1-yl] Benzoic Acid Derivatives as Potent Anti-Staphylococci and Anti-Enterococci Agents. *Antibiotics* **2022**, *11*, 939. https://doi.org/10.3390/antibiotics11070939.
9. Almalki, A.H.; Hassan, W.H.; Belal, A.; Farghali, A.; Saleh, R.M.; Allah, A.E.; Abdelwahab, A.; Lee, S.; Hassan, A.H.E.; Ghoneim, M.M.; et al. Exploring the Antimicrobial Activity of Sodium Titanate Nanotube Biomaterials in Combating Bone Infections: An In Vitro and In Vivo Study. *Antibiotics* **2023**, *12*, 799. https://doi.org/10.3390/antibiotics12050799.
10. Althobaiti, F.; Abu Ali, O.A.; Kamal, I.; Alfaifi, M.Y.; Shati, A.A.; Fayad, E.; Elbehairi, S.E.I.; Elshaarawy, R.F.M.; El-Fattah, W.A. New Ionic Liquid Microemulsion-Mediated Synthesis of Silver Nanoparticles for Skin Bacterial Infection Treatments. *Antibiotics* **2023**, *12*, 247. https://doi.org/10.3390/antibiotics12020247.
11. Nocentini, A.; Capasso, C.; Supuran, C.T. Carbonic Anhydrase Inhibitors as Novel Antibacterials in the Era of Antibiotic Resistance: Where Are We Now? *Antibiotics* **2023**, *12*, 142. https://doi.org/10.3390/antibiotics12010142.

References

1. Shaw-Taylor, L. An Introduction to the History of Infectious Diseases, Epidemics and the Early Phases of the Long-Run Decline in Mortality. *Econ. Hist. Rev.* **2020**, *73*, E1–E19. [CrossRef] [PubMed]
2. Cook, M.A.; Wright, G.D. The Past, Present, and Future of Antibiotics. *Sci. Transl. Med.* **2022**, *14*, eabo7793. [CrossRef] [PubMed]
3. Fisher, M.C.; Alastruey-Izquierdo, A.; Berman, J.; Bicanic, T.; Bignell, E.M.; Bowyer, P.; Bromley, M.; Brüggemann, R.; Garber, G.; Cornely, O.A.; et al. Tackling the Emerging Threat of Antifungal Resistance to Human Health. *Nat. Rev. Microbiol.* **2022**, *20*, 557–571. [CrossRef] [PubMed]
4. Anderson, M.; Panteli, D.; van Kessel, R.; Ljungqvist, G.; Colombo, F.; Mossialos, E. Challenges and Opportunities for Incentivising Antibiotic Research and Development in Europe. *Lancet Reg. Health Eur.* **2023**, *33*, 100705. [CrossRef] [PubMed]

Disclaimer/Publisher's Note: The statements, opinions and data contained in all publications are solely those of the individual author(s) and contributor(s) and not of MDPI and/or the editor(s). MDPI and/or the editor(s) disclaim responsibility for any injury to people or property resulting from any ideas, methods, instructions or products referred to in the content.

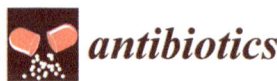

Article

Size-Controlled Ammonium-Based Homopolymers as Broad-Spectrum Antibacterials

Meltem Haktaniyan [1], Richa Sharma [1] and Mark Bradley [1,2,*]

[1] EaStCHEM, School of Chemistry, University of Edinburgh, Joseph Black Building, West Mains Road, Edinburgh EH9 3FJ, UK; meltemhaktaniyan@gmail.com (M.H.); cftri.ftbe.richa@gmail.com (R.S.)

[2] Precision Healthcare University Research Institute, Queen Mary University of London, Whitechapel, Empire House, London E1 1HH, UK

* Correspondence: m.bradley@qmul.ac.uk

Abstract: Ammonium group containing polymers possess inherent antimicrobial properties, effectively eliminating or preventing infections caused by harmful microorganisms. Here, homopolymers based on monomers containing ammonium groups were synthesized via Reversible Addition Fragmentation Chain Transfer Polymerization (RAFT) and evaluated as potential antibacterial agents. The antimicrobial activity was evaluated against Gram-positive (*M. luteus* and *B. subtilis*) and Gram-negative bacteria (*E. coli* and *S. typhimurium*). Three polymers, poly(diallyl dimethyl ammonium chloride), poly([2-(methacryloyloxy)ethyl]trimethylammonium chloride), and poly(vinyl benzyl trimethylammonium chloride), were examined to explore the effect of molecular weight (10 kDa, 20 kDa, and 40 kDa) on their antimicrobial activity and toxicity to mammalian cells. The mechanisms of action of the polymers were investigated with dye-based assays, while Scanning Electron Microscopy (SEM) showed collapsed and fused bacterial morphologies due to the interactions between the polymers and components of the bacterial cell envelope, with some polymers proving to be bactericidal and others bacteriostatic, while being non-hemolytic. Among all the homopolymers, the most active, non-Gram-specific polymer was poly([2-(methacryloyloxy)ethyl]trimethylammonium chloride), with a molecular weight of 40 kDa, with minimum inhibitory concentrations between 16 and 64 µg/mL, showing a bactericidal mode of action mediated by disruption of the cytoplasmic membrane. This homopolymer could be useful in biomedical applications such as surface dressings and in areas such as eye infections.

Keywords: antimicrobial; bactericidal; quaternary ammonium; RAFT polymerization

1. Introduction

Infection and contamination caused by microorganisms has a long, global, historical precedence, with diseases such as tuberculosis (TB), leprosy, syphilis, and "plagues" causing enormous levels of death and social challenge. The reduced effectiveness of existing antibiotics due to abuse, misuse, or overuse has led to huge increases in antimicrobial resistance and is, for example, a major problem in the area of TB, with drug-resistant and extreme drug-resistant organisms. According to a systematic analysis of the global burden associated with drug-resistant infections (excluding TB), it was estimated that 1.27 million deaths were attributable to resistant bacteria (notably *E. coli*, *S. aureus*, and *K. pneumonia*) [1]. Thus, antimicrobial agents or materials that act by alternative processes and mechanisms are important in eradicating pathogenic microorganisms. Over the past few decades, antimicrobial polymers have emerged as promising agents in surface coatings [2–5] and as materials that might, in certain situations, replace existing antimicrobials, e.g., for skin infections and topical wound dressings [6–8]. As such, huge efforts have been made in the synthesis and application of polymers as broad-spectrum antimicrobials [9–13].

Bacteria are generally classified into two groups, either Gram-positive or Gram-negative, based on their distinguishable cell envelopes. Although the inner or cytoplasmic

Citation: Haktaniyan, M.; Sharma, R.; Bradley, M. Size-Controlled Ammonium-Based Homopolymers as Broad-Spectrum Antibacterials. *Antibiotics* **2023**, *12*, 1320. https://doi.org/10.3390/antibiotics12081320

Academic Editor: Charlotte A. Huber

Received: 31 July 2023
Revised: 8 August 2023
Accepted: 14 August 2023
Published: 16 August 2023

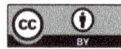

Copyright: © 2023 by the authors. Licensee MDPI, Basel, Switzerland. This article is an open access article distributed under the terms and conditions of the Creative Commons Attribution (CC BY) license (https://creativecommons.org/licenses/by/4.0/).

membranes of both bacteria resemble each other, the outer envelopes are highly distinctive, with a thick, crosslinked peptidoglycan surrounding the cytoplasmic membrane in Gram-positive bacteria. In Gram-negative bacteria, a thinner peptidoglycan layer, with an additional outer membrane layer containing phospholipids and lipopolysaccharides, is found [14]. As might be imagined, the interaction between cationic polymers and bacteria happens due to a variety of reasons, depending on the bacterium in question. Thus, the lipopolysaccharides within the outer layer of the cell membrane in Gram-negative bacteria are formally negatively charged at physiological pH [14–16] and will interact with positively charged polymers. The cell membranes of Gram-positive bacteria are likewise formally "negatively charged", in this case due to high levels of teichoic and lipoteichoic acids [17,18]. In addition, it is well known that cationic materials bind or target specific bacterial components, such as conventional cationic antibiotics including polymyxin, which binds Lipid A [19,20], brevibacillin, which binds lipoteichoic acid [21], and nisin, which binds lipids on the cytoplasmic membranes of Gram-positive bacteria to disturb peptidoglycan synthesis [22]. As such, the rationale for cationic polymers (with their enormous diversity) being able to interact with microorganisms is strong. In addition, cationic antimicrobial polymers are chemically robust compared to conventional antibiotics [23], and their applicability in wound healing [24], contact lenses [25], and as surface coatings in biomedical devices [26,27] makes them attractive tools in the fight against pathogens.

An important class of cationic antimicrobial polymers are those that contain ammonium groups [28–30], which have often been added to enhance the antimicrobial activity of existing materials [31–33] and have been shown to impart algistatic [34], bacteriostatic or bactericidal [35], tuberculostatic [36], sporostatic [5], fungistatic [37] or fungicidal [38], and virucidal [39] activity. The antimicrobial mode of action of ammonium-group-containing polymers is not fully understood but is believed to start with the binding of the cationic groups of the polymer onto the various negatively charged bacteria cell envelope components (mentioned above) via electrostatic interactions, leading to the disorganization of its structure and the leakage of low-molecular-weight components [40,41]. The strength of the antimicrobial activity of the ammonium polymers depends on the molecular weight of the polymer [42,43], the position of the cationic center (i.e., side chain or main chain) [44], the morphology and architecture of the polymer [45], the polymer's hydrophobic/hydrophilic balance [46,47], and perhaps the nature of the counter anion [48].

Ammonium-group-containing polymers are typically synthesized either directly from ammonium-group-bearing monomers or the quaternization of the amine groups of polymers by alkyl halides/reductive amination or protonation. Over the past few decades, controlled living polymerization techniques have enabled the fine regulation of the molecular weight distributions of synthesized polymers. One such method is Reversible Addition Fragmentation Chain Transfer Polymerization (RAFT), a powerful technique that allows the design and building of complex, versatile polymer architectures and is applicable to a wide range of monomers and solvents, including water [49]. Importantly, it does not use toxic metal salts, making it a perfect method for the synthesis of polymers for biomedical applications [50]. Antimicrobial polymers offer broad chemical scope, as they can be readily prepared from numerous monomers, with control of the molecular weights of polymers [51–53]. Although antibacterial polymers with ammonium groups as copolymers have been reported extensively [46,47,52], few reports have looked at the antimicrobial activity of the homopolymers of ammonium-based monomers that have been used here [36,38,54–58]. Among the cationic polymers, poly(2-(dimethylamino)ethyl methacrylate (PDMAEMA) is probably the most commonly used material (the amine becoming an ammonium ion upon protonation) for use in biomedical applications, with its incorporation into films, surface coatings, and synthesis via various polymerization techniques, such as Atom Transfer Radical Polymerization (ATRP), RAFT, etc. A report [36] on polymers (again cationic via physiological protonation) synthesized through RAFT polymerization, including poly(2-(dimethylamino)ethyl methacrylate) (4.5 kDa, 6.1 kDa, and 11.2 kDa), poly(2-(dimethylamino)ethyl acrylate) (11 kDa and 3.2 kDa), and poly(2-

aminoethylmethacrylate) (11.2 kDa), showed antimicrobial activity against *M. smegmatis* and Gram-negative (*E. coli* and *P. putida*) bacteria. PDMAEMAs selectively killed mycobacteria over Gram-negative bacteria, while the membrane lytic activity of PDMAEMA was comparatively low, giving a good selectivity window.

Cationic polymers can show cytotoxic effects [59] due to their interactions with the cell membrane via non-specific electrostatic interactions [60–62]. It has been shown that polycations possessing a higher molecular weight may exhibit greater toxicity; however, this was based upon a restricted range of polymers [63]. Amine- and guanidine-functionalized copolymers showed a correlation between the number of cationic groups and their minimum inhibitory concentration, although the degree of polymerization breadth made it complex to ascertain the effect of the larger and smaller polymers within the ensemble. Increased ratios of cationic groups can induced hemolysis [64] and an investigation to determine the cytotoxicity of PDMAEMAs (43 kDa–915 kDa) showed that the smallest polymer (43 kDa) exhibited extremely high toxicity on human brain microvascular endothelial cells [65], while the cytotoxicity and cellular membrane disruption of HepG2 cells by rhodamine B end-labeled PDMAEMAs (11–48 kDa) synthesized via ATRP showed that the shorter polymers (Mw < 17 kDa) showed reduced toxicity [60].

In this study, we focused on ammonium group containing homopolymers synthesized via RAFT polymerization. Specifically, we explored the impact of molecular weight on the antimicrobial activity, cytotoxicity, and biocompatibility, as well as their antimicrobial mode of action. A key advantage of these polymers is the fact that there is no need for modification, such as quaternization which typically requires alkylating agents to drive full functionalization. At the outset, five different monomers were polymerized via RAFT polymerization to give 20 kDa polymers, and the antimicrobial activity of the homopolymers was analyzed on Gram-negative (*S. typhimurium*, *E. coli*) and Gram-positive (*B. subtilis*, *M. luteus*) bacteria. Poly(diallyl dimethyl ammonium chloride) (PDADMAC) showed the best inhibition across all the bacterial strains and, due to their limited toxicity, poly([2-(methacryloyloxy)ethyl]trimethylammonium chloride) and poly(vinyl benzyl trimethylammonium chloride) were also selected, to investigate the effect of molecular weight (10, 20, and 40 kDa) on their antimicrobial activity and mechanisms of action.

2. Results and Discussion

2.1. Synthesis and Characterization of the Homopolymers

It is known that the antimicrobial activity of cationic polymers can be dependent on the type of monomer used and their hydrophobic content, charge density, molecular weight, and/or architecture [43,44,46,48]. The selected monomers have been reported as cationic blocks for copolymers to prepare surface coatings, hydrogels, and for gene delivery. Five cationic homopolymers, using commercially available ammonium-group-containing monomers, were hereby synthesized by RAFT polymerization, as described in Figure 1. The monomers were chosen as having either quaternary ammonium groups (diallyldimethyl ammonium chloride, [2-(methacryloyloxy)ethyl]trimethylammonium chloride, vinylbenzyl trimethylammonium chloride, 3-[(methacryloylamino)propyl]trimethylammonium chloride) or a tertiary amine (2-(dimethylamio)ethyl methacrylate, which will be protonated at physiological pH (average pKa of 7.5)) [66].

PDMAEMAs and their antibacterial actions have been studied in the literature [51,55]. It has been reported that lower-molecular-weight polymers can penetrate into Gram-positive bacteria more efficiently than their higher-molecular-weight counterparts, with cationic polyacrylates (5–10 kDa) optimal for antimicrobial activity against *S. aureus* [67]; however, there is little else known about the effect of their molecular weights on their activity or toxicity in biomedical applications. Here, we synthesized homopolymers using five different monomers, initially looking at polymers with a molecular weight of 20 kDa, before the synthesis of the chosen polymers with three different molecular weights (10, 20, and 40 kDa) to explore their antibacterial activity/mechanism and toxicity towards mammalian cells. GPC analysis of the polymers typically showed narrow, unimodal peaks with the polymerizations carried out in an aqueous environment, with the exception of 2-(dimethylamino)ethyl methacrylate, which was polymerized in ethanol (see Table 1).

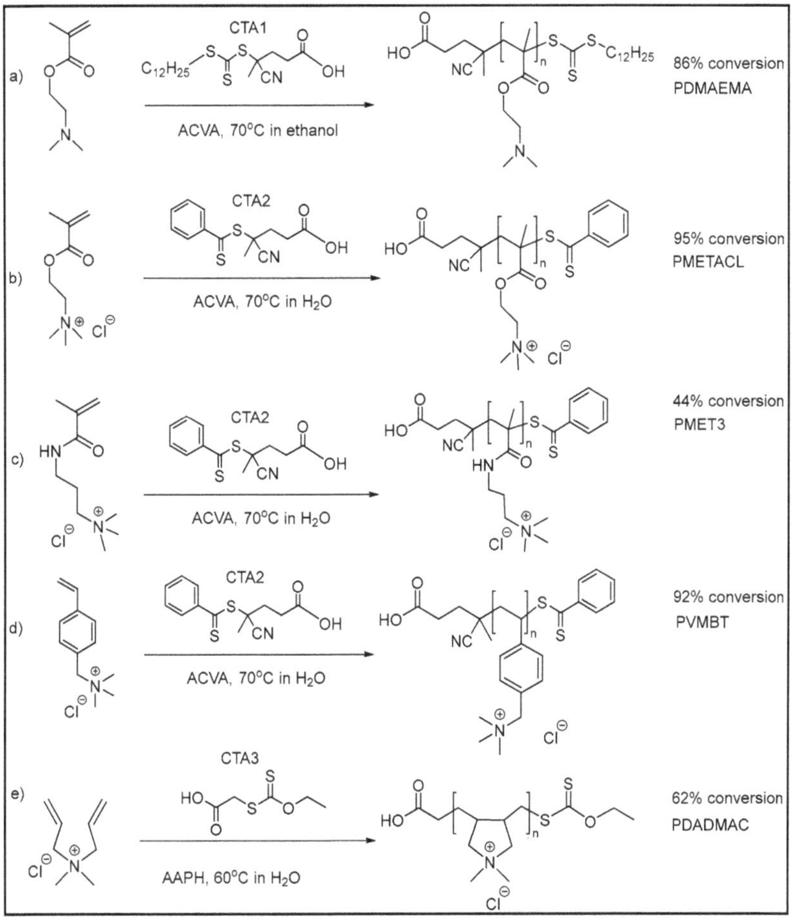

Figure 1. RAFT polymerization of quaternary ammonium-group-bearing monomers with final monomer conversion levels. (**a**) 2-(dimethylamino)ethyl methacrylate; (**b**) [2 (methacryloyloxy)ethyl]trimethylammonium chloride); (**c**) [3 (methacryloylamino)propyl]trimethylammonium chloride; (**d**) vinylbenzyl trimethylammonium chloride; and (**e**) diallyldimethylammonium chloride. Chain transfer agents: CTA1:4-cyano-4-[(dodecylsulfanylthiocarbonyl)sulfanyl]pentanoic acid, CTA2:4-cyano-4-(phenylcarbonothioylthio)pentanoic acid, CTA3:S-ethoxythiocarbonyl mercaptoacetic acid. Initiators: ACVA: 4,4-azobis(4-cyanovaleric acid), AAPH:2,2'-azobis(2-methylpropionamidine)dihydrochloride.

The polymerization of [2-(methacryloyloxy)ethyl]trimethylammonium chloride in water with 4-cyano-4-[(dodecyl sulfanyl thiocarbonyl)sulfanyl]pentanoic acid) (CTA1) was not achieved due to the limited solubility of CTA1 in aqueous environments. Water was the best solvent for the chain transfer agent 4-cyano-4-(phenylcarbonothioylthio) pentanoic acid (CTA2) with [2-(methacryloyloxy)ethyl]trimethylammonium chloride and gave the polymer in 5 h with 95% monomer conversion. GPC analysis showed a narrow, unimodal peak for the polymers (Mn calc 39.7 kDa, Mn GPC 37 kDa, Mw 39 kDa, PDI 1.03). It is worth noting that this is the first reported homopolymer synthesis of poly

[2-(methacryloyloxy)ethyl]trimethylammonium chloride (PMEATCL) in the presence of the chain transfer agent 4-cyano-4-(phenylcarbonothioylthio)pentanoic acid and the water-soluble azo initiator 4,4-azobis (4-cyanovaleric acid). Similarly, the polymerization of vinyl benzyl trimethylammonium chloride was achieved with high conversion of the monomer to the polymer under similar conditions (Mn calc: 37.5 kDa, Mn GPC 23 kDa, Mw GPC 27 kDa, PDI 1.18). Meanwhile, 10 and 20 kDa polymers of PVMBT and PMETACL were synthesized by changing the [chain transfer agent]/[initiator] ratios. The polymerization of 3-[(methacryloylamino)propyl]trimethylammonium chloride was carried out under similar conditions; however, only 44% conversion was obtained after 24 h reaction (giving a polymer of approximately 20 kDa). GPC analysis of PVMBT and PMET3 showed polymers smaller than those calculated, perhaps explained by the structural differences in these homopolymers and the standard polymers used in GPC calibration (polyethylene glycols).

Table 1. Cationic homopolymers synthesized via RAFT polymerization. Monomer to initiator ratios, chain transfer agent to initiator ratios, calculated molecular weights (obtained from monomer conversions as analyzed by ^{1}H NMR and molecular weight obtained by GPC), and PDI values.

Code	Polymer	CTA	[M]/[I]	[CTA]/[I]	Mn Calc.	Mn-GPC	Mw-GPC	PDI
P1	PDMAEMA	1	167	6	23.0 kDa	22 kDa	28 kDa	1.29
P2	PMETACL	2	100	5	17.1 kDa	17 kDa	20 kDa	1.19
P3	PMET3	2	215	5	23.1 kDa	14 kDa	16 kDa	1.18
P4	PVMBT	2	190	7	20.8 kDa	14 kDa	16 kDa	1.11
P5	PDADMAC	3	175	3.3	17.5 kDa	18 kDa	24 kDa	1.36

The RAFT polymerization of diallyldimethylammonium chloride was challenging due to poor monomer reactivity; indeed, monomers such diallyldimethylammonium chloride are typically classified as "less activated" and require xanthate- or dithiocarbamate-based chain transfer agents [68]. Thus, the water-soluble xanthate-based chain transfer agent S-ethoxythiocarbonyl mercaptoacetic acid (CTA3) was synthesized [69] by reacting potassium ethyl xanthogenate with bromoacetic acid (91% yield) (see Figure S1), and the polymerization was carried out at 60 °C in the presence of the chain transfer agent and the water-soluble azo initiator 2,2′-azobis(2-methylpropionamidine)dihydrochloride. GPC analysis showed a narrow, unimodal peak for the polymer (Mn 18 kDa and Mw 25 kDa (PDI of 1.40) at 62% conversion (after 24 h). Figure 1 shows the details of the polymerization conditions and GPC analysis of the polymers (NMR spectra of the synthesized polymers are provided in the Supplementary Materials, Figures S2–S6).

2.2. Minimum Inhibitory Concentrations of the Polymers

The minimum inhibitory concentrations (MIC) of the polymers were determined against Gram-negative (B. subtilis, E. coli) and Gram-positive (M. luteus, S. typhimurium) bacteria by the resazurin-based microtiter viability assay. The blue dye, resazurin (7-hydroxy-3H-phenoxazin-3-one-10-oxide), can be irreversibly reduced to the pink, and highly red fluorescent, resorufin, by oxidoreductase within viable cells (resorufin can be further reduced to a colorless and non-fluorescent molecule, hydroresorufin). Briefly, serially diluted polymers were added to bacterial cultures to assess the concentration at which bacterial growth ceased. Color changes were observed visibly and spectrometrically. All assays were carried out in triplicate and the results of this are shown in Table 2. The MICs varied in the range of 16–64 µg/mL (Table 2). Expressing the data in terms of molarity (based on the average molecular weights of the polymers) displays their comparative strengths in an alternative manner and perhaps enables a fairer comparison between polymers with different molecular weights, and with conventional antibiotics, which have much lower molecular weights. As can be seen from Table 2, PDADMAC showed the best inhibition against all bacteria screened.

Table 2. Minimum inhibitory concentrations of the synthesized homopolymers. Concentrations in µM are based on the average molecular weight of the polymer.

Polymer	Code	B. subtilis		E. coli		M. luteus		S. typhimurium	
		µg/mL	µM	µg/mL	µM	µg/mL	µM	µg/mL	µM
PDMAEMA	P1	32	1.6	32	1.6	32	1.6	32	1.6
PMETACL	P2	64	1.9	64	1.9	64	1.9	64	1.9
PMET3	P3	32	1.4	32	1.5	16	0.7	64	2.8
PVBMT	P4	32	0.9	64	1.7	64	1.7	64	1.7
PDADMAC	P5	16	0.9	16	0.9	16	0.9	32	1.8
Standard Antibiotics		Clindamycin		Gentamicin		Gentamicin		Chloramphenicol	
		4	9.4	0.5	1.1	0.5	1.1	1	3.1

The toxicity of the homopolymers was analyzed on HeLa cells via an MTT assay 1.25–10 µM (25–200 µg/mL—see Figure S7). This showed that PMETACL and PVBMT were the least toxic cytotoxic polymers (to HeLa cells), and since neither of these homopolymers has been investigated previously, with respect to antimicrobial activity, they were selected alongside PDADMAC for further investigation.

2.3. Investigation of the Molecular Weight and Antimicrobial Activity

The antimicrobial activity of cationic polymers is influenced by several factors, including the molecular weight, the hydrophobicity/hydrophilicity balance, the positions of cationic units, and the polymer architecture [13,70]. Literature [71] suggests that the larger the polymer (Mw > 100 kDa), the greater the biocidal effects, until supposed permeability limitations come into play and activity falls. However, such studies have typically used polydisperse polymers. Here, we targeted monodisperse polymers with molecular weights between 10 and 40 kDa, rationalizing that smaller polymers would be more likely to penetrate into bacteria while the largest polymers might be expected to interact with the outer membranes of Gram–negative bacteria, although the cumulative effect of additional monomer units could contribute to the antibacterial properties of the polymers. Small polymers have advantages over small molecules as, due to their mechanisms of action, they are unlikely to be subjected to classic resistance mechanisms. In this context, three different molecular weights of PDADMAC, PMETACL, and PVBMT were synthesized via RAFT polymerization (Table 3) (for GPC analysis of polymers see Figure S8).

Table 3. Properties of PDADMAC, PMETACL, and PVMBT synthesized with different molecular weights (approx. 10 kDa, 20 kDa, and 40 kDa) via RAFT polymerization using CTA2 for the PMETACLs and PVMBTs and CTA3 for the PDADMACs in aqueous media.

Polymer	Mn Calc.	Mn-GPC	Mw-GPC	PDI
PMETACl-10	10.4 kDa	11 kDa	14 kDa	1.24
PMETACl-20	17.1 kDa	17 kDa	20 kDa	1.19
PMETACl-40	39.7 kDa	39 kDa	40 kDa	1.03
PDADMAC-10	11.9 kDa	11 kDa	15 kDa	1.36
PDADMAC-20	17.5 kDa	18 kDa	24 kDa	1.36
PDADMAC-40	36.8 kDa	35 kDa	48 kDa	1.37
PVMBT-10	13.7 kDa	6 kDa	7 kDa	1.20
PVMBT-20	20.8 kDa	14 kDa	16 kDa	1.11
PVMBT-40	37.4 kDa	23 kDa	27 kDa	1.18

The minimum inhibitory concentration of the low (10 kDa), medium (20 kDa), and high (40 kDa) molecular weights of a particular polymer at three different concentrations were evaluated (see Table 4) and showed that the higher-molecular-weight polymers were more effective in inhibiting bacterial growth, an effect confirmed by an agar diffusion assay against all four tested bacterial species (see Figure S9, Table S1).

Table 4. Effect of molecular weight on the polymers' MICs as determined by a resazurin assay. The molecular weights corresponding to the nominal low (10 kDa), medium (20 kDa), and high (40 kDa) polymers are given in Table 3 (n = 3). The three polymers in bold were explored in more detail as they showed good levels of antibacterial activity and low cytotoxicity.

Polymer Mn	Polymer Name	MICs for Different Target Microorganisms							
		B. subtilis		E. coli		M. luteus		S. typhimurium	
		µg/mL	µM	µg/mL	µM	µg/mL	µM	µg/mL	µM
10 kDa	PDADMAC-10	16	1.4	32	2.7	32	2.7	64	5.4
17 kDa	**PDADMAC-20**	16	0.9	16	0.9	16	0.9	32	1.8
40 kDa	PDADMAC-40	16	0.4	16	0.4	16	0.4	32	0.9
12 kDa	PMETACL-10	64	6.2	64	6.2	64	6.2	64	6.2
18 kDa	PMETACL-20	64	3.7	64	3.7	64	3.7	64	3.7
37 kDa	**PMETACL-40**	32	0.9	32	0.9	32	0.9	64	1.7
14 kDa	PVMBT-10	64	4.7	64	4.7	64	4.7	128	9.3
21 kDa	PVMBT-20	32	1.5	32	1.5	64	3.1	64	3.1
37 kDa	**PVMBT-40**	32	0.9	32	10.9	32	0.9	64	1.7

Among the tested polymers, PDADMAC-40 showed the best inhibition of all bacteria strains, with an MIC in the range of 0.43–0.86 µM (16–32 µg/mL). However, it is worth mentioning that increased polymer chain length was also found to lead to enhanced cytotoxicity, with PDADMAC-40 being highly cytotoxic to HeLa cells even at the lowest concentration (1.25 µM) tested. Importantly, PDADMAC-20, PMETACL-40, and PVMBT-40 showed similar MIC values (0.9 µM), but were much less cytotoxic.

2.4. Antimicrobial Mechanisms of the Polymers

A live/dead assay was used for the assessment of bacterial membrane integrity after treatment with the polymers, with double staining using SYTO 9 and propidium iodide (PI). Figure 2 shows images of bacteria after a 4-h incubation period with each of the three polymers (PDADMAC-20, PMEATCL-40, and PVMBT-40) at 2× MIC (Figure 2). The loss of membrane integrity (structural disturbance of the membrane) signified the bactericidal action of the compounds, the generally accepted mechanism for ammonium-group-bearing polymers [13].

In order to understand the mechanism of action, E. coli and M. luteus were treated with the most active polymers (PDADMAC-20, PVMBT-40, and PMETACL-40) and analyzed by SEM to observe the bacterial morphology. As shown in Figure 3, the distortion of the bacteria suggested that the polymers were disrupting/distorting the bacterial envelopes of both Gram-positive and Gram-negative bacteria, with changes in membrane roughness, shrinking, and involutions. The E. coli "outer envelope" showed wrinkles and deep hollows, while a misshaped and raptured membrane of M. luteus was observed. Moreover, pores were found on the surface of M. luteus, suggesting the permeabilization of the plasma membrane and leakage of cellular content. These phenomena suggest that these polymers kill bacteria by destroying their cell membranes.

2.5. Membrane Depolarization Assays

Perturbation of the bacterial outer membrane (Gram-negative bacteria) was assessed using the fluorescent probe (1-N-phenyl-naphthylamine) (NPN) that enters and binds damaged membranes. Supported by the SEM images, the assay results suggested that the outer membrane of E. coli was depolarized by the polymers, with PVMBT-40 giving a 10-fold increase in fluorescence (Figure 4). Presumably, the ammonium groups accumulate on the membranes via electrostatic interactions, and the hydrophobic aryl groups interdigitate with the lipophobic membrane, promoting the interlacing of the polymer, leading to enhanced permeability. Gram-positive bacteria have a thick layer of crosslinked peptidoglycan decorated with negatively charged teichoic acid, surrounding their cytoplasmic membranes. Cationic polymers can accumulate onto this via electrostatic interactions and then penetrate deep into the peptidoglycan layer by virtue of nano-sized pores or defects. These accumulated cationic polymers can then disturb the integrity of the cytoplasmic membrane, leading to bacterial death. This effect of the polymers on Gram-positive bacteria (*B. subtilis*) was measured by the polymer-induced leakage of the fluorescent dye calcein. Analysis (Figure 5) showed that the polymers accessed the cytoplasmic membrane, even in the presence of the thick cell wall. PDADMAC-20 and PMETACL-40 showed a similar fluorescence increase to Triton X-100 (1% *v/v*), with PDADMAC-20 acting faster than PMEATCL-40, presumably due to its lower molecular weight. The more hydrophilic polymer chains of PMEATCL-40 penetrated into the peptidoglycan layer more efficiently than PVMBT-40.

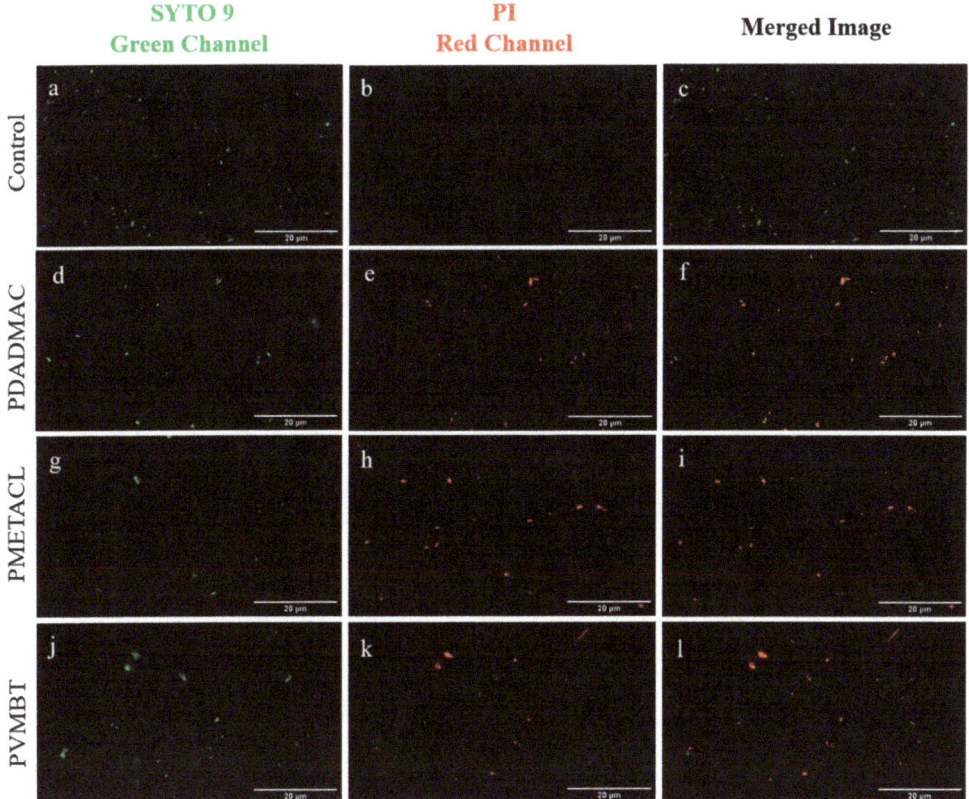

Figure 2. Fluorescent microscopy images of *E. coli* stained using a live/dead assay (live are shown in green (SYTO 9) and dead are shown in red (PI)). Control bacteria (**a**–**c**) and bacteria following treatment with the three lead polymers (PDADMAC (**d**–**f**); PMETACL (**g**–**i**) and PVMBT (**j**–**l**)). Bacteria were imaged on a Zeiss Axiovert 200M, with a 40× objective, in the FITC channel (λex 488 nm) (**a,d,g,i**) and the Texas red channel (λex 561 nm) (**b,e,f,j**) with the merged images shown (**c,f,h,k**). Red fluorescence indicates loss of membrane integrity and signifies the bactericidal action of the compound (scale bar: 20 μm).

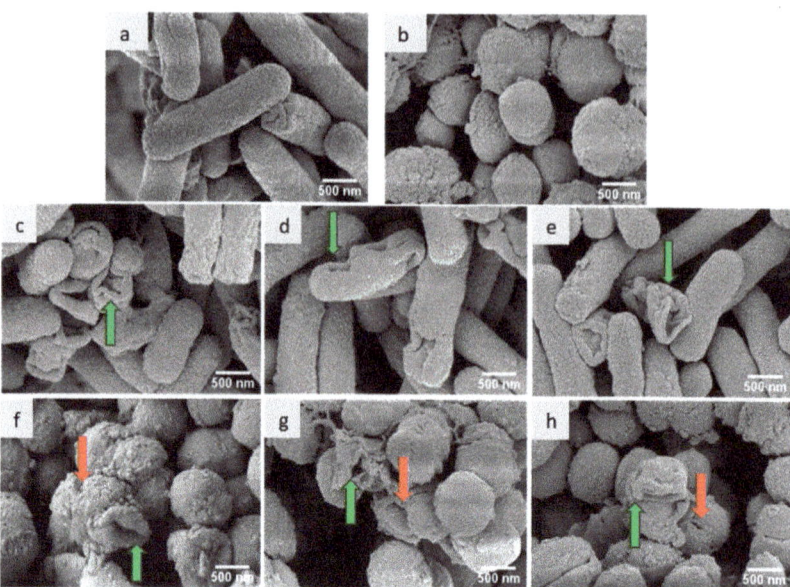

Figure 3. SEM images of (**a**) untreated *E. coli*; (**c**) PDADMAC-20-treated *E. coli*; (**d**) PVMBT-40-treated *E. coli*; and (**e**) PMETACL-40-treated *E. coli*. (**b**) Untreated *M. luteus*; (**f**) PDADMAC-20-treated *M. luteus*; (**g**) PVMBT-40-treated *M. luteus*; and (**h**) PMETACL-40-treated *M. luteus*. Green arrows indicate bacteria with impaired membranes. Red arrows indicate the pores on the bacterial surface of *M. luteus*. Scale bars: 500 nm.

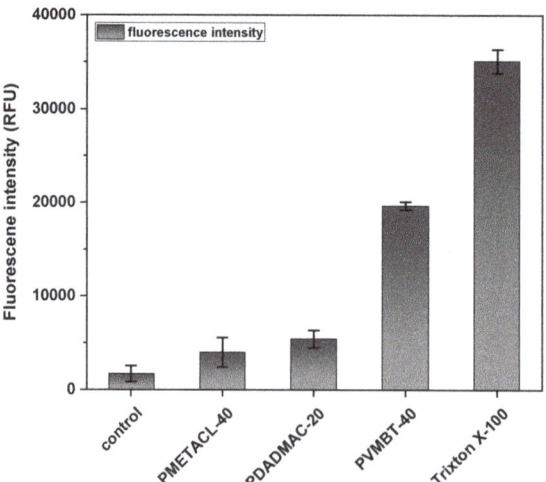

Figure 4. Permeabilization of the outer membrane of *E. coli* was measured using a 1-N-phenyl-naphthylamine (NPN) assay in the presence of polymers PVMBT-40, PDADMAC-20, and PMETACL-40 after 20 min. Bacteria were incubated with NPN for 30 min to stabilize the fluorescence (data are not shown) and polymers added at 4× MIC (3.6 µM). Bacteria without polymer treatment were used as a negative control, while Triton X-100 (1% v/v)-treated bacteria served as the positive control (n = 3).

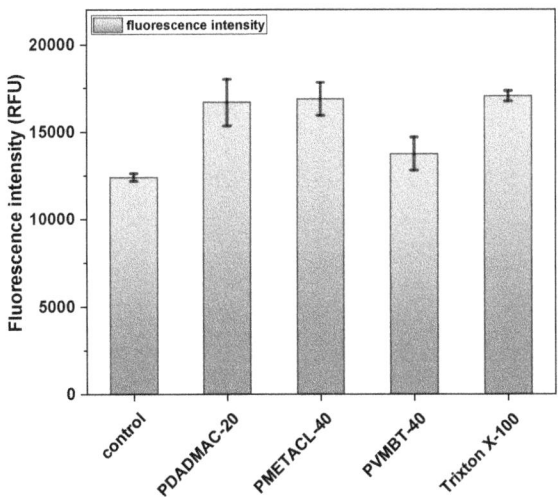

Figure 5. Permeabilization of the membrane of *B. subtilis* by polymers PVMBT-40, PDADMAC-20, and PMEATCL-40 (at 4× MIC) and the increase in fluorescence of calcein monitored over 30 min. Calcein-AM-loaded bacteria without polymer treatment were used as a negative control, while Triton X-100 (1% v/v)-treated bacteria served as the positive control (n = 3).

2.6. Cytotoxicity and Hemolytic Activity of Polymers

As shown above, the higher-molecular-weight polymers showed better antimicrobial activity. An MTT cytotoxicity assay showed that the homopolymers (see Figure 6) displayed greater toxicity with increasing concentration and the higher-molecular-weight polymers were more toxic than the corresponding lower-molecular-weight analogues (Figure S10) [60]. This is due to the multiple positively charged segments, interacting with components of the negatively charged membrane (in both extracellular and intracellular compartments), ultimately initiating apoptosis [60,63]. Much of this will be entropic- and polymer-flexibility driven—once bound, the adjacent cations will be in proximity to bind additional elements of the cell membrane. Figure 6 shows HeLa cell viability after incubation with polymers for 24 h, with the three homopolymers of PMETACL being the least toxic (Figure S10), even at 1280 µM (far beyond the antibacterial MIC of the polymer (16–32 µg/mL); over half the cells were viable).

The hemolytic activity was investigated as a biocompatibility indicator (PDADMAC-20, PMETACL-40, and PVMBT-40 (as seen in Figure 7)); all showed limited hemolysis, even at the highest concentrations used (1280 µM).

A practical approach to assessing selectivity towards bacterial vs. mammalian cells is to measure the HC_{50}/MIC ratio, where HC_{50} is the polymer concentration required to lyse 50% of red blood cells [51], with many of the polymers described herein selective against bacteria over mammalian cells across the concentration range evaluated (Table 5).

Table 5. Selective toxicity of PDADMAC-20, PMETACL-40, and PVMBT-40.

Polymer	MIC (µg/mL)				HC_{50} mg/mL	Selectivity HC_{50}/MIC
	E. coli	B. subtilis	M. luteus	S. typhimurium		
PDADMAC-20	16	16	16	32	>26	>800
PVMBT-40	32	32	32	64	>51	>800
PMETACL-40	32	32	32	64	>51	>800

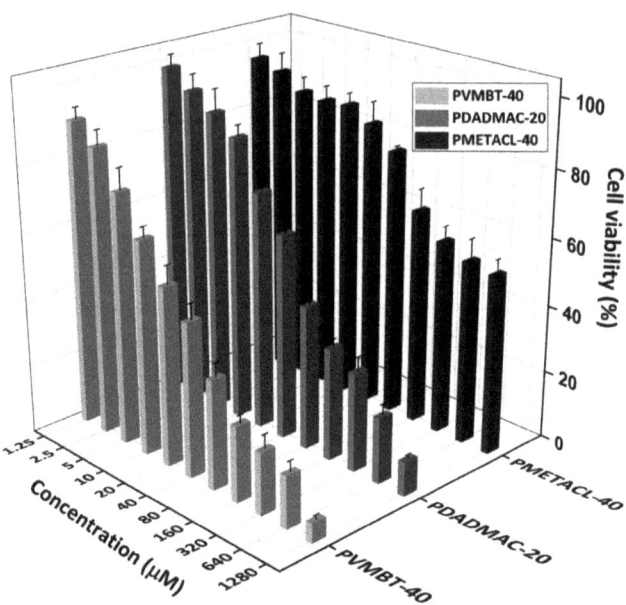

Figure 6. MTT cytotoxicity assay of the polymers PDADMAC-20, PMETACL-40, and PVMBT-40 at 1.25–1280 μM on HeLa cells for 24 h. Results are presented as relative cell viability compared to that of the untreated negative control (100% cell viability). The error bars are standard deviation of the mean (n = 3).

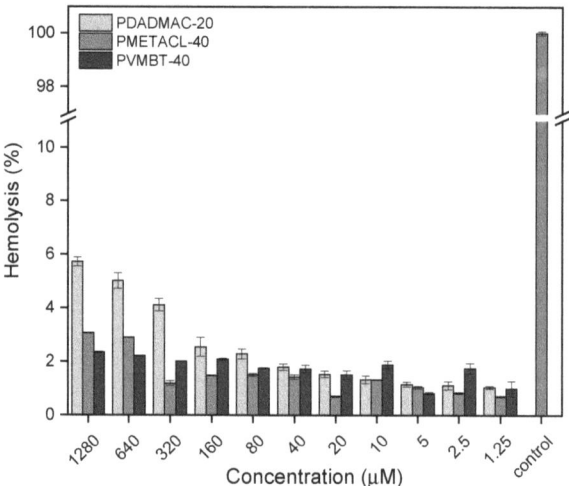

Figure 7. The hemolytic activity (sheep erythrocytes) of the polymers PDADMAC-20, PMETACL-40, and PVMBT-40. A hemolysis test was used to assess the biocompatibility of polymers with varying concentrations of the polymers. The amount of leaked hemoglobin (% hemolysis) was measured relative to a positive control (Triton X-100 (1% v/v) defined as giving 100% lysis of red blood cells and a negative control (PBS-treated red blood cells) giving no lysis.

3. Materials and Methods

All monomers and common chemical reagents, 2,2-azobis(2-methylpropionamidine)dihydrochloride (AAPH, 97%), potassium ethyl xanthogenate (96%), bromoacetic acid (97%),

4,4′-azobis(4-cyanopentanoic acid) (ACVA), 4-cyano-4-[(dodecylsulfanylthiocarbonyl)sulfanyl]pentanoic acid (CTA1), 4-cyano-4-(phenylcarbonothioylthio)pentanoic acid (CTA2), NaOH, anhydrous acetonitrile, ethanol, acetone, hexane, and deuterated solvents (D_2O, $CDCl_3$) were purchased from Sigma Aldrich (St. Louis, MO, USA), Fluorochem (Glossop, UK), Fisher Scientific (Hampton, NH, USA), or Alfa Easer (Haverhill, MA, USA) and used as received, unless otherwise noted. Except for diallyldimethylammonium chloride (65% wt. in H_2O), all monomers were passed through a basic alumina column to remove inhibitors before polymerization reactions. The chain transfer agent, S-ethoxythiocarbonyl mercaptoacetic acid (CTA3), was synthesized according to the literature [69]. Deionized (DI) water was from a Milli-Q system. Dulbecco's Modified Eagle Medium (DMEM), Opti-MEM (OMEM), 0.25% trypsin−EDTA, fetal bovine serum (FBS), and streptomycin (5000 µg/mL)/penicillin (5000 U/mL) were obtained from ThermoFisher Scientific, Horsham, UK, while 3-[4,5-dimethylthiazol-2-yl]-2,5 diphenyltetrazolium bromide was purchased from Alfa Easer. Phosphate buffer solution (PBS) was prepared from PBS tablets (Oxoid Ltd., ThermoFisher Scientific, Horsham, UK). Defibrinated sheep blood (SB054-100 mL) was provided by TCS Biosciences. The LIVE/DEAD™ BacLight™ Bacterial Viability Kit for microscopy was purchased from Sigma-Aldrich. Calcein-AM was purchased from Sigma-Aldrich. N-Phenyl-1-naphthylamine (98%) was purchased from Thermo Scientific. *Escherichia coli* (DH5α), *Salmonella typhimurium* SL1344, *Micrococcus luteus* (ATCC 4698), and *Bacillus subtilis* (ATCC 6051) were used as Gram-positive and Gram-negative test strains. Microbial culture broths and agar medium (Invitrogen, Inchinnan, UK; Fisher Scientific, UK; and Merck, Inchinnan, UK), buffers, and water were sterilized by autoclaving before use. Polymer solutions were filter-sterilized (0.22 µ, Millipore Inc., Burlington, MA, USA) before use.

3.1. Methods

3.1.1. General Synthesis of Homopolymers via Reversible Addition Fragmentation Chain Transfer Polymerization

Monomers were subjected to free radical polymerization to determine the reaction conditions and understand the compatibility of monomers, initiators, and solvent. Subsequently, all monomers were subjected to RAFT polymerization with a suitable chain transfer agent. During the polymerization reactions, aliquots were taken to follow monomer conversion (by ^{1}H NMR spectrometry in D_2O or $CDCl_3$). The experimental molecular weights of the polymers were calculated based on the integration of the disappearing vinyl protons of the responsible monomer and the appearance of the methylene peak of the formed polymer via ^{1}H NMR. Theoretical molecular weights were calculated according to the literature [50] based on the formula below, where $[M]_0$, and $[CTA]_0$ are the initial concentrations of the monomer and chain transfer agent; p is the monomer conversion; and Mw_M and Mw_{CTA} are the molar masses of the monomer and chain transfer agent, respectively.

$$M_{n,th} = \left(\frac{[M]_0 \cdot Mw_M}{[CTA]_0}\right) + Mw_{CTA}$$

The monomer DADMAC was polymerized using the initiator 2,2′-azobis (2-methylpropionamidine) dihydrochloride (AAPH) and the xanthate-type chain transfer agent S-ethoxythiocarbonyl mercaptoacetic acid (CTA3) at 60 °C. The other monomers were polymerized using the initiator 4,4-azobis (4-cyanovaleric acid) (ACVA) and either 4-cyano-4-(phenylcarbonothioylthio) pentanoic acid (CTA2) or 4-cyano-4-[(dodecyl sulfanyl thiocarbonyl)sulfanyl]pentanoic acid) (CTA1) at 70 °C as the chain transfer agents. In order to synthesize the desired different molecular weights of the polymers, the chain transfer and initiator concentrations in the reaction were tuned while the monomer concentrations were kept constant (Figure 1).

3.1.2. P1-RAFT Polymerization of Poly(2-(dimethylamino)ethyl methacrylate)

First, 2-(dimethylamino)ethyl methacrylate (5 mL), radical initiator 4,4′-azobis(4-cyanopentanoic acid) (ACVA), (0.0084 g), chain transfer agent CTA1-(4-cyano-4-[(dodecylsulfanyl thiocarbonyl)sulfanyl] pentanoic acid) (0.0726 g), and 10 mL ethanol were mixed in a septum sealable glass tube (50 mL). The solution was degassed by argon bubbling for 30 min. The polymerization was carried out at 70 °C for 24 h. The polymer was purified by removal of the ethanol, redissolution in THF, and precipitation using n-hexane. The polymer was dried under vacuum at 40 °C for 2 days to give a yellow-colored polymer (78% yield).

3.1.3. P2-RAFT Polymerization of Poly([2-(methacryloyloxy)ethyl]trimethylammonium chloride)

First, [2-(methacryloyloxy)ethyl]trimethylammonium chloride) (6 g, 75% wt in H_2O), initiator 4,4-azobis (4-cyanovaleric acid) (8 mg), raft agent CTA2 (40 mg), and water (17.9 mL) were mixed in a 50 mL Schlenk flask and the reaction solution was purged with nitrogen for 30 min. The polymerization reaction was carried out at 70 °C for 24 h. Aliquots were taken at different time intervals to check monomer to polymer conversion via ^1H NMR analysis. The resulting polymer was purified by precipitation using acetone, redissolved in methanol, and again precipitated using acetone and dried under vacuum at 40 °C to give a salmon-colored polymer (94% yield). This polymer was synthesized with three different molecular weights by changing the chain transfer agent to initiator ratio.

3.1.4. P3-RAFT Polymerization of Poly[3-(methacryloylamino)propyl]trimethylammonium chloride

First, [3-(methacryloylamino)propyl]trimethylammonium chloride (13 g 50% wt in H_2O), initiator 4,4-azobis(4-cyanovaleric acid) (8 mg), CTA2 (40 mg), and water (17.5 mL) were mixed in a 100 mL flask and the reaction solution was purged with nitrogen for a 30 min. It was then placed into a preheated oil bath at 70 °C for 24 h. The resulting polymer was purified by precipitation with excess acetone, redissolved in methanol, re-precipitated with acetone, and dried under vacuum at 40 °C (51% yield).

3.1.5. P4-RAFT Polymerization of Poly(vinylbenzyl trimethylammonium chloride)

The monomer (4 g), 4,4-azobis(4-cyanovaleric acid) (ACVA) as an initiator (7.84 mg), CTA2 (28 mg), and water (25 mL) were mixed in a 50 mL Schlenk flask and purged with nitrogen for 30 min. The polymerization reaction was carried out at 70 °C for 24 h. The resulting polymer was purified by precipitation using THF and dried under vacuum at 40 °C (89% yield). This polymer was synthesized with three different molecular weights by changing the changing the chain transfer agent to initiator ratio.

3.1.6. P5-RAFT Polymerization of Poly(diallydimethyl ammonium chloride)

The polymerization of diallyldimethyl ammonium chloride was carried out by the protocol of Demarteau [72]. Diallyldimethyl ammonium chloride (10 mL, 65% wt in H_2O), initiator 2,2′-azobis (2-methylpropionamidine)dihydrochloride (AAPH) (0.019 g), CTA3 (0.041 g), and water (8 mL) were mixed in a 50 mL Schlenk tube. Then, the reaction mixture was degassed by bubbling with argon for 30 min and placed in preheated oil bath at 60 °C for 24 h. The resulting polymer was precipitated in a mixture of acetone/ethanol (1:1) three times and dried under vacuum at 40 °C (70% yield). This polymer was synthesized with three different molecular weights by changing the chain transfer agent to initiator ratio.

The synthesized polymers were numbered as follows: PDMAEMA (P1), PMETACL (P2), PMET3 (P3), PVBMT (P4), and PDADMAC (P5).

3.1.7. Synthesis of Chain Transfer Agent S-Ethoxythiocarbonyl Mercaptoacetic Acid (CTA3)

Water-soluble xanthate-type chain transfer agent CTA3 was synthesized according to the literature [69]. Sodium hydroxide (1.25 g, 62.4 mmol) was dissolved in chilled water (50 mL) and then bromoacetic acid (1 eq, 4.37 g, 62.4 mmol) was added until a clear solution was obtained. Potassium ethyl xanthogenate (1 eq, 5 g, 62.4 mmol) was then added to the mixture over 30 min. The solution was stirred at room temperature for 24 h and then acidified with 4 M HCl. The resulting mixture was extracted with chloroform (3 × 50 mL). The organic extracts were dried over anhydrous magnesium sulfate, filtered, and concentrated under vacuum. The solid was washed with hexane and dried under vacuum to give white crystals. ^{1}H NMR (500 MHz, D$_2$O) δ 4.63 (q, J = 7.1 Hz, 2H, CH$_2$), 3.93 (s, 2H, CH$_2$), 1.34 (t, J = 7.1 Hz, 3H, CH$_3$). ^{13}C NMR (126 MHz, D$_2$O) δ 213.95, 172.80, 71.72, 37.32, 12.79) (Figure S1b). LC-MS (ESI) for C$_5$H$_8$O$_3$S$_2$: [M−H]$^+$ calcd.: 179.1; found: 179.1. Data were consistent with the literature [69].

3.2. Characterization of Homopolymers

3.2.1. Nuclear Magnetic Resonance Spectroscopy

All monomers, polymers, and RAFT agents were analyzed on a Bruker AVA500 spectrometer in CDCl$_3$ or D$_2$O at either 500 MHz (H^1 NMR) or 125 MHz (C^{13}).

3.2.2. Molecular Weight Determination of Polymers by GPC analysis

Aqueous-based GPC analysis of the polymers was carried out on an Agilent Technologies 1100 system, 8 μm Agilent PL Aquagel-OH 30, and 8 μm Agilent PL Aquagel-OH 40 columns with an RI detector. The eluent was 0.50 M acetic acid, 0.30 M NaH$_2$PO$_4$, at pH 2.5, with a flow rate of 1.0 mL min^{-1} at 25 °C. Calibration was achieved using InfinityLab EasiVial poly(ethylene oxide) standards with Mn values ranging from 1.1 to 905 kDa. GPC analysis of poly (2-(dimethylamino)ethyl methacrylate) (PDMAEMA) was carried out on an Agilent 1260 Infinity system on two PL-GEL mixed-c columns (5 μm) with both UV and RI detectors. The eluent used was THF at a flow rate of 1.0 mL min^{-1} at 35 °C. Molecular weights were obtained relative to poly(methyl methacrylate) standards.

3.3. Antimicrobial Activity of the Polymers

3.3.1. Primary Screening: Determination of Minimum Inhibitory Concentration

Antibacterial activity was assessed using a resazurin colorimetric assay [73]. Five μL of a cryopreserved glycerol stock of the bacterial culture (*Escherichia coli*, *Salmonella typhimurium*, *Micrococcus luteus*, and *Bacillus subtilis*) was streaked onto Luria–Bertani, nutrient agar, tryptic soy agar, and nutrient agar plates, respectively. A single bacterial colony was transferred to 5 mL of the respective broth medium and incubated at 37 °C and grown until the mid-log phase. The culture was diluted and the concentration adjusted to 0.5 McFarland standard with sterile Mueller–Hinton broth (2 × 10^7 CFU/mL). The resazurin solution was prepared in a brown glass vial by dissolving 34 mg of resazurin in sterile distilled water (5 mL) with vortexing for 1 h to ensure homogeneity. A single 96-well microtiter plate (Corning, black 96-well flat-bottomed plates) was dedicated to each bacterial species to prevent contamination. The design of the assay was prepared with two rows and two columns from each end filled with sterile water to avoid edge effects. The assay was adapted from previously reported protocols [73]. Two columns of broth sterility controls, 1 column of a growth control, 2 columns of polymer sterility controls (P1-5 with one polymer in each well), 1 column of a positive antibiotic control, and, lastly, 2 columns of polymer test samples (P1-5 with one polymer in each well) were used. All wells were filled with 100 μL of Mueller–Hinton broth. The broth sterility and growth control columns contained 100 μL of sterile water; the polymer sterility control and test wells contained 100 μL of polymers (final concentration 128 μg/mL) in the designated wells. Antibiotic wells, all at 64 μg/mL, contained chloramphenicol (for S. *typhimurium*), gentamicin (for E. *coli* and M. *luteus*), and clindamycin (for B. *subtilis*). Five μL of the diluted bacterial suspension (2 × 10^7 CFU/mL) was added into all wells (except the broth sterility and polymer sterility control columns) and mixed thoroughly. After overnight incubation at 37 °C, resazurin solution (5 μL, 6.75 mg/mL) was added to all wells and incubated at 37 °C for another 4 h. Changes in color from blue (resazurin, no bacterial growth) to pink (resorufin, bacterial growth) were recorded at 595 nm on a microplate reader (BioTek Synergy HT). The lowest concentration that did not show a color change was considered as the minimum inhibitory concentration (MIC). Each assay was performed in triplicate.

3.3.2. Effect of Molecular Weight on Antimicrobial Activity of Polymers

In order to determine the effect of the molecular weight on the antibacterial activity, three differently sized polymers were synthesized for PDADMAC, PMETACL, and PVBMT.

Zone diffusion assays and growth kinetics: Agar plates were inoculated by spreading 100 µL bacteria (1×10^6 CFU/mL), 1-cm-diameter wells were punched into the agar, and 100 µL of polymer solution (at $2\times$ MIC) was added into the wells and the zones of inhibition were measured after 8 h.

3.4. Live/Dead Assay

Bacterial cultures (5 mL) grown to the late log phase were harvested by centrifugation. The cell pellet was resuspended in 5 mL 0.85% NaCl, aliquoted (each aliquot was 1 mL), and incubated with $4\times$ MIC concentrations of the selected polymers for 4 h at 37 °C. The live cell control consisted of an aliquot incubated with only 0.85% NaCl. After incubation, all samples were washed with 0.85% NaCl twice. A Live/Dead BacLight Bacterial Viability Kit (Invitrogen) was used to check cell viability. The assay was performed according to the kit instructions. Component A (200 µL of a 3.34 mM solution in DMSO) was mixed in equal proportions with Component B (200 µL of a 20 mM solution in DMSO) and 3 µL of this combined dye mixture was added to 1 mL of all bacterial samples before incubation for 30 min in the dark. Samples were analyzed using an AxioVert 200M inverted fluorescent microscope to analyze for green (λex 488 nm, λem 520 nm) and red (λex 561 nm, λem 646 nm) fluorescence.

3.5. Bacterial Membrane Integrity Assays

Outer membrane permeabilization assay: The method for the determination of the outer membrane depolarization assay was adapted from the literature [74]. First, 1-N-phenyl-1-naphthylamine was dissolved in acetone (3 mM). Gram-negative bacteria *E. coli* were grown to 1.0 OD. Cells were harvested by centrifugation, washed, and resuspended to 0.1 OD in 5 mM HEPES with 5 mM glucose at pH 7.2. Then, 10 µL of NPN stock was added to each 1 mL of bacteria to give a concentration of NPN of 30 µM. Next, 200 µL of bacterial suspension was added to each well of a 96-well plate as five replicates at 37 °C, followed by analysis on a fluorescent microplate spectrometer (BioTek Synergy HT) over 30 min (every 1 min) (λex 350 nm λem 429 nm). Then, 10 µL of polymer solution ($4\times$ MIC) was added to each well. Moreover, 1% v/v Triton X-100 was used as a positive control, while a bacterial suspension without polymer was used as a negative control. The increase in the fluorescence of NPN was monitored at 5-min intervals and the fluorescence values after 30 min plotted. All experiments were repeated three times independently.

Cytoplasmic depolarization assay: The method for the determination of the inner membrane depolarization assay was adapted from the literature [75]. A stock solution of calcein-AM was prepared in DMSO (1 mM) and stored in the dark at -20 °C. *B. subtilis* was cultured in media overnight and centrifuged ($3000\times g$—5 min) to give a pellet. The pellet was washed with PBS and resuspended to a 0D600 of 1.0 with PBS containing 10% (v/v) broth. The bacteria were incubated with 3 µM calcein-AM for 1 h at 37 °C. The dye-loaded cells were collected by centrifugation ($3000\times g$—5 min) and suspended to 0.1 OD in PBS. Then, 200 µL of bacterial suspension was added to sterile black-wall 96-well plates (three replicates) and monitored for 30 min (λex 622 nm, λem 670 nm) on a fluorescence plate reader. Then, 10 µL of polymer solution ($4\times$ MIC) was added to each well. Bacteria without polymers were used as a negative control, while 1% v/v Triton X-100 was used as a positive control. All experiments were repeated three times independently.

3.6. Scanning Electron Microscopy

Aliquots (10 mL of OD 0.5 of Gram-positive (*M. luteus*) and Gram-negative (*E. coli*)) of bacteria were incubated with 0.85% NaCl (control) and the polymers PDAMAC-mid (20 kDa), PVMBT-high (40 kDa), and PMETACL-high (40 kDa) (all 2× MIC) for two hours. After pelleting, the bacteria were fixed in a solution of 3% glutaraldehyde in 0.1 M sodium cacodylate buffer (pH 7.3) for 2 h and washed (3 × 10 min changes of 0.1 M sodium cacodylate buffer). Samples were then post-fixed in 1% osmium tetroxide (in 0.1 M sodium cacodylate buffer) for 45 min, before further 3 × 10 min washes were performed in 0.1 M sodium cacodylate buffer. Dehydration in graded concentrations of acetone (50%, 70%, 90%, and 3 × 100%—each for 10 min) was followed by critical point drying using liquid carbon dioxide. After mounting on aluminum stubs with carbon tabs attached, the specimens were sputter-coated with 20 nm thickness of gold–palladium and viewed using a Hitachi S-4700 scanning electron microscope.

3.7. MTT Assay

In vitro cytotoxicity tests were carried out using an MTT assay on HeLa cells, based on a previously published protocol, with some modifications [76]. Cells were grown in complete medium (Dulbecco's Modified Eagle Medium, DMEM, Gibco) supplemented with 2 mM L-glutamine, 10% fetal bovine serum, and 1% antibiotics (penicillin 100 U/mL and streptomycin 100 µg/mL) until sub-confluent at 37 °C and 5% CO_2 in a cell incubator (HERAcell ®150, Kendro, Hereaeus Group, Hagen, Germany). HeLa cells were used at passage numbers below 15 and tested for mycoplasma contamination regularly. For cytotoxicity tests, cells were seeded in a 96-well plate at the density of 1×10^4 cells per well and cultured in a 100 µL of growth medium. After 24 h, the culture medium was replaced with polymer solutions (50 µL) prepared in growth media at increasing concentrations. The cells were further incubated for 24 h under the same conditions. After the incubation of cells with polymers containing media, all the solutions were carefully removed from the wells and 100 µL MTT solution (5 mg of MTT dissolved in 1 mL PBS and 9 mL serum-free DMEM without phenol-red) was added to each well in a light-protected environment. After 4 h, unreacted dye was removed by aspiration. Cells were carefully washed with PBS twice. Then, 100 µL of solubilizing solution (a mixture of 2-propanol and dimethyl sulfoxide in a 1:1 volume ratio) was added to each well to dissolve the formed formazan crystals. The solution was shaken for at least 30 min to ensure the dissolution of all crystals before measuring the absorbance at 570 nm on a BioTek Synergy H1 plate reader. Cells treated with complete medium only were taken as a positive control (100% viability) and cells treated with DMSO (100%) were taken as a negative control. All tests were repeated three times. The relative cell viability (%) with respect to the control was determined using the formula below:

$$\text{Cell viability}(\%) = \left(\frac{OD_{\text{sample}} - OD_{\text{negative control}}}{OD_{\text{positive control}} - OD_{\text{negative control}}} \right) \times 100$$

where OD is the optical density at 570 nm.

The test was applied in the range of 1.25 µM to 1280 µM for the polymers (PDADMACs, PMEATCLs, and PVMBTs).

3.8. Hemolysis Assays

Assays were carried out following previously published protocols [77]. Sheep red blood cells (RBCs) were diluted 1:20 in PBS (pH 7.4), pelleted by centrifugation, and washed three times in PBS (20 mL, 1000 g, 10 min). The RBCs were then resuspended to 5% (v/v) in PBS. Different concentrations of PDAMAC-mid (20 kDa), PVMBT-high (40 kDa), and PMETACL-high (40 kDa) (150 µL, in the range of 1.25–1280 µM) were prepared, followed by the addition of the 5% RBC suspension (150 µL). PBS buffer was used as a negative control, and Triton X-100 (1% v/v in PBS) was used as a positive hemolysis control. Tubes were incubated at 37 °C for 1 h with 300 rpm shaking in an incubator. Samples were then centrifuged (2000× g, 4 min), and 100 µL aliquots of supernatants were transferred into a 96-well microplate, where absorbance values were read at 405 nm using a plate reader. The hemolysis percentage was calculated using the absorbance values and the formula below:

$$\text{Hemolysis}(\%) = \left(\frac{A_{\text{polymer}} - A_{\text{negative}}}{A_{\text{positive}} - A_{\text{negative}}}\right) \times 100$$

where A_{polymer} is the absorbance of the polymer-treated cells' supernatant, A_{negative} is the absorbance of the negative control (1% v/v Triton X-100-treated cells' supernatant), and A_{positive} is the absorbance of the positive control (PBS-treated cells' supernatant). All experiments were performed as independent triplicates, each consisting of triplicates.

4. Conclusions

In this study, five quaternary homopolymers were screened on Gram-negative and Gram-positive bacteria to detect the most active antimicrobial polymer. Selected polymers (PDADMACs, PVMBTs, and PMETACLs) were synthesized with varying molecular weights (~10, ~20, and ~40 kDa) and with the higher-molecular-weight polymers showing (on a mole/mole bases) higher activity (lower MIC values). PVMBT (40 kDa) and PMETACL (40 kDa) and PDADMACs (20 kDa) showed good growth inhibition against both Gram-positive (B. subtilis, M. luteus) and Gram-negative (S. typhimurium, E. coli) bacteria, with MIC values as low as 0.9 µM. The antimicrobial action mechanisms of the polymers were determined using dye permeabilization assays and visualization by SEM, which showed the formation of "holes" on the bacteria and a highly distorted cell envelope. Cytotoxic evaluations of the polymers were carried out using MTT and hemolysis assays, and the best polymers showed great selectivity towards bacteria over eukaryotic cells. Overall, the polymer PMETACL, in its higher-molecular-weight form, showed strong inhibition of bacterial growth (MIC = 0.9–1.8 µM (16–32 µg/mL)), with a bactericidal mode of action against both Gram-negative and Gram-positive bacteria, and it also showed low mammalian cell toxicity, making it a potential candidate for biomedical applications.

Supplementary Materials: The following supporting information can be downloaded at: https://www.mdpi.com/article/10.3390/antibiotics12081320/s1. Figure S1. (a) ^{1}H NMR spectra of chain transfer agent 3 recorded in D_2O, with peak assignments, (b) ^{13}C NMR of the chain transfer agent 2 recorded in D_2O, with peak assignments. Figure S2. ^{1}H NMR spectra of poly(2-(dimethylamino)ethyl methacrylate) recorded in $CDCl_3$, with peak assignments. E, D represent the peaks of the polymer's main chain; A, B, C represent the peaks of the polymer's side chain. Figure S3. ^{1}H NMR spectra of poly([2-(methacryloyloxy)ethyl]trimethylammonium chloride) recorded in D_2O, with peak assignments. E, D represent the peaks of the polymer's main chain; A, B, C represent the peaks of the polymer's side chain. Inset (F, G, H) shows the region of the RAFT agent. Figure S4. ^{1}H NMR spectra of poly[3-(methacryloylamino)propyl]trimethylammonium chloride recorded in D_2O, with peak assignments. E, D represent the peaks of the polymer's main chain; A, B, C represent the peaks of the polymer's side chain. Inset (F, G, H) shows the region of the RAFT agent. Figure S5. ^{1}H NMR spectra of poly(vinylbenzyl trimethylammonium chloride) recorded in D_2O, with peak assignments. E, D represent the peaks of the polymer's main chain; A, B, C represent the peaks of the polymer's side chain. Figure S6. ^{1}H NMR spectra of poly(diallyldimethyl ammonium chloride) recorded in D_2O, with peak assignments. C and D represent the peaks of the polymer's main chain; A and B represent the peaks of the polymer's side chain. Figure S7. Assessment of HeLa cell viability in the presence of five homopolymers (Mw ~20 kDa) using an MTT assay. Figure S8. GPC analysis of three different molecular weight of PDADMACs, PMETCLs, PVMBTs with elution using an aqueous buffer of 0.50 M acetic acid and 0.30 M NaH_2PO_4 (pH 2.5) at a flow rate of 1.0 mL min^{-1} at 25 °C. Peaks relative to poly(ethylene glycol) standards. Figure S9. Agar plates were inoculated with the target bacterial species, wells of 1 cm diameter were punched into the plates, and 100 µL of polymer solutions (at 2× MIC) were added into the wells and incubated overnight before the zones of inhibition were measured. Figure S10. Cytotoxicity of different molecular weights of the polymers (PDADMACs, PVMBTs, and PMEATCLs). Table S1. Zones of inhibition (agar well diffusion assay) in cm.

Author Contributions: Validation, M.H and R.S; Formal analysis, M.H. and R.S.; Investigation, M.H.; Writing—original draft, M.H and R.S.; Writing—review and editing, M.H., R.S. and M.B.; Visualization, M.H.; Supervision, M.B. All authors have read and agreed to the published version of the manuscript.

Funding: This research was funded by a PhD scholarship from the Turkish Ministry of National Education Study Abroad Programme, and the Royal Society (United Kingdom) and the Science and Engineering Research Board (SERB, India) [grant number NIF/R1/192688] for a Newton International Fellowship.

Institutional Review Board Statement: Not applicable.

Informed Consent Statement: Not applicable.

Data Availability Statement: The data is contained in the manuscript or supplemantary materials.

Conflicts of Interest: The authors declare no conflict of interest.

Abbreviations

RAFT: Reversible Addition Fragmentation Chain Transfer Polymerization; SEM: Scanning Electron Microscopy; PDMAEMA: poly(2-(dimethylamino)ethyl methacrylate); PMETACL: poly([2-(methacryloyloxy)ethyl]trimethylammonium chloride); PDADMAC: poly(diallyl dimethyl ammonium chloride); PMET3: poly[3-(methacryloylamino)propyl]trimethylammonium chloride; PVMB: poly(vinyl benzyl trimethylammonium chloride); PI: propidium iodide.

References

1. Collabrators, A.R. Articles Global Burden of Bacterial Antimicrobial Resistance in 2019: A Systematic Analysis. *Lancet* **2022**, *399*, 629–655. [CrossRef]
2. Wang, X.; Jing, S.; Liu, Y.; Liu, S.; Tan, Y. Diblock Copolymer Containing Bioinspired Borneol and Dopamine Moieties: Synthesis and Antibacterial Coating Applications. *Polymer* **2017**, *116*, 314–323. [CrossRef]
3. Vishwakarma, A.; Dang, F.; Ferrell, A.; Barton, H.A.; Joy, A. Peptidomimetic Polyurethanes Inhibit Bacterial Biofilm Formation and Disrupt Surface Established Biofilms. *JACS* **2021**, *143*, 9440–9449. [CrossRef] [PubMed]
4. Yu, X.; Yang, Y.; Yang, W.; Wang, X.; Liu, X.; Zhou, F.; Zhao, Y. One-Step Zwitterionization and Quaternization of Thick PDMAEMA Layer Grafted through Subsurface-Initiated ATRP for Robust Antibiofouling and Antibacterial Coating on PDMS. *J. Colloid Interface Sci.* **2022**, *610*, 234–245. [CrossRef] [PubMed]
5. Tabriz, A.; Azeem, M.; Rehman, U.; Bilal, M.; Niazi, K. Quaternized Trimethyl Functionalized Chitosan Based Antifungal Membranes for Drinking Water Treatment Quaternized Trimethyl Functionalized Chitosan Based Antifungal Membranes for Drinking Water Treatment. *Carbohydr. Polym.* **2018**, *207*, 17–25. [CrossRef]
6. Wulandari, E.; Budhisatria, R.; Soeriyadi, A.H.; Willcox, M.; Boyer, C.; Wong, E.H.H. Polymer Chemistry Combating Multidrug-Resistant Bacteria. *Polym. Chem.* **2021**, *12*, 7038–7047. [CrossRef]
7. Leong, J.; Shi, D.; Pang, J.; Tan, K.; Yang, C.; Yang, S.; Wang, Y.; Ngow, Y.S.; Kng, J.; Balakrishnan, N.; et al. Potent Antiviral and Antimicrobial Polymers as Safe and Effective Disinfectants for the Prevention of Infections. *Adv. Healthc. Mater.* **2022**, *11*, 2101898. [CrossRef]
8. Maria, O.; Keshari, S.; Dash, M.; Lupascu, F.; Pânzariu, A.; Tuchilus, C.; Ghetu, N.; Danciu, M.; Dubruel, P.; Pieptu, D.; et al. New Antimicrobial Chitosan Derivatives for Wound Dressing Applications. *Carbohydr. Polym.* **2016**, *141*, 28–40. [CrossRef]
9. Dundas, A.A.; Sanni, O.; Dubern, J.; Dimitrakis, G.; Hook, A.L.; Irvine, D.J.; Williams, P.; Alexander, M.R. Validating a Predictive Structure—Property Relationship by Discovery of Novel Polymers Which Reduce Bacterial Biofilm Formation. *Adv. Mater.* **2019**, *31*, 1903513. [CrossRef]
10. Mukherjee, S.; Barman, S.; Mukherjee, R.; Haldar, J. Amphiphilic Cationic Macromolecules Highly Effective Against Multi-Drug Resistant Gram-Positive Bacteria and Fungi With No Detectable Resistance. *Front. Bioeng. Biotechnol.* **2020**, *8*, 55. [CrossRef]
11. Fu, Y.; Yang, Y.; Xiao, S.; Zhang, L.; Huang, L.; Chen, F.; Fan, P.; Zhong, M.; Tan, J.; Yang, J. Mixed Polymer Brushes with Integrated Antibacterial and Antifouling Properties. *Prog. Org. Coatings* **2019**, *130*, 75–82. [CrossRef]
12. Wang, H.; Wang, L.; Zhang, P.; Yuan, L.; Yu, Q.; Chen, H. High Antibacterial Efficiency of PDMAEMA Modified Silicon Nanowire Arrays. *Colloids Surf. B Biointerfaces* **2011**, *83*, 355–359. [CrossRef] [PubMed]
13. Haktaniyan, M.; Bradley, M. Polymers Showing Intrinsic Antimicrobial Activity. *Chem. Soc. Rev.* **2022**, *51*, 8584–8611. [CrossRef] [PubMed]

14. Li, J.; Koh, J.J.; Liu, S.; Lakshminarayanan, R.; Verma, C.S.; Beuerman, R.W. Membrane Active Antimicrobial Peptides: Translating Mechanistic Insights to Design. *Front. Neurosci.* **2017**, *11*, 73. [CrossRef] [PubMed]
15. Silhavy, T.J.; Kahne, D.; Walker, S. The Bacterial Cell Envelope. *Cold Spring Harb. Perspect. Biol.* **2010**, *2*, a000414. [CrossRef]
16. Huang, K.C.; Mukhopadhyay, R.; Wen, B.; Gitai, Z.; Wingreen, N.S. Cell Shape and Cell-Wall Organization in Gram-Negative Bacteria. *Biophys. Comput. Biol.* **2008**, *105*, 19282–19287. [CrossRef]
17. Brown, S.; Santa Maria, J.P.; Walker, S. Wall Teichoic Acids of Gram-Positive Bacteria. *Annu. Rev. Microbiol.* **2013**, *67*, 313–336. [CrossRef]
18. Schneewind, O.; Missiakas, D. Lipoteichoic Acids, Phosphate-Containing Polymers in the Envelope of Gram-Positive Bacteria. *J. Bacteriol.* **2014**, *196*, 1133–1142. [CrossRef]
19. Khondker, A.; Rheinstädter, M.C. How Do Bacterial Membranes Resist Polymyxin Antibiotics? *Commun. Biol.* **2020**, *3*, 77. [CrossRef]
20. Jiang, X.; Yang, K.; Yuan, B.; Han, M.; Zhu, Y.; Roberts, K.D.; Patil, N.A.; Li, J.; Gong, B.; Hancock, R.E.W.; et al. Molecular Dynamics Simulations Informed by Membrane Lipidomics Reveal the Structure-Interaction Relationship of Polymyxins with the Lipid A-Based Outer Membrane of Acinetobacter Baumannii. *J. Antimicrob. Chemother.* **2020**, *75*, 3534–3543. [CrossRef]
21. Yang, X.; Huang, E.; Yousef, A.E. Brevibacillin, a Cationic Lipopeptide That Binds to Lipoteichoic Acid and Subsequently Disrupts Cytoplasmic Membrane of Staphylococcus Aureus. *Microbiol. Res.* **2017**, *195*, 18–23. [CrossRef] [PubMed]
22. Heesterbeek, D.A.C.; Martin, N.I.; Velthuizen, A.; Duijst, M.; Ruyken, M.; Wubbolts, R.; Rooijakkers, S.H.M.; Bardoel, B.W. Complement-Dependent Outer Membrane Perturbation Sensitizes Gram-Negative Bacteria to Gram-Positive Specific Antibiotics. *Sci. Rep.* **2019**, *9*, 3074. [CrossRef] [PubMed]
23. Santos, M.R.; Fonseca, A.C.; Mendonça, P.V.; Branco, R.; Serra, A.C.; Morais, P.V.; Coelho, J.F. Recent Developments in Antimicrobial Polymers: A Review. *Materials* **2016**, *9*, 599. [CrossRef] [PubMed]
24. Dias, F.G.G.; de Freitas Pereira, L.; Parreira, R.L.T.; Veneziani, R.C.S.; Bianchi, T.C.; de Paula Fontes, V.F.N.; de Carlos Galvani, M.; Cerce, D.D.P.; Martins, C.H.G.; Rinaldi-Neto, F.; et al. Evaluation of the Antiseptic and Wound Healing Potential of Polyhexamethylene Guanidine Hydrochloride as Well as Its Toxic Effects. *Eur. J. Pharm. Sci.* **2021**, *160*, 105739. [CrossRef]
25. Kumar, S.; Pillai, R.; Reghu, S.; Vikhe, Y.; Zheng, H.; Koh, C.H.; Chan-park, M.B. Novel Antimicrobial Coating on Silicone Contact Lens Using Glycidyl Methacrylate and Polyethyleneimine Based Polymers. *Macromol. Rapid Commun.* **2020**, *41*, 20000175. [CrossRef]
26. Gultekinoglu, M.; Karahan, S.; Kart, D.; Sagiroglu, M.; Erta, N.; Ozen, A.H.; Ulubayram, K. Polyethyleneimine Brushes Effectively Inhibit Encrustation on Polyurethane Ureteral Stents Both in Dynamic Bioreactor and in Vivo. *Mater. Sci. Eng. C* **2017**, *71*, 1166–1174. [CrossRef]
27. Peng, J.; Liu, P.; Peng, W.; Sun, J.; Dong, X.; Ma, Z. Poly (Hexamethylene Biguanide) (PHMB) as High-Efficiency Antibacterial Coating for Titanium Substrates. *J. Hazard. Mater.* **2021**, *411*, 125110. [CrossRef]
28. Rahman, M.A.; Jui, M.S.; Bam, M.; Cha, Y.; Luat, E.; Alabresm, A.; Nagarkatti, M.; Decho, A.W.; Tang, C. Facial Amphiphilicity-Induced Polymer Nanostructures for Antimicrobial Applications. *ACS Appl. Mater. Interfaces* **2020**, *12*, 21221–21230. [CrossRef]
29. Venkateswaran, S.; Wu, M.; Gwynne, P.J.; Hardman, A.; Lilienkampf, A.; Pernagallo, S.; Blakely, G.; Swann, D.G.; Gallagher, M.P.; Bradley, M. Bacteria Repelling Poly(Methylmethacrylate-Co-Dimethylacrylamide) Coatings for Biomedical Devices Devices. *J. Mater. Chem. B* **2014**, *2*, 6723–6729. [CrossRef]
30. Dizman, B.; Elasri, M.O.; Mathias, L.J. Synthesis and Characterization of Antibacterial and Temperature Responsive Methacrylamide Polymers. *Macromolecules* **2006**, *39*, 5738–5746. [CrossRef]
31. Hoque, J.; Akkapeddi, P.; Yadav, V.; Manjunath, G.B.; Uppu, D.S.S.M.; Konai, M.M.; Yarlagadda, V.; Sanyal, K.; Haldar, J. Broad Spectrum Antibacterial and Antifungal Polymeric Paint Materials: Synthesis, Structure—Activity Relationship, and Membrane-Active Mode of Action. *Appl. Mater.* **2015**, *7*, 1804–1815. [CrossRef]
32. Wee, V.; Ng, L.; Pang, J.; Tan, K.; Leong, J.; Voo, Z.X.; Hedrick, J.L. Antimicrobial Polycarbonates: Investigating the Impact of Nitrogen- Containing Heterocycles as Quaternizing Agents. *Macromolecules* **2014**, *47*, 1285–1291.
33. Oh, J.; Kim, S.; Oh, M.; Khan, A. Antibacterial Properties of Main-Chain Cationic Polymers Prepared through Amine–Epoxy 'Click' Polymerization. *RSC Adv.* **2020**, *10*, 26752–26755. [CrossRef] [PubMed]
34. Yandi, W.; Mieszkin, S.; Callow, M.E.; Callow, J.A.; Finlay, J.A.; Liedberg, B.; Ederth, T. Antialgal Activity of Poly(2-(Dimethylamino)Ethyl Methacrylate) (PDMAEMA) Brushes against the Marine Alga Ulva. *Biofouling* **2017**, *33*, 169–183. [CrossRef]
35. Ji, W.; Koepsel, R.R.; Murata, H.; Zadan, S.; Campbell, A.S.; Russell, A.J. Bactericidal Specificity and Resistance Profile of Poly(Quaternary Ammonium) Polymers and Protein-Poly(Quaternary Ammonium) Conjugates. *Biomacromolecules* **2017**, *18*, 2583–2593. [CrossRef]
36. Phillips, D.J.; Harrison, J.; Richards, S.J.; Mitchell, D.E.; Tichauer, E.; Hubbard, A.T.M.; Guy, C.; Hands-Portman, I.; Fullam, E.; Gibson, M.I. Evaluation of the Antimicrobial Activity of Cationic Polymers against Mycobacteria: Toward Antitubercular Macromolecules. *Biomacromolecules* **2017**, *18*, 1592–1599. [CrossRef] [PubMed]
37. Yang, Y.; Cai, Z.; Huang, Z.; Tang, X.; Zhang, X. Antimicrobial Cationic Polymers: From Structural Design to Functional Control. *Polym. J.* **2018**, *50*, 33–44. [CrossRef]

38. De Jesús-Téllez, M.A.; De la Rosa-García, S.; Medrano-Galindo, I.; Rosales-Peñafiel, I.; Gómez-Cornelio, S.; Guerrero-Sanchez, C.; Schubert, U.S.; Quintana-Owen, P. Antifungal Properties of Poly[2-(Dimethylamino)Ethyl Methacrylate] (PDMAEMA) and Quaternized Derivatives. *React. Funct. Polym.* **2021**, *163*, 104887. [CrossRef]
39. Keum, H.; Kim, D.; Whang, C.-H.; Kang, A.; Lee, S.; Na, W.; Jon, S. Impeding the Medical Protective Clothing Contamination by a Spray Coating of Trifunctional Polymers. *ACS Omega* **2022**, *7*, 10526–10538. [CrossRef]
40. Qiu, H.; Si, Z.; Luo, Y.; Feng, P.; Wu, X.; Hou, W.; Zhu, Y.; Chan-Park, M.B.; Xu, L.; Huang, D. The Mechanisms and the Applications of Antibacterial Polymers in Surface Modification on Medical Devices. *Front. Bioeng. Biotechnol.* **2020**, *8*, 910. [CrossRef]
41. Kwaśniewska, D.; Chen, Y.L.; Wieczorek, D. Biological Activity of Quaternary Ammonium Salts and Their Derivatives. *Pathogens* **2020**, *9*, 459. [CrossRef] [PubMed]
42. Ikeda, T.; Hirayama, H.; Yamaguchi, H.; Tazuke, S. Polycationic Biocides with Pendant Active Groups: Molecular Weight Dependence of Antibacterial Activity. *Antimicrob. Agents Chemother.* **1986**, *30*, 132–136. [CrossRef] [PubMed]
43. Hj, M.Á. The Effect of Molecular Weight on the Antibacterial Activity of N,N,N-Trimethyl Chitosan (TMC). *Int. J. Mol. Sci.* **2019**, *20*, 1743. [CrossRef]
44. Guo, J.; Qin, J.; Ren, Y.; Wang, B.; Cui, H.; Ding, Y.; Mao, H.; Yan, F. Antibacterial Activity of Cationic Polymers: Side-Chain or Main-Chain Type? *Polym. Chem.* **2018**, *9*, 4611–4616. [CrossRef]
45. Santos, M.R.E.; Mendonça, P.V.; Almeida, M.C.; Branco, R.; Serra, A.C.; Morais, P.V.; Coelho, J.F.J. Increasing the Antimicrobial Activity of Amphiphilic Cationic Copolymers by the Facile Synthesis of High Molecular Weight Stars by Supplemental Activator and Reducing Agent Atom Transfer Radical Polymerization. *Biomacromolecules* **2019**, *20*, 1146–1156. [CrossRef] [PubMed]
46. Pham, P.; Oliver, S.; Wong, E.H.H.; Boyer, C. Effect of Hydrophilic Groups on the Bioactivity of Antimicrobial Polymers. *Polym. Chem.* **2021**, *12*, 5689–5703. [CrossRef]
47. Phuong, P.T.; Oliver, S.; He, J.; Wong, E.H.H.; Mathers, R.T.; Boyer, C. Effect of Hydrophobic Groups on Antimicrobial and Hemolytic Activity: Developing a Predictive Tool for Ternary Antimicrobial Polymers. *Biomacromolecules* **2020**, *21*, 5241–5255. [CrossRef]
48. Copolymer, P.; Xue, Y.; Xiao, H. Antibacterial/Antiviral Property and Mechanism of Dual-Functional Quaternized Pyridinium-Type Copolymer. *Polymers* **2015**, *7*, 2290–2303. [CrossRef]
49. Roka, N.; Kokkorogianni, O.; Kontoes-Georgoudakis, P.; Choinopoulos, I.; Pitsikalis, M. Recent Advances in the Synthesis of Complex Macromolecular Architectures Based on Poly(N-Vinyl Pyrrolidone) and the RAFT Polymerization Technique. *Polymers* **2022**, *14*, 701. [CrossRef]
50. Nothling, M.D.; Fu, Q.; Reyhani, A.; Allison-Logan, S.; Jung, K.; Zhu, J.; Kamigaito, M.; Boyer, C.; Qiao, G.G. Progress and Perspectives Beyond Traditional RAFT Polymerization. *Adv. Sci.* **2020**, *7*, 2001656. [CrossRef]
51. Paslay, L.C.; Abel, B.A.; Brown, T.D.; Koul, V.; Choudhary, V.; McCormick, C.L.; Morgan, S.E. Antimicrobial Poly(Methacrylamide) Derivatives Prepared via Aqueous RAFT Polymerization Exhibit Biocidal Efficiency Dependent upon Cation Structure. *Biomacromolecules* **2012**, *13*, 2472–2482. [CrossRef] [PubMed]
52. Sathyan, A.; Kurtz, I.; Rathore, P.; Emrick, T.; Schiffman, J.D. Using Catechol and Zwitterion-Functionalized Copolymers to Prevent Dental Bacterial Adhesion. *ACS Appl. Bio Mater.* **2023**, *6*, 2905–2915. [CrossRef] [PubMed]
53. Song, F.; Zhang, L.; Chen, R.; Liu, Q.; Liu, J.; Yu, J.; Liu, P.; Duan, J.; Wang, J. Bioinspired Durable Antibacterial and Antifouling Coatings Based on Borneol Fluorinated Polymers: Demonstrating Direct Evidence of Antiadhesion. *ACS Appl. Mater. Interfaces* **2021**, *13*, 33417–33426. [CrossRef]
54. Keely, S.; Rawlinson, L.A.B.; Haddleton, D.M.; Brayden, D.J. A Tertiary Amino-Containing Polymethacrylate Polymer Protects Mucus-Covered Intestinal Epithelial Monolayers against Pathogenic Challenge. *Pharm. Res.* **2008**, *25*, 1193–1201. [CrossRef]
55. Rawlinson, L.A.B.; O'Gara, J.P.; Jones, D.S.; Brayden, D.J. Resistance of Staphylococcus Aureus to the Cationic Antimicrobial Agent Poly(2-(Dimethylamino Ethyl)Methacrylate) (PDMAEMA) Is Influenced by Cell-Surface Charge and Hydrophobicity. *J. Med. Microbiol.* **2011**, *60*, 968–976. [CrossRef] [PubMed]
56. Vitro, I.; Skóra, M. Studies on Antifungal Properties of Methacrylamido Propyl Trimethyl Ammonium Chloride Polycations and Their Toxicity. *Microbiol. Spectr.* **2023**, *11*, e0084423. [CrossRef]
57. Grace, J.L.; Huang, J.X.; Cheah, S.E.; Truong, N.P.; Cooper, M.A.; Li, J.; Davis, T.P.; Quinn, J.F.; Velkov, T.; Whittaker, M.R. Antibacterial Low Molecular Weight Cationic Polymers: Dissecting the Contribution of Hydrophobicity, Chain Length and Charge to Activity. *RSC Adv.* **2016**, *6*, 15469–15477. [CrossRef] [PubMed]
58. Lin, S.; Wu, J.H.; Jia, H.Q.; Hao, L.M.; Wang, R.Z.; Qi, J.C. Facile Preparation and Antibacterial Properties of Cationic Polymers Derived from 2-(Dimethylamino)Ethyl Methacrylate. *RSC Adv.* **2013**, *3*, 20758–20764. [CrossRef]
59. Lv, H.; Zhang, S.; Wang, B.; Cui, S.; Yan, J. Toxicity of Cationic Lipids and Cationic Polymers in Gene Delivery. *J. Control. Release* **2006**, *114*, 100–109. [CrossRef]
60. Cai, J.; Yue, Y.; Rui, D.; Zhang, Y.; Liu, S.; Wu, C. Effect of Chain Length on Cytotoxicity and Endocytosis of Cationic Polymers. *Macromol. Res.* **2011**, *44*, 2050–2057. [CrossRef]
61. Correia, J.S.; Mirón-barroso, S.; Hutchings, C.; Ottaviani, S.; Castellano, L. How Does the Polymer Architecture and Position of Cationic Charges Affect Cell Viability? *Polym. Chem.* **2022**, *14*, 303–317. [CrossRef] [PubMed]
62. Online, V.A. A Polyion Complex Micelle with Heparin for Growth Factorfactor Delivery and Uptake into Cells. *J. Mater. Chem. B* **2013**, *1*, 1635–1643. [CrossRef]

63. Monnery, B.D.; Wright, M.; Cavill, R.; Hoogenboom, R.; Shaunak, S.; Steinke, J.H.G.; Thanou, M. Cytotoxicity of Polycations: Relationship of Molecular Weight and the Hydrolytic Theory of the Mechanism of Toxicity. *Int. J. Pharm.* **2017**, *521*, 249–258. [CrossRef]
64. Locock, K.E.S.; Michl, T.D.; Valentin, J.D.P.; Vasilev, K.; Hayball, J.D.; Qu, Y.; Traven, A.; Griesser, H.J.; Meagher, L.; Haeussler, M. Guanylated Polymethacrylates: A Class of Potent Antimicrobial Polymers with Low Hemolytic Activity. *Biomacromolecules* **2013**, *14*, 4021–4031. [CrossRef] [PubMed]
65. Layman, J.M.; Ramirez, S.M.; Green, M.D.; Long, T.E. Influence of Polycation Molecular Weight on Poly(2-Dimethylaminoethyl Methacrylate)-Mediated DNA Delivery in Vitro. *Biomacromolecules* **2009**, *10*, 1244–1252. [CrossRef] [PubMed]
66. Samsonova, O.; Pfeiffer, C.; Hellmund, M.; Merkel, O.M.; Kissel, T. Low Molecular Weight PDMAEMA-Block-PHEMA Block-Copolymers Synthesized via RAFT-Polymerization: Potential Non-Viral Gene Delivery Agents. *Polymers* **2011**, *3*, 693–718. [CrossRef]
67. Foster, L.L.; Yusa, S.I.; Kuroda, K. Solution-Mediated Modulation of Pseudomonas Aeruginosa Biofilm Formation by a Cationic Synthetic Polymer. *Antibiotics* **2019**, *8*, 61. [CrossRef]
68. Perrier, S. 50th Anniversary Perspective: RAFT Polymerization-A User Guide. *Macromolecules* **2017**, *50*, 7433–7447. [CrossRef]
69. Cao, J.; Siefker, D.; Chan, B.A.; Yu, T.; Lu, L.; Saputra, M.A.; Fronczek, F.R.; Xie, W.; Zhang, D. Interfacial Ring-Opening Polymerization of Amino-Acid-Derived N-Thiocarboxyanhydrides toward Well-Defined Polypeptides. *ACS Macro Lett.* **2017**, *6*, 836–840. [CrossRef]
70. Druvari, D.; Koromilas, N.D.; Bekiari, V.; Bokias, G.; Kallitsis, J.K. Polymeric Antimicrobial Coatings Based on Quaternary Ammonium Compounds. *Coatings* **2018**, *8*, 8. [CrossRef]
71. Kenawy, E.R.; Worley, S.D.; Broughton, R. The Chemistry and Applications of Antimicrobial Polymers: A State-of-the-Art Review. *Biomacromolecules* **2007**, *8*, 1359–1384. [CrossRef] [PubMed]
72. Demarteau, J.; De Añastro, F.; Shaplov, A.S. Polymer Chemistry. *Polym. Chem.* **2020**, *11*, 1481–1488. [CrossRef]
73. Teh, C.H.; Nazni, W.A.; Nurulhusna, A.H.; Norazah, A.; Lee, H.L. Determination of Antibacterial Activity and Minimum Inhibitory Concentration of Larval Extract of Fly via Resazurin-Based Turbidometric Assay. *BMC Microbiol.* **2017**, *17*, 36. [CrossRef] [PubMed]
74. Mukherjee, A.; Barman, R.; Das, B.; Ghosh, S. Highly Efficient Biofilm Eradication by Antibacterial Two-Dimensional Supramolecular Polymers. *Chem. Mater.* **2021**, *33*, 8656–8665. [CrossRef]
75. Wu, C.L.; Peng, K.L.; Yip, B.S.; Chih, Y.H.; Cheng, J.W. Boosting Synergistic Effects of Short Antimicrobial Peptides with Conventional Antibiotics against Resistant Bacteria. *Front. Microbiol.* **2021**, *12*, 747760. [CrossRef]
76. Singhsa, P.; Diaz-Dussan, D.; Manuspiya, H.; Narain, R. Well-Defined Cationic N-[3-(Dimethylamino)Propyl]Methacrylamide Hydrochloride-Based (Co)Polymers for SiRNA Delivery. *Biomacromolecules* **2018**, *19*, 209–221. [CrossRef]
77. Azuma, R.; Nakamichi, S.; Kimura, J.; Yano, H.; Kawasaki, H.; Suzuki, T.; Kondo, R.; Kanda, Y.; Shimizu, K.I.; Kato, K.; et al. Solution Synthesis of N,N-Dimethylformamide-Stabilized Iron-Oxide Nanoparticles as an Efficient and Recyclable Catalyst for Alkene Hydrosilylation. *ChemCatChem* **2018**, *10*, 2378–2382. [CrossRef]

Disclaimer/Publisher's Note: The statements, opinions and data contained in all publications are solely those of the individual author(s) and contributor(s) and not of MDPI and/or the editor(s). MDPI and/or the editor(s) disclaim responsibility for any injury to people or property resulting from any ideas, methods, instructions or products referred to in the content.

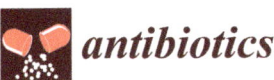

Article

Tricyclic Fused Lactams by Mukaiyama Cyclisation of Phthalimides and Evaluation of their Biological Activity

Lewis T. Ibbotson [1], Kirsten E. Christensen [1], Miroslav Genov [2], Alexander Pretsch [2], Dagmar Pretsch [2] and Mark G. Moloney [1,*]

[1] The Department of Chemistry, Chemistry Research Laboratory, University of Oxford, 12 Mansfield Road, Oxford OX1 3TA, UK
[2] Oxford Antibiotic Group, The Oxford Science Park, Magdalen Centre, Oxford OX4 4GA, UK
* Correspondence: mark.moloney@chem.ox.ac.uk

Abstract: We report that phthalimides may be cyclized using a Mukaiyama-type aldol coupling to give variously substituted fused lactam (1,2,3,9b-tetrahydro-5H-pyrrolo[2,1-a]isoindol-5-one) systems. This novel process shows a high level of regioselectivity for o-substituted phthalimides, dictated by steric and electronic factors, but not for m-substituted phthalimides. The initial aldol adduct is prone to elimination, giving 2,3-dihydro-5H-pyrrolo[2,1-a]isoindol-5-ones, and the initial cyclisation can be conducted in such a way that aldol cyclisation-elimination is achievable in a one-pot approach. The 2,3-dihydro-5H-pyrrolo[2,1-a]isoindol-5-ones possess cross conjugation and steric effects which significantly influence the reactivity of several functional groups, but conditions suitable for epoxidation, ester hydrolysis and amide formation, and reduction, which provide for ring manipulation, were identified. Many of the derived lactam systems, and especially the eliminated systems, show low solubility, which compromises biological activity, although in some cases, antibacterial and cytotoxic activity was found, and this new class of small molecule provides a useful skeleton for further elaboration and study.

Keywords: pyrrolidinone; aldol; antibacterial

Citation: Ibbotson, L.T.; Christensen, K.E.; Genov, M.; Pretsch, A.; Pretsch, D.; Moloney, M.G. Tricyclic Fused Lactams by Mukaiyama Cyclisation of Phthalimides and Evaluation of their Biological Activity. *Antibiotics* **2023**, *12*, 9. https://doi.org/10.3390/antibiotics12010009

Academic Editor: Charlotte A. Huber

Received: 25 November 2022
Revised: 14 December 2022
Accepted: 15 December 2022
Published: 21 December 2022

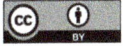

Copyright: © 2022 by the authors. Licensee MDPI, Basel, Switzerland. This article is an open access article distributed under the terms and conditions of the Creative Commons Attribution (CC BY) license (https://creativecommons.org/licenses/by/4.0/).

1. Introduction

The critical importance of natural products in the development of pharmaceutically active compounds has been thoroughly documented, and although popularity of this approach has waned in recent years in favour of combinatorial and rational design, there have been strong calls for its reinvigoration [1]. These calls are particularly relevant for antibacterial agents, for which there is a serious deficit of new candidates in the drug pipeline [2,3], at a time when there is considerable urgency to expand therapeutics as a result of the rapid emergence of resistant bacterial strains [4]. The challenges peculiar to antibacterial drug discovery [5–8] imply that natural products often provide biologically validated start points suitable for immediate elaboration in the quest for new pharmaceutically useful agents [9,10]. It has recently been recognised that existing strategies for the discovery of new antibacterials have not been effective [11], probably as a result at least in part of overreliance of combinatorial approaches leading to structurally narrow libraries [12,13], and there is an urgent need for the identification of novel leads for expanding the antibacterial drug development pipeline [14,15]. The work of Waldmann [16,17] and Danishefsky [18] has reiterated the importance of natural products as a starting point for drug discovery, and our contribution to this area has been to show that chemical libraries modelled on natural products [19], including equisetin [20], reutericyclin [21], kibdelomycin [22], and streptolydigin [23], which all possess a core tetramate unit, or oxazolomycin [24] and pramanicin [25], which possess an α-hydroxypyroglutamate core, may exhibit significant antibacterial activity and provide useful opportunities for further optimisation. Critical to the success of this work has been the finding that C-acyl or C-carboxamide side chains may be introduced under mild conditions to tetramate and pyroglutamate skeletons [19] and that this leads to enhanced antibacterial activity. It would appear, therefore, that an α, α, α-tricarbonyl unit comprises, at least in part, the active pharmacophore, and this was corroborated by the finding that the core tetramate without an α, α, α-tricarbonyl unit had little intrinsic antibacterial activity [26].

The recent discovery of pyrrolizilactone [27], UCS1025A and B [28–30] and CJ-16264 [31], is of interest since all are comprised of a common lactam-lactone fused ring core and C-acyl decalin side chain. Studies of the biosynthesis [32], synthesis [33–36], and SAR [37] of UCS1025A suggest that the core skeleton might offer an opportunity for development, not least because of its similarity with bioactive tetramates, which are also appended with decalins [38]. Of significance is the antibacterial bioactivity of these systems, with MIC values of typically 1–15 ug/mL against Gram-positive MDR strains and some Gram-negative ones [31]. Limited SAR analysis with three CJ-16,264 stereoisomers shows MIC values of 2–16 ug/mL against MRSA, *E. faecelis*, and *E. faecium* [39]. As a result, the development of methodology for their total synthesis has attracted attention [40,41] and the total synthesis of myceliothermophins C, D, and E [42], a related structural type, has also recently been achieved. The synthesis of the azabicyclo[3.3.0]octane core provides a key background [43] and an unusual approach to the pyrrolizidine core from an 8-membered ring by transannular cyclisation has been reported [44]. Of particular interest was the elegant ring cyclisation methodology originally reported by Lambert [34] and developed later by both Hoye [35,45] and Christmann [33,46,47], since this provided rapid entry to the core lactam system from maleimides by an aldol-like ring closure, using in situ generated silyl enolates as nucleophiles. We have recently reported that this approach is suitable for substituted maleimides, and can be used to access a small library of novel pyrrolidinones [48]; of interest was their lack of antibacterial activity, but a similar phenomenon had been observed for unsubstituted tetramates [19]. We report here that the aldol cyclisation may be further extended to phthalimides, and that this gives rise to a range of functionalised systems whose biological activity has been assessed.

2. Results and Discussion

Substituted phthalic anhydrides **1a–d** (Scheme 1) and **2a–e** (Scheme 2) and γ-aminobutyric acid (GABA) were condensed by heating without solvent to 170 °C for 6 h, during which the molten mixture slowly turned to a straw yellow colour, using the previously reported procedure [49–53], and successfully gave a range of substituted systems in excellent yields. Upon completion of the reaction, the cooled solid mass was dissolved in dichloromethane and washed using 0.5 N HCl, giving the desired products **3a–d** and **4a–e** in excellent yields (Schemes 1 and 2, and Table 1). Esterification of acids **3a–d** and **4a–e** to their corresponding methyl esters **5a–d** and **6a–e** using thionyl chloride and MeOH at rt over 16 h gave the products in quantitative yields in many cases (Table 1); however, this was ineffective for **4b** due to its unexpectedly low solubility, and synthesis of **6b** required direct condensation of methyl γ-aminobutanoate hydrochloride with the anhydride in toluene with DIPEA under reflux for 16 h, giving the desired product **6b** (quantitative yield), the structure of which was confirmed by single crystal X-ray diffraction (Figure S1, Supporting Information (SI)) [54–57]. Protection of the free hydroxyl group of hydroxyphthalimide **5d** as the OBn and OMe ethers **5e** and **5f** was achieved using standard procedures in excellent yields. Benzylation of **3a** using thionyl chloride/benzyl alcohol gave benzyl ester **7** in up to 60% yield (Scheme 1) and conversion to anilide **7b** and 8-amidoquinoline **7c** using the appropriate amine was similarly possible.

Reagents and conditions: (a) $H_2NCH_2CH_2CH_2CO_2H$, 170 °C, 6 h; (b) MeOH, $SOCl_2$, rt, 16 h; (c) BnBr, K_2CO_3, acetone, rt, 16 h; (d) MeI, K_2CO_3, DMF, 2h; (e) BnOH, $SOCl_2$, rt, 16 h or NaH, BnBr, DMF, rt, 16 h; (f) EDC, $PhNH_2$; (g) $SOCl_2$ then 8-aminoquinoline; (h) TBDMSiOTf (3 equiv.), TEA or DIPEA (3 equiv.), DCM, rt, 16h; (i) TBDMSiOTf (1.1 eq), DIPEA (3 eq), DCM, rt, 16h.; (j) TFA, H_2O (9:1), 30 min, r.t.

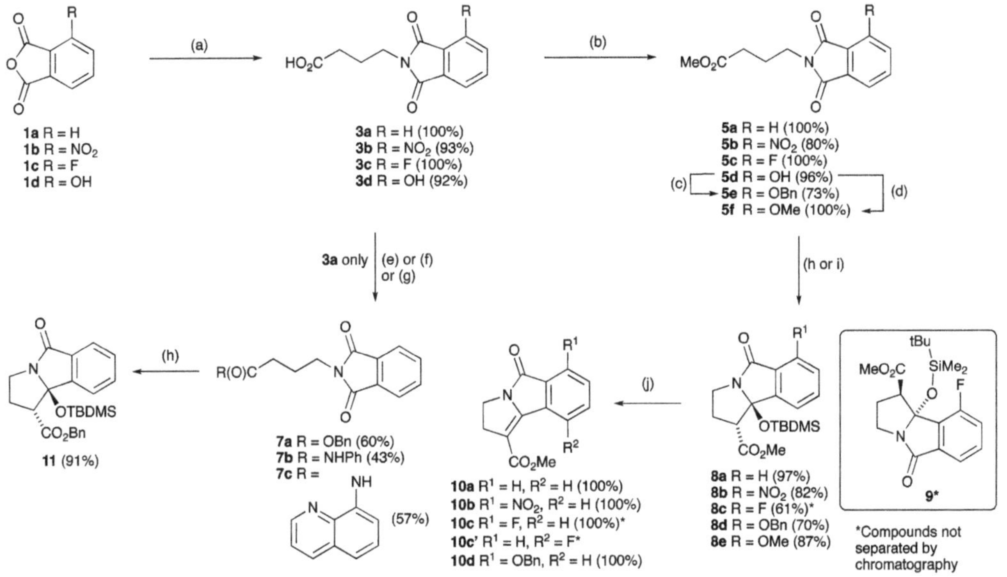

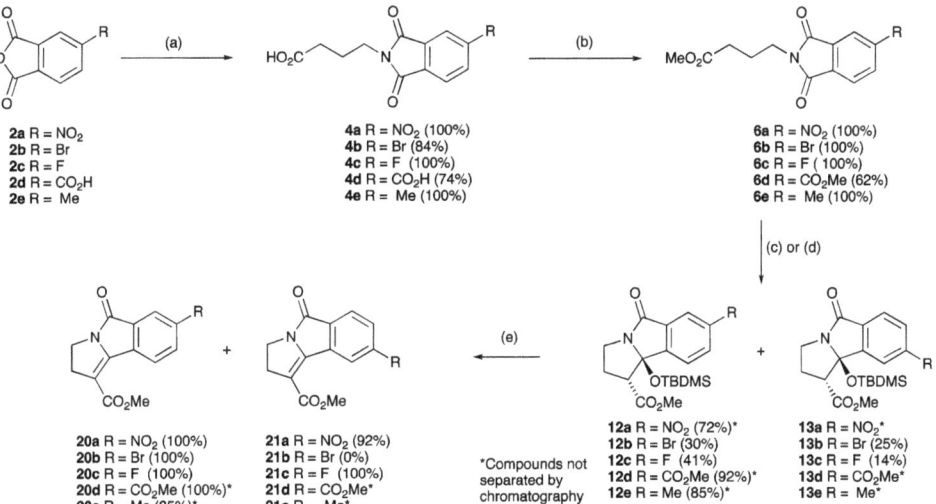

Scheme 1. Synthesis and ring closure of substituted phthalimides.

Reagents and conditions: (a) $H_2NCH_2CH_2CH_2CO_2H$, 170 °C, 6 h; (b) MeOH, $SOCl_2$, rt, 16 h; (c) TBDMSOTf (3 equiv.), TEA or DIPEA (3 equiv.), DCM, rt, 16h; (d) TBDMSOTf (1.1 eq), TEA or DIPEA (3 eq), DCM, rt, 16h.; (e) TFA, H_2O, 30 min, r.t.

Scheme 2. Synthesis and ring closure of substituted phthalimides.

Table 1. Yields for Phthalimides 3,4, Esters 5,6 and Lactams 8, 12 and 13 (Schemes 1 and 2).

R	Phthalimide	Temperature (°C)	Yield (%)	Ester	Yield (%)	Lactam	Yield (%)
H	3a	170	100	5a	100	8a	97
NO_2	3b	175	93	5b	80	8b	82
F	3c	170	100	5c	100	8c/9	61 *
OH	3d	195	92	5d	96	-	-
OBn	-	-	-	5e	73	8d	70
OMe	-	-	-	5f	100	8e	87
NO_2	4a	175	100	6a	100	12a,13a	72 *
Br	4b	170	84	6b	0 (100)	12b,13b	55 *
F	4c	170	100	6c	100	12c,13c	55 *
CO_2H	4d	205	74	-	-	-	-
CO_2Me	-	-	-	6d	62	12d,13d	92 *
CH_3	4e	170	100	6e	100	12e,13e	85 *

* Yields are the total for both isomers.

With the required phthalimides in hand, **5a** was treated with N,N-diisopropylethylamine (DIPEA) and t-butyldimethylsilyl triflate (TBDMSOTf) according to a modification of the literature's procedure [34], and purification using flash column chromatography afforded the silyl containing tricyclic pyrrolizidinone **8a** with a good yield of 97% (Scheme 1 and Table 1). This material was readily characterised by standard spectroscopic techniques; of interest were the non-equivalent silyl dimethyl groups that had shifted upfield to −0.08 and −0.51 ppm due to the anisotropy of the adjacent aromatic ring, consistent with ring closure. The stereochemistry was confirmed by a combination of one and single crystal X-ray diffraction (Figure S1, ESI) [54–57]; the *trans*-relationship of the methyl ester and silyloxy moiety were evident, placing the methyl ester into a pseudoaxial position, and with one of the silyl methyl groups located over the aromatic ring, accounting for the shielding observed in the NMR spectrum. While the structure of **8a** was further confirmed by LRMS and HRMS, with the major mass ions being 362 [MH$^+$] and 384 [MNa$^+$] as expected, importantly these signals were accompanied by a mass ion of 132 less than the desired product at 230 [MH+]; this was consistent with in situ desilyloxylation giving **10a**. In fact, the cyclisation of **5a** was found to be unreliable, instead often giving **10a** directly and quantitatively by in situ elimination. Synthesis of similar tetrahydro-1H-pyrrolo[2,1-a]isoindoles [58–60] and their unsaturated systems [61–63] has been reported. In order to understand the progress of this reaction, varying equivalents of TBDMSOTf were used with phthalimides **5a,b** and it was found that while the formation of the products **8a,b** was achievable in high yields with 1.1 equivalents of TBDMSOTf, nearly quantitative direct conversion of **8a** to unsaturated pyrrolizidinones **10a,b** could be achieved using 2.0 equivalents of TBDMSOTf (Table S1, ESI).

Application of these cyclisation conditions to phthalimides **5b–f** successfully gave cyclised products **8b–e** in good to excellent yield (Schemes 1 and 2 and Table 1). TLC and ^{1}H NMR spectroscopic analysis indicated formation of only a single regioisomer, except for **5c** which gave an isomeric mixture of **8c** also containing **9** (ratio 7:1). Structural assignment was confirmed in the case of **8b,c**, **9** and **12a** by single crystal X-ray diffraction (Figure S1, ESI) [54–57]. The mode of cyclisation appeared to be dictated by the sterically bulky substituents on the aromatic ring, but in the case of **5c** was biased by both the small size and electronegativity of the fluorine substituent which also gave the alternative isomer **9**. Substituted phthalimides **6a–e** were subjected to the same ring-closing conditions, giving good to excellent yields of products **12a–e** and **13a–e** (Schemes 1 and 2, and Table 1), usually as an approximately equal mixture of isomers, which proved to be difficult to separate by flash column chromatography, and arising by ring closure onto either phthalimide carbonyl group. While the cyclisations using methyl esters were very high yielding and reliable reactions, of interest was whether reactions of substrates with bulkier esters would be as effective; benzyl ester variant **7a** in fact cyclised to **11** with an excellent yield of 91% using the standard conditions (1.1 eq TBDMSOTf, 3 eq DIPEA) fully diastereoselectively, as the *trans-* isomer (Scheme 1), although both anilide **7b** and quinoline **7c** did not.

The solventless phthalimide synthesis proved to be very effective with phthalic anhydride and glutamic acid, giving the desired diacid product **14a** in 60% yield (Scheme 3) [64–66]. However, this material was not easily soluble, but L-glutamic acid 5-methyl ester along with phthalic anhydride gave the desired and much more soluble product **14b** in 72% yield after heating at 175 °C for 6 h; this reaction remained effective on a multigram scale. In addition, L-glutamic dimethyl ester hydrochloride and phthalic anhydride under the same conditions gave the product **14c** in a yield of 30%; the same product could be prepared by esterification of diacid **14a** and with a similar yield (38%). This approach was similarly suitable for L-glutamic acid 5-benzyl ester, which gave the product **14d** with a yield of 38% [67,68]. The most effective method for the monomethyl esterification of benzyl glutamate **14e** used MeI, Cs_2CO_3, DMF, which gave the desired product **14f** in 40% yield. This approach could also be used for imide formation with phthalic anhydride and 2-aminophenylacetic acid via solventless conditions to give **15a**, followed by esterification which gave the desired ester **15b** with a yield of 38% (Scheme 4); however, a better alternative proved to be direct condensation of the methyl ester of aminophenylacetic acid to give **15b** and in quantitative yield. Nitrile **18**, was also readily available, prepared as shown (Scheme 4).

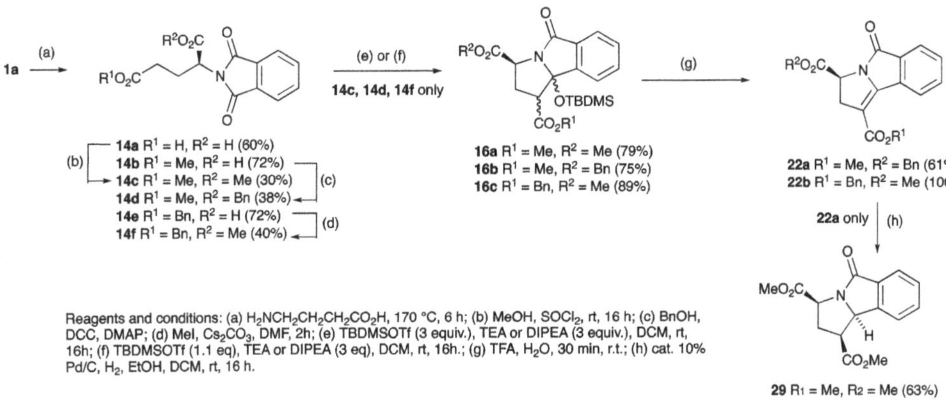

Scheme 3. Synthesis and ring closure of glutamyl substituted phthalimides.

Cyclisation of these analogues was examined using the conditions optimised above. The L-dimethyl ester glutamic acid appended phthalimide **14c** cyclised in excellent yield of 79% to give **16a** as a diastereomeric mixture (Scheme 3); one of these was successfully crystallised and the structure for the major one determined by single crystal X-ray diffraction (Figure S1, ESI). This clearly shows that the two methyl esters are *cis*-related, with all substituents in a pseudoaxial-like arrangement [54–57]. The cyclisation of **14d** under the same conditions gave a single diastereomer of **16b**, most likely due to the greater steric hindrance of the two substituents, the structure of which was confirmed by single crystal X-ray diffraction (Figure S1, ESI) [54–57]. Benzyl glutamate **14f** was subjected to TBDMSOTf mediated cyclisations, but gave poor yields of **16c** of around 35% when using 1.1 eq of TBDMSOTf, although this improved to much higher yields (89%) with 3.0 eq of TBDMSOTf, as a mixture of inseparable diastereomers (*d.r* of 1:0.6), the major of which was assumed to have the same stereochemistry as **16a**, based on comparison to established NMR spectroscopic data. When compound **15b** (Scheme 4) was subjected to standard cyclisation conditions, product **17** was successfully obtained as a single stereoisomer in 39% yield. Of interest is that nitrile **18** also readily cyclised to the analogous product **19** as a mixture of diastereomers; a related material has previously been reported by photocyclisation [69].

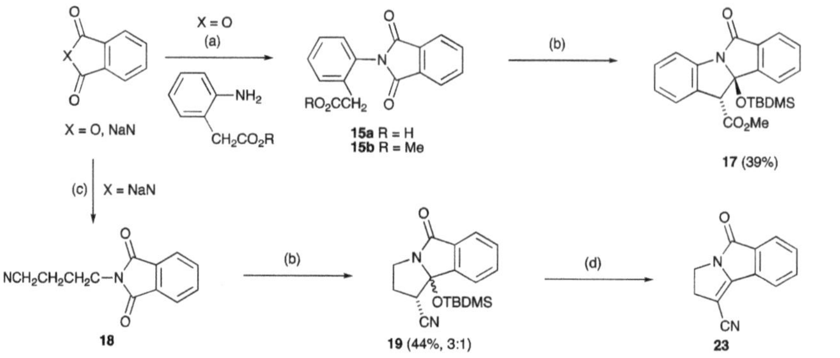
X = O
(a)
X = O, NaN
NH_2
CH_2CO_2R
RO_2CCH_2
15a R = H
15b R = Me
(b)
OTBDMS
CO_2Me
17 (39%)
(c)
X = NaN
$NCH_2CH_2CH_2C$—N
18
(b)
OTBDMS
CN
19 (44%, 3:1)
(d)
CN
23

Reagents and conditions: (a) 150 °C, 6 h; (b) TBDMSOTf (1.1 equiv.), DIPEA (3 equiv.), DCM, rt, 16h; (c) $BrCH_2CH_2CH_2CN$, DMF, 100 °C, 16 h (93%); (d) TFA, H_2O, 30 min, r.t.

Scheme 4. Synthesis and ring closure of substituted phthalimides.

Since TFA elimination reactions had been previously reported on silyloxyethers [60,70–73], similar reactions were then carried on **8a–d** and **12a–e, 13a–e**, giving quantitative conversions to the eliminated products **10a–d**, **20a–e**, **21a–e**, **22a–b** (Schemes 1–4). When the diastereomeric mixture of **19** was stirred in TFA/H_2O (9:1) for 30 min, only the *trans*- isomer reacted, leaving the *cis*-isomer unconverted, consistent with a fast antiperiplanar elimination; the structure of the unsaturated product **23** was confirmed by single crystal X-ray diffraction (Scheme 4 and Figure S2, (SI)) [54–57]. Moreover, it was found that the eliminated cyclised products could also be obtained directly by using TBDMSOTf (2 equiv.) for the ring closure reaction of both phthalimides **5a,b,c,e** and **14c,f** adducts and in excellent yield (Scheme 5).

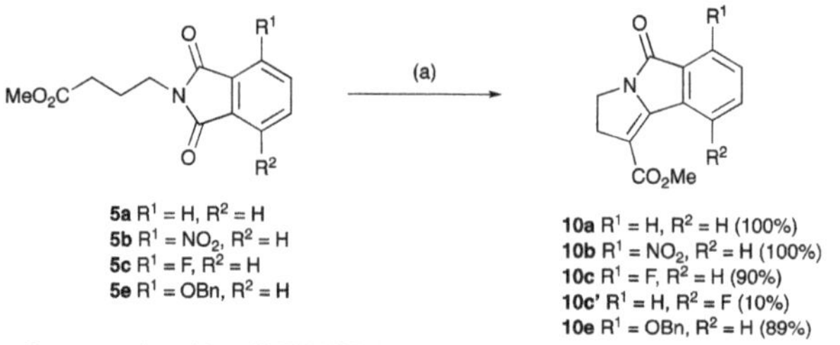
MeO_2C
R^1
R^2
(a)
CO_2Me
5a R^1 = H, R^2 = H
5b R^1 = NO_2, R^2 = H
5c R^1 = F, R^2 = H
5e R^1 = OBn, R^2 = H
10a R^1 = H, R^2 = H (100%)
10b R^1 = NO_2, R^2 = H (100%)
10c R^1 = F, R^2 = H (90%)
10c' R^1 = H, R^2 = F (10%)
10e R^1 = OBn, R^2 = H (89%)

Reagents and conditions: (a) TBDMSOTf (2.0 equiv.), DIPEA (3.0 equiv.), DCM, rt, 16h.

Scheme 5. One-pot ring closure and elimination of substituted phthalimides.

Hoye described the mechanism of this ring-closing process as an intramolecular Mukaiyama-like addition in which formation of a silyl ketene acetal is followed by addition to one of the imide carbonyls via in situ silyl activation [45], and Christmann proposed the intermediacy of a *bis*-silylketene acetal formed in situ from the starting carboxylic acid [46]. Although the Mukaiyama aldol addition [74] is very well known [75–80], Mukaiyama-type additions to imides are not; however, a one-pot approach, in which silyl ketene acetals are intermediates, has been described for addition to imines [81]. We propose a similar mechanism for a Mukaiyama-imide aldol addition involving the formation of the silyl ketene acetal followed either by coordination of the imide carbonyl giving a 5,6-bicyclic transition state that undergoes aldol addition (Route A), or cyclisation involving separate imide activation by a second molecule of TBDMSOTf (Route B) (Figure 1).

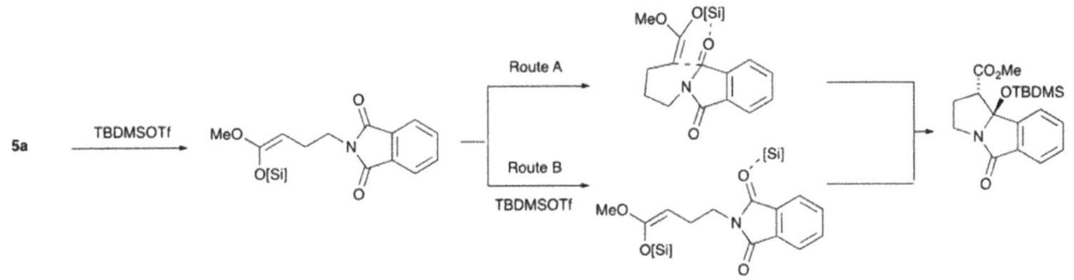

Figure 1. Possible mechanism for aldol ring closure.

With the pyrrolidinones in hand, of interest was an examination of their further reactivity; it was expected that this might not be straightforward, since low solubility was found for many compounds, especially the planar derivatives such as **10, 20** and **21**. Additionally, the high level of cross-conjugation along with significant steric effects in these densely functionalised systems was expected to significantly modify their chemical behaviour. Functionalisation of the (electron deficient) carbon-carbon double bond of the unsaturated system of cyclised adducts, for which there was some precedent literature [82], was examined [83] using 35% aqueous hydrogen peroxide in the presence of 4-methyl morpholine. The unsubstituted variant **10a** proved to be unreactive under these conditions, although when dissolved in dichloromethane with *m*CPBA and left stirring for 16 h at room temperature, α-ketoester **24** was obtained in low yield (Scheme 6). Such a product would be expected to arise by initial epoxidation of the double bond, followed by a further attack by *m*CPBA leading to a ring opening. However, it was found that if this reaction was conducted in the presence of calcium carbonate, successful epoxidation was achieved, giving **25**. This approach proved not to be successful for **10b**, since 1.2 equivalents of *m*CPBA gave not the expected epoxide but adduct **26** (Scheme 6), whose structure was confirmed by careful NMR spectroscopic analysis. Catalytic hydrogenation gave highly efficient conversion of lactams **10a–d, 20a–e, 21a–e** to lactams **27a–j**, in a reaction in which the strong yellow colour of the starting material was fully discharged, consistent with the removal of the extended conjugation (Table 2 and Scheme 7). In the case of the nitro derivatives **10b, 20a**, and **21a**, concomitant reduction to the amine derivatives **27b–d** occurred. The structures of **27b** and **27f** were confirmed by single crystal X-ray diffraction (Figure S2, ESI) [54–57]. Reduction of **10d** also involved hydrogenolysis and afforded phenol **27h**. Glutamate derivatives **22a,b** were subjected to the same hydrogenation conditions and gave *cis*-dimethyl esters **29a,b** (Scheme 3), whose stereochemistry was shown from nOe analysis.

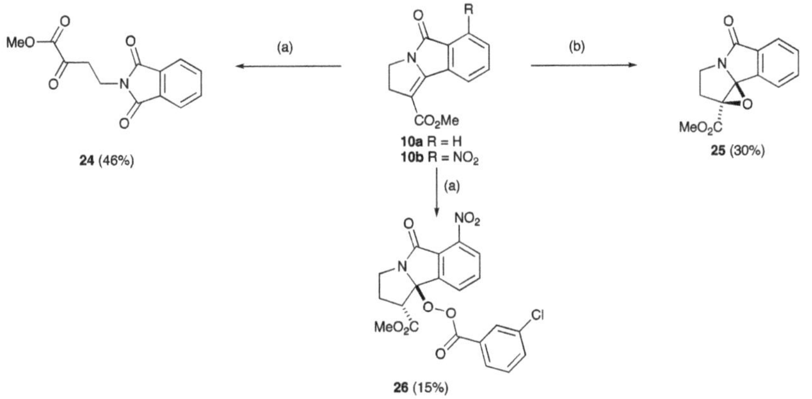

Reagents and conditions: (a) *m*CPBA (1.2 equiv.), DCM, rt, 16h.; (b) *m*CPBA (1.2 equiv.), Ca$_2$CO$_3$ (1.2 equiv.), DCM, rt, 16h.

Scheme 6. Elaboration of 2,3-dihydro-5*H*-pyrrolo[2,1-*a*]isoindol-5-ones.

Table 2. Reduction of unsaturated bicyclic lactams 10a–d, 20a–e, 21a–e.

Substrate	Product	R^1	R^2	R^3	R^4	Yield (%)
10a	27a	H	H	H	H	100
10b	27b	NH$_2$	H	H	H	100
20a	27c	H	NH$_2$	H	H	100
21a	27d	H	H	NH$_2$	H	100
10c	27e	F	H	H	H	50
10c'	27f	H	H	H	F	14
20c	27g	H	F	H	H	100
10d	27h	OH	H	H	H	86
20e	27i	H	Me	H	H	95
21e	27j	H	H	Me	H	95

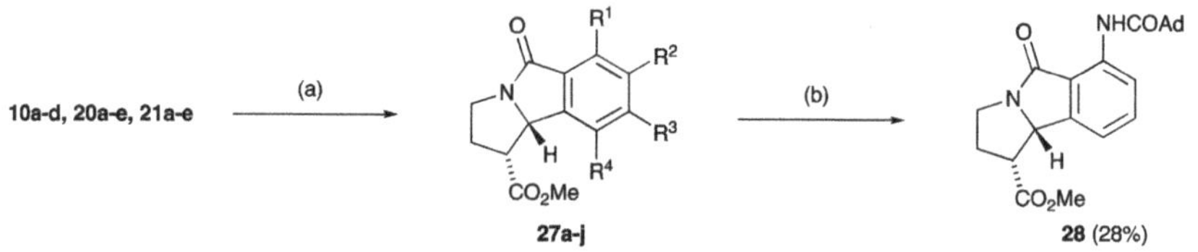

Reagents and conditions: (a) cat. 10% Pd/C, H$_2$, EtOH, DCM, rt, 16 h (see Table 2); (b) AdCOCl, DIPEA, DCM, 16h, rt

Scheme 7. Reduction of 2,3-dihydro-5H-pyrrolo[2,1-a]isoindol-5-ones.

With **27b** in hand, conversion to corresponding amide **28** using 1-adamantanecarbonyl chloride (Scheme 8) was made, as this group had given some of the highest levels of antibacterial activity seen for tetramates [19]; although this reaction proceeded successfully, the yield was low (28%), and this most likely arose by the combination of an electronically and sterically deactivated amine with a hindered acid chloride.

Of interest was whether this approach might be able to be adjusted to allow the ready introduction of ring substituents on the core skeleton, including C-H functionalisation, since related systems had been shown to be amenable to such manipulation [84]. Since the use of 8-aminoquinoline as a directing group for C-H activation is now well-known [85–87], 8-hydroxyquinoline ester **30** was prepared via N,N'-dicyclohexylcarbodiimide coupling with 8-hydroxyquinoline (64%), and although this could be effectively cyclised to **31** under standard conditions, in subsequent reactions **31** did not undergo remote C-H arylation. However, **31** when treated with TFA:H$_2$O afforded the desired unsaturated system **32** quantitatively (Scheme 8). While ester hydrolysis of **8a** and **11** was found to be straightforward, giving acids **33** and **34**, the attempted DCC/DMAP coupling of **33** with 8-aminoquinoline proved to be unsuccessful, giving only the rearranged N-acylurea intermediate; 1-ethyl-3-(3-dimethylaminopropyl)carbodiimide (EDC) along with 1-hydroxybenzotriazole (HOBt) gave a similar outcome. It was also found that **10a** could be hydrolysed directly under basic conditions in excellent yield to give **33** directly, and that this, when treated with TFA, water, and methanol, gave acid **34** in quantitative yield (Scheme 8). With **34** in hand, amide formation was examined (Scheme 8) but the products **35a–c** could be obtained only in modest yield, and aniline was completely unreactive. This likely reflects the unusual electronic character of the extended conjugated push-pull system in the starting material. Alternatively, **36** could be obtained by direct reduction of acid **34** or by hydrolysis of **27a** in good yield (Scheme 8) and conversion to the picolyl amide **37** under a variety of conditions gave a modest yield of product.

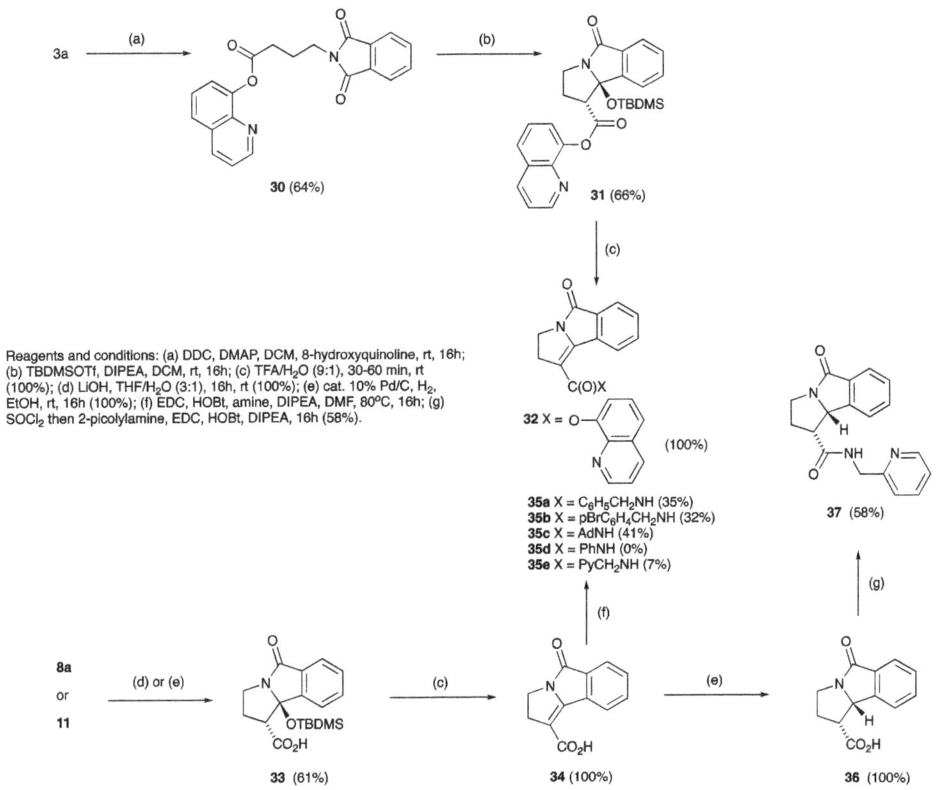
3a
(a)
30 (64%)
(b)
OTBDMS
31 (66%)
(c)
Reagents and conditions: (a) DDC, DMAP, DCM, 8-hydroxyquinoline, rt, 16h; (b) TBDMSOTf, DIPEA, DCM, rt, 16h; (c) TFA/H2O (9:1), 30-60 min, rt (100%); (d) LiOH, THF/H2O (3:1), 16h, rt (100%); (e) cat. 10% Pd/C, H2, EtOH, rt, 16h (100%); (f) EDC, HOBt, amine, DIPEA, DMF, 80°C, 16h; (g) SOCl2 then 2-picolylamine, EDC, HOBt, DIPEA, 16h (58%).
C(O)X
32 X = O–
(100%)
35a X = C6H5CH2NH (35%)
35b X = pBrC6H4CH2NH (32%)
35c X = AdNH (41%)
35d X = PhNH (0%)
35e X = PyCH2NH (7%)
37 (58%)
(f)
(g)
8a
or
11
(d) or (e)
(c)
(e)
OTBDMS
CO2H
33 (61%)
34 (100%)
36 (100%)

Scheme 8. Elaboration of lactam systems.

3. Bioassays

The compounds were tested using a primary 96-well plate screening assay against MRSA (Gram+) and *E. coli* (Gram−) bacterial strains and MIC values and along with the calculated molecular weights, ClogP, tPSA along with HBD and HBA (Table S2, ESI). The only systems showing activity were **12e/13e, 31,** and **32**. This probably reflects the high level of hydrophobicity of the silyloxy ethers and the particularly low solubility of the unsaturated systems, even though their cheminformatic descriptors are broadly desirable. This outcome suggests that some fragments might be suitable for further elaboration to identify better antibacterial activity. Some compounds were also tested for cytotoxic activity against four different cell lines: HeLa, HEK 293, CaCo, and MDCK (Table S3 (SI)). Nearly all the compounds that were tested showed some weak activity, but **35c** was found to be moderately active against HeLa and HEK 293 with lesser activity against CaCo and MDCK. Once again, the low solubility of these compounds under assay conditions is likely to be an important limitation of this compound class.

4. Materials and Methods

Full experimental details are provided in the Supplementary Materials File S1.

5. Conclusions

We have shown that phthalimides may be effectively cyclized using a Mukaiyama-type aldol coupling leading to variously substituted fused lactam (1,2,3,9b-tetrahydro-5*H*-pyrrolo[2,1-*a*]isoindol-5-one) systems. This novel process shows a high level of regioselectivity for *o*-substituted phthalimides, dictated by steric and electronic factors, but not for *m*-substituted phthalimides. The initial aldol adduct is prone to elimination, and the cyclisation can be conducted in such a way that aldol cyclisation-elimination is achievable in one pot. The eliminated skeletal systems (2,3-dihydro-5*H*-pyrrolo[2,1-*a*]isoindol-5-one) possess cross-conjugation and steric effects which significantly influence the reactivity of several functional groups, but conditions suitable for epoxidation, ester hydrolysis and amide formation, and reduction, were identified. Many of the derived lactam systems, and especially the eliminated systems, show low solubility, which compromises biological activity, although in some cases, antibacterial and cytotoxic activity was found and this new class of small molecule provides a useful skeleton for further elaboration and study. We have earlier shown that a core bicyclic tetramate displays no intrinsic antibacterial activity [26], but that this can be restored after appropriate heterocyclic ring substitution [19]. The work herein shows that the core tetrahydro-5*H*-pyrrolo[2,1-*a*]isoindol-5-one system is now synthetically readily available, and further investigation is needed to develop the understanding of both its medicinal chemistry and biological activity.

Supplementary Materials: The following supporting information can be downloaded at: https://www.mdpi.com/article/10.3390/antibiotics12010009/s1. File S1: Supporting Information (SI). References [88–96] occur only in the supplementary materials.

Author Contributions: Conceptualization, M.G.M. and L.T.I.; methodology K.E.C., M.G., A.P., D.P., M.G.M. and L.T.I.; formal analysis, K.E.C., M.G., A.P., D.P., M.G.M. and L.T.I.; writing—original draft preparation, M.G.M.; writing—review and editing, K.E.C., M.G.M. and L.T.I. All authors have read and agreed to the published version of the manuscript.

Funding: This research received no external funding.

Institutional Review Board Statement: Not applicable.

Informed Consent Statement: Not applicable.

Acknowledgments: We are grateful for the award of beamtime to the Block Allocation Group award (MT20876) used to collect the Single Crystal Synchrotron X-ray diffraction data on the I19 beamline at Diamond Light Source.

Conflicts of Interest: The authors declare no conflict of interest.

References and Notes

1. Newman, D.J.; Cragg, G.M. Natural products as sources of new drugs over the 30 years from 1981 to 2010. *J. Nat. Prod.* **2012**, *75*, 311–335. [CrossRef] [PubMed]
2. Boucher, H.W.; Talbot, G.H.; Benjamin, D.K.; Bradley, J.; Guidos, R.J.; Jones, R.N.; Murray, B.E.; Bonomo, R.A.; Gilbert, D. 10 × '20 Progress—Development of new drugs active against gram-negative bacilli: An update from the Infectious Diseases Society of America. *Clin. Infect. Dis.* **2013**, *56*, 1685–1694. [CrossRef] [PubMed]
3. Butler, M.S.; Cooper, M.A. Antibiotics in the clinical pipeline in 2011. *J. Antibiot.* **2011**, *64*, 413–425. [CrossRef] [PubMed]
4. O'Neill, J. *Antimicrobial Resistance: Tackling a Crisis for the Health and Wealth of Nations*; Review on Antimicrobial Resistance: London, UK, 2014.
5. Singh, S.B. Confronting the challenges of discovery of novel antibacterial agents. *Biorg. Med. Chem. Lett.* **2014**, *24*, 3683–3689. [CrossRef] [PubMed]
6. Silver, L.L. Challenges of antibacterial discovery. *Clin. Microbiol. Rev.* **2011**, *24*, 71–109. [CrossRef]
7. Dick, T.; Young, D. How antibacterials really work: Impact on drug discovery. *Future Microbiol.* **2011**, *6*, 603–604. [CrossRef]
8. Gwynn, M.N.; Portnoy, A.; Rittenhouse, S.F.; Payne, D.J. Challenges of antibacterial discovery revisited. *Ann. N. Y. Acad. Sci.* **2010**, *1213*, 5–19. [CrossRef]
9. Walsh, C.T.; Wencewicz, T.A. Prospects for new antibiotics: A molecule-centered perspective. *J. Antibiot.* **2014**, *67*, 7–22. [CrossRef]
10. Wencewicz, T.A. New antibiotics from Nature's chemical inventory. *Bioorg. Med. Chem. Lett.* **2016**, *24*, 6227–6252. [CrossRef]
11. Payne, D.J.; Gwynn, M.N.; Holmes, D.J.; Pompliano, D.L. Drugs for bad bugs: Confronting the challenges of antibacterial discovery. *Nat. Rev. Drug Discov.* **2007**, *6*, 29–40. [CrossRef]
12. Cragg, G.M.; Grothaus, P.G.; Newman, D.J. Impact of natural products on developing new anti-cancer agents. *Chem. Rev.* **2009**, *109*, 3012–3043. [CrossRef] [PubMed]
13. Walsh, D.P.; Chang, Y.-T. Chemical genetics. *Chem. Rev.* **2006**, *106*, 2476–2530. [CrossRef] [PubMed]
14. Morel, C.; Mossialos, E. Stoking the antibiotic pipeline. *Br. Med. J.* **2010**, *340*, 1115–1118. [CrossRef] [PubMed]
15. So, A.D.; Gupta, N.; Cars, O. Tackling antibiotic resistance. *Br. Med. J.* **2010**, *340*, 1091–1092. [CrossRef] [PubMed]

16. Koch, M.A.; Waldmann, H. Protein structure similarity clustering and natural product structure as guiding principles in drug discovery. *Drug Discov. Today* **2005**, *10*, 471–483. [CrossRef] [PubMed]
17. Balamurugan, R.; Dekker, F.J.; Waldmann, H. Design of compound libraries based on natural product scaffolds and protein structure similarity clustering (PSSC). *Mol. BioSyst.* **2005**, *1*, 36–45. [CrossRef]
18. Danishefsky, S. On the potential of natural products in the discovery of pharma leads: A case for reassessment. *Nat. Prod. Rep.* **2010**, *27*, 1114–1116. [CrossRef]
19. Khan, M.K.; Wang, D.; Moloney, M.G. Functionalised Nitrogen Heterocycles and the Search for New Antibacterials and Bioactives. *Synthesis* **2020**, *52*, 1602–1616. [CrossRef]
20. Singh, S.B.; Zink, D.L.; Goetz, M.A.; Dombrowski, A.W.; Polishook, J.D.; Hazuda, D.J. Equisetin and a novel opposite stereochemical homolog phomasetin, two fungal metabolites as inhibitors of HIV-1 integrase. *Tetrahedron Lett.* **1998**, *39*, 2243–2246. [CrossRef]
21. Ganzle, M.G. Reutericyclin: Biological activity, mode of action, and potential applications. *Appl. Microbiol. Biotechnol.* **2004**, *64*, 326–332. [CrossRef]
22. Phillips, J.W.; Goetz, M.; Smith, S.; Zink, D.; Polishook, J.; Onishi, R.; Salowe, S.; Wiltsie, J.; Allocco, J.; Sigmund, J.; et al. Discovery of kibdelomycin, a potent new class of bacterial type II topoisomerase inhibitor by chemical-genetic profiling in *Staphylococcus aureus*. *Chem. Biol.* **2011**, *18*, 955–965. [CrossRef] [PubMed]
23. Tuske, S.; Sarafianos, S.G.; Wang, X.; Hudson, B.; Sineva, E.; Mukhopadhyay, J.; Birktoft, J.J.; Leroy, O.; Ismail, S.; Clark, A.D.; et al. Inhibition of Bacterial RNA Polymerase by Streptolydigin: Stabilization of a Straight-Bridge-Helix Active-Center Conformation. *Cell* **2005**, *122*, 541–552. [CrossRef] [PubMed]
24. Moloney, M.G.; Trippier, P.C.; Yaqoob, M.; Wang, Z. The Oxazolomycins: A Structurally Novel Class of Bioactive Compounds. *Curr. Drug Discov. Technol.* **2004**, *1*, 181–199. [CrossRef]
25. Schwartz, R.E.; Helms, G.L.; Bolessa, E.A.; Wilson, K.E.; Giacobbe, R.A.; Tkacz, J.S.; Bills, G.F.; Liesch, J.M.; Zink, D.L.; Curotto, J.E.; et al. Pramanicin, a novel antimicrobial agent from a fungal fermentation. *Tetrahedron* **1994**, *50*, 1675–1686. [CrossRef]
26. Jeong, Y.-C.; Moloney, M.G. Tetramic Acids as Scaffolds: Synthesis, Tautomeric and Antibacterial Behaviour. *Synlett* **2009**, 2487–2491. [CrossRef]
27. Nogawa, T.; Kawatani, M.; Uramoto, M.; Okano, A.; Aono, H.; Futamura, Y.; Koshino, H.; Takahashi, S.; Osada, H. Pyrrolizilactone, a new pyrrolizidinone metabolite produced by a fungus. *J. Antibiot.* **2013**, *66*, 621–623. [CrossRef]
28. Nakai, R.; Ishida, H.; Asai, A.; Ogawa, H.; Yamamoto, Y.; Kawasaki, H.; Akinaga, S.; Mizukami, T.; Yamashita, Y. Telomerase inhibitors identified by a forward chemical genetics approach using a yeast strain with shortened telomere length. *Chem. Biol.* **2006**, *13*, 183–190. [CrossRef]
29. Agatsuma, T.; Akama, T.; Nara, S. Matsumiya, S.; Nakai, R.; Ogawa, H.; Otaki, S.; Ikeda, S.-I.; Saitoh, Y.; Kanda, Y. UCS1025A and B, new antitumor antibiotics from the fungus Acremonium species. *Org. Lett.* **2002**, *4*, 4387–4390. [CrossRef]
30. Nakai, R.; Ogawa, H.; Asai, A.; Ando, K.; Agaisuma, T.; Maisumiya, S.; Akinaga, S.; Yamashiya, Y.; Mizukami, T. UCS1025A, a Novel Antibiotic Produced by *Acremonium* sp. *J. Antibiot.* **2000**, *53*, 294–296. [CrossRef]
31. Sugie, Y.; Hirai, H.; Kachi-Tonai, H.; Kim, Y.-J.; Kojima, Y.; Shiomi, Y.; Sugiura, A.; Suzuki, Y.; Yoshikawa, N.; Brennan, L.; et al. New Pyrrolizidinone Antibiotics CJ-16, 264 and CJ-16, 367. *J. Antibiot.* **2001**, *54*, 917–925. [CrossRef]
32. Li, L.; Tang, M.C.; Tang, S.; Gao, S.; Soliman, S.; Hang, L.; Xu, W.; Ye, T.; Watanabe, K.; Tang, Y. Genome Mining and Assembly-Line Biosynthesis of the UCS1025A Pyrrolizidinone Family of Fungal Alkaloids. *J. Am. Chem. Soc.* **2018**, *140*, 2067–2071. [CrossRef] [PubMed]
33. De Figueiredo, R.M.; Fröhlich, R.; Christmann, M. Efficient Synthesis and Resolution of Pyrrolizidines. *Angew. Chem. Int. Ed.* **2007**, *46*, 2883–2886. [CrossRef] [PubMed]
34. Lambert, T.H.; Danishefsky, S.J. Total Synthesis of UCS1025A. *J. Am. Chem. Soc.* **2006**, *128*, 426–427. [CrossRef] [PubMed]
35. Hoye, T.R.; Dvornikovs, V. Comparative Diels–Alder Reactivities within a Family of Valence Bond Isomers: A Biomimetic Total Synthesis of (±)-UCS1025A. *J. Am. Chem. Soc.* **2006**, *128*, 2550–2551. [CrossRef]
36. Nozaki, K.; Oshima, K.; Utimoto, K. Trialkylborane as an initiator and terminator of free radical reactions. Facile routes to boron enolates via α-carbonyl radicals and aldol reaction of boron enolates. *Bull. Chem. Soc. Jpn.* **1991**, *64*, 403–409. [CrossRef]
37. Nicolaou, K.C.; Pulukuri, K.K.; Rigol, S.; Buchman, M.; Shah, A.A.; Cen, N.; McCurry, M.D.; Beabout, K.; Shamoo, Y. Enantioselective Total Synthesis of Antibiotic CJ-16,264, Synthesis and Biological Evaluation of Designed Analogues, and Discovery of Highly Potent and Simpler Antibacterial Agents. *J. Am. Chem. Soc.* **2017**, *139*, 15868–15877. [CrossRef]
38. Nicolaou, K.C.; Rigol, S.; Yu, R. Total Synthesis Endeavors and Their Contributions to Science and Society: A Personal Account. *CCS Chem.* **2019**, *1*, 3–37. [CrossRef]
39. Nicolaou, K.C.; Rigol, S. A brief history of antibiotics and select advances in their synthesis. *J. Antibiot.* **2017**, *71*, 153–184. [CrossRef]
40. Nicolaou, K.C.; Shah, A.A.; Korman, H.; Khan, T.; Shi, L.; Worawalai, W.; Theodorakis, E.A. Total Synthesis and Structural Revision of Antibiotic CJ-16,264. *Angew. Chem. Int. Ed.* **2015**, *54*, 9203–9208. [CrossRef]
41. Lambert, T.H.; Danishefsky, S.J. Synthesis of UCS1025A. *Synfacts* **2006**, 0536. [CrossRef]
42. Nicolaou, K.C.; Shi, L.; Lu, M.; Pattanayak, M.R.; Shah, A.A.; Ioannidou, H.A.; Lamani, M. Total Synthesis of Myceliothermophins C, D, and E. *Angew. Chem. Int. Ed.* **2014**, *126*, 11150–11154. [CrossRef]

43. Martinez, S.T.; Belouezzane, C.; Pinto, A.C.; Glasnov, T. Synthetic strategies towards the azabicyclo 3.3.0-octane core of natural pyrrolizidine alkaloids. an overview. *Org. Prep. Proc. Int.* **2016**, *48*, 223–253. [CrossRef]
44. Uchida, K.; Ogawa, T.; Yasuda, Y.; Mimura, H.; Fujimoto, T.; Fukuyama, T.; Wakimoto, T.; Asakawa, T.; Hamashima, Y.; Kan, T. Stereocontrolled Total Synthesis of (+)-UCS1025A. *Chem. Int. Ed.* **2012**, *51*, 12850–12853. [CrossRef] [PubMed]
45. Hoye, T.R.; Dvornikovs, V.; Sizova, E. Silylative Dieckmann-Like Cyclizations of Ester-Imides (and Diesters). *Org. Lett.* **2006**, *8*, 5191–5194. [CrossRef]
46. De Figueiredo, R.M.; Oczipka, P.; Fröhlich, R.; Christmann, M. Synthesis of 4-Maleimidobutyric Acid and Related Maleimides. *Synthesis* **2008**, 1316–1318. [CrossRef]
47. De Figueiredo, R.M.; Voith, M.; Fröhlich, R.; Christmann, M. Synthesis of a Malimide Analogue of the Telomerase Inhibitor UCS1025A Using a Dianionic Aldol Strategy. *Synlett* **2007**, *3*, 391–394. [CrossRef]
48. Ibbotson, L.T.; Christensen, K.E.; Genov, M.; Pretsch, A.; Pretsch, D.; Moloney, M.G. Skeletal Analogues of UCS1025A and B by Cyclization of Maleimides: Synthesis and Biological Activity. *Synlett* **2022**, *33*, 396–400. [CrossRef]
49. Guénin, E.; Monteil, M.; Bouchemal, N.; Prangé, T.; Lecouvey, M. Syntheses of phosphonic esters of alendronate, pamidronate and neridronate. *Eur. J. Org. Chem.* **2007**, *20*, 3380–3391. [CrossRef]
50. Wu, H.; Wu, J.; Zhang, W.; Li, J.; Fang, J.; Lian, X.; Qin, T.; Hao, J.; Zhou, Q.; Wu, S. Discovery and structure-activity relationship study of phthalimide-phenylpyridine conjugate as inhibitor of Wnt pathway. *Bioorg. Med. Chem. Lett.* **2019**, *29*, 870–872. [CrossRef]
51. Dato, F.M.; Sheikh, M.; Uhl, R.Z.; Schüller, A.W.; Steinkrüger, M.; Koch, P.; Neudörfl, J.M.; Gütschow, M.; Goldfuss, B.; Pietsch, M. ω-Phthalimidoalkyl Aryl Ureas as Potent and Selective Inhibitors of Cholesterol Esterase. *ChemMedChem* **2018**, *13*, 1833–1847. [CrossRef]
52. Gabbasov, T.M.; Tsyrlina, E.M.; Spirikhin, L.V.; Yunusov, M.S. Amides of N-Deacetyllappaconitine and Amino Acids. *Chem. Nat. Compd.* **2018**, *54*, 951–955. [CrossRef]
53. Griesbeck, A.G.; Henz, A.; Kramer, W.; Lex, J.; Nerowski, F.; Oelgemöller, M.; Peters, K.; Peters, E.M. Synthesis of Medium-and Large-Ring Compounds Initiated by Photochemical Decarboxylation of ω-Phthalimidoalkanoates. *Helv. Chim. Acta* **1997**, *80*, 912–933. [CrossRef]
54. Low temperature single crystal X-ray diffraction data for **6b**, **8a**, **8b**, **8c**, **12a**, **21**, **16b**, **23**, **27f** and **27b** were collected using a Rigaku Oxford SuperNova diffractometer and data for **9** were collected at Diamond Light Source, Beamline I19-1. Raw frame data were reduced using CrysAlisPro and the structures were solved using 'Superflip' before refinement with CRYSTALS as per the CIF. Full refinement details are given in the Supporting Information (CIF); Crystallographic data have been deposited with the Cambridge Crystallographic Data Centre (CCDC 2160046-56).
55. Palatinus, L.; Chapuis, G.J. SUPERFLIP—A computer program for the solution of crystal structures by charge flipping in arbitrary dimensions. *Appl. Cryst.* **2007**, *40*, 786–790. [CrossRef]
56. Parois, P.; Cooper, R.I.; Thompson, A.L. Crystal structures of increasingly large molecules: Meeting the challenges with CRYSTALS software. *Chem. Cent. J.* **2015**, *9*, 30. [CrossRef] [PubMed]
57. Cooper, R.I.; Thompson, A.L.; Watkin, D.J. CRYSTALS enhancements: Dealing with hydrogen atoms in refinement. *J. Appl. Cryst.* **2010**, *43*, 1100–1107. [CrossRef]
58. Yoon, U.C.; Lee, C.W.; Oh, S.W.; Mariano, P.S. Exploratory studies probing the intermediacy of azomethine ylides in the photochemistry of N-phthaloyl derivatives of α-amino acids and β-amino alcohols. *Tetrahedron* **1999**, *55*, 11997–12008. [CrossRef]
59. Takahashi, Y.; Miyashi, T.; Yoon, U.C.; Oh, S.W.; Mancheno, M.; Su, Z.; Falvey, D.F.; Mariano, P.S. Mechanistic Studies of the Azomethine Ylide-Forming Photoreactions of N-(Silylmethyl)phthalimides and N-Phthaloylglycine. *J. Am. Chem. Soc.* **1999**, *121*, 3926–3932. [CrossRef]
60. Yoon, U.C.; Kim, D.U.; Lee, Y.J.; Choi, Y.S.; Lee, Y.-J.; Ammon, H.L.; Mariano, P.S. Novel and efficient azomethine ylide forming photoreactions of N-(silylmethyl) phthalimides and related acid and alcohol derivative. *J. Am. Chem. Soc.* **1995**, *117*, 2698–2710. [CrossRef]
61. Muchowski, J.M.; Nelson, P.H. The reaction of carboalkyxycyclopropyltriphenylphosphonium salts with imide anions: A three-step synthesis of ±isoretronecanol. *Tetrahedron Lett.* **1980**, *21*, 4585–4588. [CrossRef]
62. Fuchs, P.L. Carboethoxycyclopropyltriphenylphosphonium fluoroborate. *Reagent for the facile cycloalkenylation of carbonyl groups J. Am. Chem. Soc.* **1974**, *96*, 1607–1609.
63. Maury, J.; Mouysset, D.; Feray, L.; Marque, S.R.A.; Siri, D.; Bertrand, M.P. Aminomethylation of Michael Acceptors: Complementary Radical and Polar Approaches Mediated by Dialkylzincs. *Chem.—Eur. J.* **2012**, *18*, 3241–3247. [CrossRef] [PubMed]
64. Border, S.E.; Pavlović, R.Z.; Lei, Z.; Gunther, M.J.; Wang, H.; Cui, H.; Badjić, J.D. Light Triggered Transformation of Molecular Baskets into Organic Nanoparticles. *Chem.—Eur. J.* **2019**, *25*, 273–279. [CrossRef] [PubMed]
65. Jamel, N.M.; Alheety, K.A.; Ahmed, B.J. Methods of Synthesis Phthalimide Derivatives and Biological Activity—Review. *J. Pharm. Sci. Res.* **2019**, *11*, 3348–3354.
66. Wang, W.; Ding, J.; Xiao, C.; Tang, Z.; Li, D.; Chen, J.; Zhuang, X.; Chen, X. Synthesis of amphiphilic alternating polyesters with oligo (ethylene glycol) side chains and potential use for sustained release drug delivery. *Biomacromolecules* **2011**, *12*, 2466–2474. [CrossRef] [PubMed]

67. Chen, M.H.; Goel, O.P.; Magano, J.; Rubin, J.R.; Company, W.-L.; Arbor, A. An efficient stereoselective synthesis of [3S(1S,9S)]-3-[[[9-(benzoylamino)octahydro-6,10-dioxo-6H-pyridazino-(1,2-a)(1,2)-diazepin-1-yl]-carbonyl]amino]-4-oxobutanoic acid, an interleukin converting enzyme (ICE) inhibitor. *Bioorg. Med. Chem. Lett.* **1999**, *9*, 1587–1592. [CrossRef]
68. King, F.E.; Clark-Lewis, J.W.; Wade, R.; Swindin, W.A. Syntheses from phthalimido-acids. Part VII. Oxazolones and other intermediates in the synthesis of phthalylpeptides, and an investigation on maleic acid. *J. Chem. Soc.* **1957**, *166*, 873–880. [CrossRef]
69. McKay, A.F.; Garmaise, D.L.; Gaudry, R.; Baker, H.A.; Paris, G.Y.; Kay, R.W.; Just, G.E.; Schwartz, R. Bacteriostats. II.1 The Chemical and Bacteriostatic Properties of Isothiocyanates and their Derivatives. *J. Am. Chem. Soc.* **1959**, *81*, 4328–4335. [CrossRef]
70. Schlessinger, R.H.; Poss, M.A.; Richardson, S. Total synthesis of (+)-rosaramicin aglycone and its diacetate. *J. Am. Chem. Soc.* **1986**, *108*, 3112–3114. [CrossRef]
71. Baker, R.; Cummings, W.J.; Hayes, J.F.; Kumar, A. Enantiospecific synthesis of the C-9 to C-18 fragment of macbecins I and II. *J. Chem. Soc. Chem. Commun.* **1986**, *1*, 1237–1239. [CrossRef]
72. Robins, M.J.; Samano, V.; Johnson, M.D. Nucleic acid-related compounds. 58. Periodinane oxidation, selective primary deprotection, and remarkably stereoselective reduction of tert-butyldimethylsilyl-protected ribonucleosides. Synthesis of 9-(.beta.-D-xylofuranosyl)adenine or 3'-deuterioadenosine from adenosine. *J. Org. Chem.* **1990**, *55*, 410–412. [CrossRef]
73. Martin, S.F.; Dodge, J.A.; Burgess, L.E.; Hartmann, M. A formal total synthesis of (+)-macbecin I. *J. Org. Chem.* **1992**, *57*, 1070–1072. [CrossRef]
74. Mukaiyama, T.; Kobayashi, S. Tin(II) Enolates in the Aldol, Michael, and Related Reactions. *Org. React.* **1994**, *46*, 1–103.
75. Banno, K. New Cross Aldol Reactions. Titanium Tetrachloride-promoted Reactions of Silyl Enol Ethers with Carbonyl Compounds Containing A Functional Group. *Bull. Chem. Soc. Jpn.* **1976**, *49*, 2284–2291. [CrossRef]
76. Kalita, H.R.; Borah, A.J.; Phukan, P. Efficient allylation of aldehydes with allyltributylstannane catalyzed by CuI. *Tetrahedron Lett.* **2007**, *48*, 5047–5049. [CrossRef]
77. Downey, C.W.; Johnson, M.W. A tandem enol silane formation-Mukaiyama aldol reaction mediated by TMSOTf. *Tetrahedron Lett.* **2007**, *48*, 3559–3562. [CrossRef]
78. Mahrwald, R. Diastereoselection in Lewis-acid-mediated aldol additions. *Chem. Rev.* **1999**, *99*, 1095–1120. [CrossRef] [PubMed]
79. Phukan, P. Mukaiyama aldol reactions of silyl enolates catalyzed by iodine. *Syn. Commun.* **2004**, *34*, 1065–1070. [CrossRef]
80. Han, J.H.; Kim, S.B.; Mukaiyama, T. A New Catalyst System for the Aldol Type Condensation of Silyl Enol Ethers and Ketene Silyl Acetals. *Bull. Korean Chem. Soc.* **1994**, *15*, 529–531. [CrossRef]
81. Wade Downey, C.; Ingersoll, J.A.; Glist, H.M.; Dombrowski, C.M.; Barnett, A.T. One-Pot Silyl Ketene Acetal-Formation Mukaiyama–Mannich Additions to Imines Mediated by Trimethylsilyl Trifluoromethanesulfonate. *Eur. J. Org. Chem.* **2015**, *2015*, 7287–7291. [CrossRef]
82. Cottrell, I.F.; Davis, P.J.; Moloney, M.G. Stereoselective oxygenation of bicyclic lactams. *Tetrahedron Asymmetry* **2004**, *15*, 1239–1242. [CrossRef]
83. Tan, S.W.B.; Chai, C.L.L.; Moloney, M.G. Mimics of pramanicin derived from pyroglutamic acid and their antibacterial activity. *Org. Biomol. Chem.* **2017**, *15*, 1889–1912. [CrossRef] [PubMed]
84. Verho, O.; Maetani, M.; Melillo, B.; Zoller, J.; Schreiber, S.L. Stereospecific palladium-catalyzed C–H arylation of pyroglutamic acid derivatives at the C3 position enabled by 8-aminoquinoline as a directing group. *Org. Lett.* **2017**, *19*, 4424–4427. [CrossRef]
85. Rej, S.; Ano, Y.; Chatani, N. Bidentate directing groups: An efficient tool in C–H bond functionalization chemistry for the expedient construction of C–C bonds. *Chem. Rev.* **2020**, *120*, 1788–1887. [CrossRef] [PubMed]
86. Liu, Z.; Wang, Y.; Wang, Z.; Zeng, T.; Liu, P.; Engle, K.M. Catalytic intermolecular carboamination of unactivated alkenes via directed aminopalladation. *J. Am. Chem. Soc.* **2017**, *139*, 11261–11270. [CrossRef] [PubMed]
87. Corbet, M.; De Campo, F. 8-Aminoquinoline: A Powerful Directing Group in Metal-Catalyzed Direct Functionalization of C-H Bonds. *Angew. Chem.—Int. Ed.* **2013**, *52*, 9896–9898. [CrossRef] [PubMed]
88. Ko, K.S.; Park, G.; Yu, Y.; Pohl, N.L. Protecting-Group-Based Colorimetric Monitoring of Fluorous-Phase and Solid-Phase Synthesis of Oligoglucosamines. *Org. Lett.* **2008**, *10*, 5381–5384. [CrossRef] [PubMed]
89. Caswell, L.R.; Yang, K.C.C. Nitrophthaloyl and aminophthaloyl derivatives of amino acids. *J. Chem. Eng. Data* **1968**, *13*, 291–292. [CrossRef]
90. Staubli, A.; Ron, E.; Langer, R. Hydrolytically degradable amino acid-containing polymers. *J. Am. Chem. Soc.* **1990**, *112*, 4419–4424. [CrossRef]
91. Richards, J.C.; Spenser, I.D. The stereochemistry of the enzymic decarboxylation of L-arginine and of L-ornithine. *Can. J. Chem.* **1982**, *60*, 2810–2820. [CrossRef]
92. Tomar, R.; Bhattacharya, D.; Babu, S.A. Assembling of medium/long chain-based β-arylated unnatural amino acid derivatives via the Pd(II)-catalyzed sp3 β-C-H arylation and a short route for rolipram-type derivatives. *Tetrahedron* **2019**, *75*, 2447–2465. [CrossRef]
93. Vatulina, G.G.; Tuzhilkova, T.N.; Matveeva, T.V.; Krasnov, V.P.; Burde, N.L.; Alekseeva, L.V. Search for radioprotectors in the series of glutamic acid derivatives. *Chem. Pharm. J.* **1986**, *20*, 647–653. [CrossRef]
94. Robl, J.A. Peptidomimetic synthesis: Utilization of N-acyliminium ion cyclization chemistry in the generation of 7, 6-and 7, 5-fused bicyclic lactams. *Tetrahedron Lett.* **1994**, *35*, 393–396. [CrossRef]

95. Fife, T.H.; Duddy, N.W. Intramolecular aminolysis of esters. Cyclization of esters of (o-aminophenyl) acetic acid. *J. Am. Chem. Soc.* **1983**, *105*, 74–79. [CrossRef]
96. Kim, G.; Keum, G. A new route to quinolone and indole skeletons via ketone-and ester-imide cyclodehydration reactions. *Heterocycles* **1997**, *45*, 1979–1988. [CrossRef]

Disclaimer/Publisher's Note: The statements, opinions and data contained in all publications are solely those of the individual author(s) and contributor(s) and not of MDPI and/or the editor(s). MDPI and/or the editor(s) disclaim responsibility for any injury to people or property resulting from any ideas, methods, instructions or products referred to in the content.

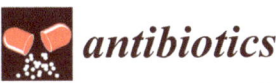

Article

Synergistic Antifungal Activity of Synthetic Peptides and Antifungal Drugs against *Candida albicans* and *C. parapsilosis* Biofilms

Leandro P. Bezerra [1], Cleverson D. T. Freitas [1,*], Ayrles F. B. Silva [1], Jackson L. Amaral [1], Nilton A. S. Neto [1], Rafael G. G. Silva [2], Aura L. C. Parra [1], Gustavo H. Goldman [3], Jose T. A. Oliveira [1], Felipe P. Mesquita [4] and Pedro F. N. Souza [1,4,*]

[1] Department of Biochemistry and Molecular Biology, Federal University of Ceará, Fortaleza 60451, CE, Brazil; leandro.bioquimica@gmail.com (L.P.B.); ayrlesbrandao@gmail.com (A.F.B.S.); jacksoncesarc@gmail.com (J.L.A.); niltonararipeneto@hotmail.com (N.A.S.N.); alchaconp@unal.edu.co (A.L.C.P.); jtaolive@ufc.br (J.T.A.O.)
[2] Department of Biology, Federal University of Ceará, Fortaleza 60451, CE, Brazil; rafaelguimaraes@ufc.br
[3] Faculty of Pharmaceutical Sciences of Ribeirão Preto, University of São Paulo, São Paulo P.O. Box 05508-000, SP, Brazil; ggoldman@usp.br
[4] Drug Research and Development Center, Department of Physiology and Pharmacology, Federal University of Ceará, Rua Coronel, Nunes de Melo 100, Caixa, Fortaleza 60430-275, CE, Brazil; felipe_mesquita05@hotmail.com
* Correspondence: cleversondiniz@hotmail.com (C.D.T.F.); pedrofilhobio@gmail.com (P.F.N.S.)

Abstract: *C. albicans* and *C. parapsilosis* are biofilm-forming yeasts responsible for bloodstream infections that can cause death. Synthetic antimicrobial peptides (SAMPs) are considered to be new weapons to combat these infections, alone or combined with drugs. Here, two SAMPs, called *Mo*-CBP$_3$-PepI and *Mo*-CBP$_3$-PepIII, were tested alone or combined with nystatin (NYS) and itraconazole (ITR) against *C. albicans* and *C. parapsilosis* biofilms. Furthermore, the mechanism of antibiofilm activity was evaluated by fluorescence and scanning electron microscopies. When combined with SAMPs, the results revealed a 2- to 4-fold improvement of NYS and ITR antibiofilm activity. Microscopic analyses showed cell membrane and wall damage and ROS overproduction, which caused leakage of internal content and cell death. Taken together, these results suggest the potential of *Mo*-CBP$_3$-PepI and *Mo*-CBP$_3$-PepIII as new drugs and adjuvants to increase the activity of conventional drugs for the treatment of clinical infections caused by *C. albicans* and *C. parapsilosis*.

Keywords: antibiofilm activity; candidiasis; synergism; synthetic peptides; antifungal drugs

1. Introduction

Biofilms are established by microbial cells on an inert or living surface, promoting the development of microcolonies with polymeric matrices and enhancing the resistance to various antimicrobial agents [1,2]. *Candida* species are biofilm-forming yeasts responsible for up to 15% of hospital-acquired cases of sepsis [3]. A mature biofilm produced by *Candida* spp. consists of an extracellular matrix composed of glycoproteins (55%), carbohydrates (25%), lipids (15%), and nucleic acids (5%) [4]. The National Institute of Health (NIH) in the USA considers biofilms to be a public health problem and estimated that they can be responsible for 80% of the difficulties in curing human infections [1,2,4,5]. The most susceptible people are immunocompromised patients, AIDS+ patients, patients under chemotherapy treatment or immunosuppressive therapies, and patients fitted with medical devices (catheters, pacemakers, and heart valves) [6,7].

C. albicans and *C. parapsilosis* are common opportunistic fungal pathogens that asymptomatically colonize the mucosal surfaces and skin of healthy individuals. However, in some circumstances they can cause an infection called candidiasis [8]. In addition, *C. albicans* and *C. parapsilosis* are responsible for bloodstream infections termed candidemia, which are common in immunocompromised patients, including those in intensive care units [9]. Currently, the treatment of infections caused by *C. albicans* and *C. parapsilosis* involves the use of antifungal agents that interrupt different metabolic pathways of the cell. However, some studies have reported *Candida* resistance to these antifungal molecules [10–12]. A study by Katiyar and collaborators [13] described *Candida* clinical isolates that contain genes responsible for resistance to some commercial antifungal agents [13]. To counter this problem, synthetic antimicrobial peptides (SAMPs) have been described as new alternatives, either alone or combined with commercial antifungal drugs, to control *Candida* infection and overcome the pathogens' resistance [1]. SAMPs have some important antimicrobial characteristics found in natural antimicrobial peptides, such as positive net charge, α-helical structure, low molecular weight (600–1200 Da), high hydrophobic ratio (40–60%) and amphipathicity [1,14].

Recently, our research group designed, characterized, and evaluated the antimicrobial activity of two synthetic peptides, called *Mo*-CBP$_3$-PepI (CPIAQRCC) and *Mo*-CBP$_3$-PepIII (AIQRCC). These peptides were designed based on the structure of *Mo*-CBP$_3$, a chitin-binding protein purified from *Moringa oleifera* seeds [15,16]. The anticandidal activity and mechanism of action of these peptides were evaluated by Oliveira et al. (2019) and Lima et al. (2020). Therefore, the aim of this study was to evaluate the antifungal activity and action mechanism of *Mo*-CBP$_3$-PepI and *Mo*-CBP$_3$-PepIII, alone or combined with NYS and ITR, against *C. albicans* and *C. parapsilosis* biofilms.

2. Results

2.1. Antibiofilm Activity of Synthetic Peptides and Two Commercial Drugs

The activities of *Mo*-CBP$_3$-PepI and *Mo*-CBP$_3$-PepIII (50 μg mL^{-1}) against *C. albicans* and *C. parapsilosis* biofilms are shown in Figure 1. The biofilm formation of *C. albicans* was inhibited 10% by *Mo*-CBP$_3$-PepI, whereas *Mo*-CBP$_3$-PepIII did not show any activity. Interestingly, the commercial drugs ITR and NYS inhibited biofilm formation by only 7% and 40%, respectively (Figure 1A). Regarding the synergistic effect, the combination of both peptides *Mo*-CBP$_3$-PepI and *Mo*-CBP$_3$-PepIII with ITR or NYS significantly enhanced the inhibition of *C. albicans* biofilm formation. For instance, the two peptides combined with NYS increased the inhibition of *C. albicans* biofilm formation by 40% to 80% (Figure 1A). ITR and NYS inhibited *C. parapsilosis* biofilm formation by 45% and 43%, respectively. In contrast, *Mo*-CBP$_3$-PepI and *Mo*-CBP$_3$-PepIII inhibited this by only 15% and 25%, respectively (Figure 1B). On the other hand, combinations of *Mo*-CBP$_3$-PepI + ITR, *Mo*-CBP$_3$-PepIII + ITR, *Mo*-CBP$_3$-PepI + NYS, and *Mo*-CBP$_3$-PepIII + NYS inhibited the biofilm formation by about 98%, 96%, 79%, and 82%, respectively (Figure 1B).

Regarding the degradation of mature *C. albicans* biofilm, ITR and NYS decreased the biofilm mass by about 50% and 30%, while *Mo*-CBP$_3$-PepI and *Mo*-CBP$_3$-PepIII only degrading it by 60% and 30%, respectively (Figure 1C). Remarkably, the combinations *Mo*-CBP$_3$-PepI + ITR and *Mo*-CBP$_3$-PepIII + ITR did not have any effect (Figure 1C). However, the combinations *Mo*-CBP$_3$-PepI + NYS and *Mo*-CBP$_3$-PepIII + NYS degraded 85% and 50% of the mature *C. albicans* biofilm (Figure 1C). Concerning the degradation of mature *C. parapsilosis* biofilm, only the combination Mo-CBP3-PepI + NYS showed activity, reducing the biofilm biomass by 50% (Figure 1D).

2.2. Analysis of Candida Biofilm Morphology

Scanning electron microscopy (SEM) was used to evaluate damage to *C. albicans* and *C. parapsilosis* biofilms after all treatments (Figures 2 and 3). The control cells did not show any damage or alterations on the surface; only spherical-shaped cells were observed without cracks or scars. The treatment with peptides or drugs caused only mild damage, such as wrinkles and slight changes to the morphology of cells, which had a very similar appearance to the control (Figures 2 and 3). In contrast, the combination of both peptides with the two drugs caused a significant reduction in the mature biofilm compared to control, and it was possible to see damage such as small blebs, new buds, scars, and rings of truncated bud scars. *Mo*-CBP$_3$-PepI + NYS and *Mo*-CBP$_3$-PepIII + NYS were by far the most lethal to *C. albicans* and *C. parapsilosis*. In those treatments, the cells were greatly damaged, with high roughness levels, severe alterations in morphology, and a clear indication of cell lysis leading to loss of cytoplasm (Figures 2 and 3).

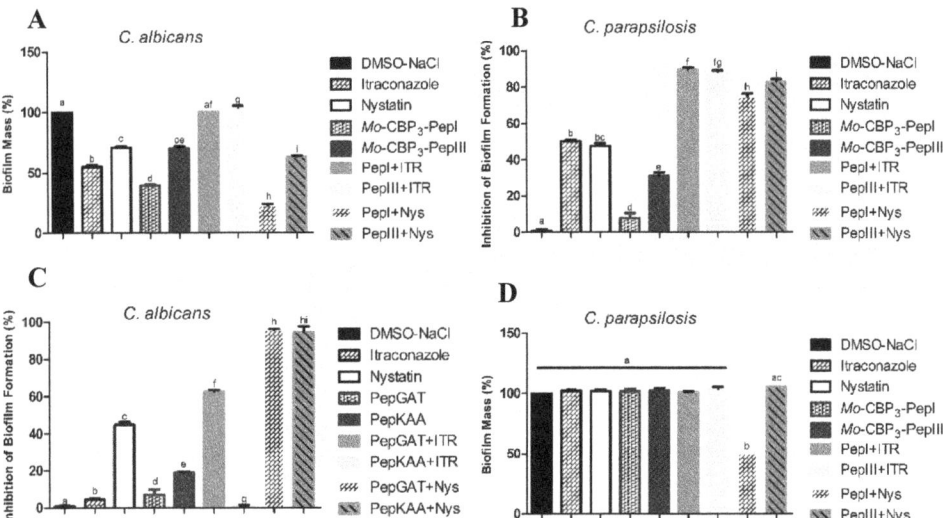

Figure 1. (**A,B**) Inhibitory activity of biofilm formation and (**C,D**) degradation of mature biofilm of *C. albicans* and *C. parapsilosis*. DMSO-NaCl was used as a negative control and ITR and NYS as positive controls. The letters represent the mean ± standard deviation of three replicates. Different lowercase letters indicate a statistically significant difference compared to DMSO-NaCl by analysis of variance ($p < 0.05$).

Because *Mo*-CBP$_3$-PepI + NYS showed the best inhibitory activity against biofilm formation, this sample was chosen to investigate alteration of mature biofilms of *C. albicans* and *C. parapsilosis* (Figure 4). The control biofilm (treated with DMSO-NaCl) did not present any damage, while the biofilms treated with NYS or *Mo*-CBP$_3$-PepI presented mild damage, such as altered morphology and wrinkles, distortion, and apparent reduction in biomass compared to the controls. However, *Mo*-CBP$_3$-PepI + NYS was highly lethal to mature *C. albicans* and *C. parapsilosis* biofilms (Figure 4). These biofilms had a large reduction in biomass, as well as severe cell damage, such as depression-like cavities and damage to the cell wall, alterations in cell shape, wrinkles and scars, and loss of internal content (Figure 4).

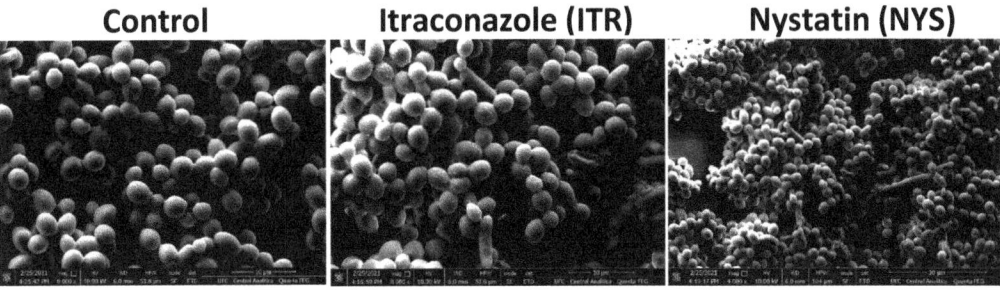

Figure 2. *Cont.*

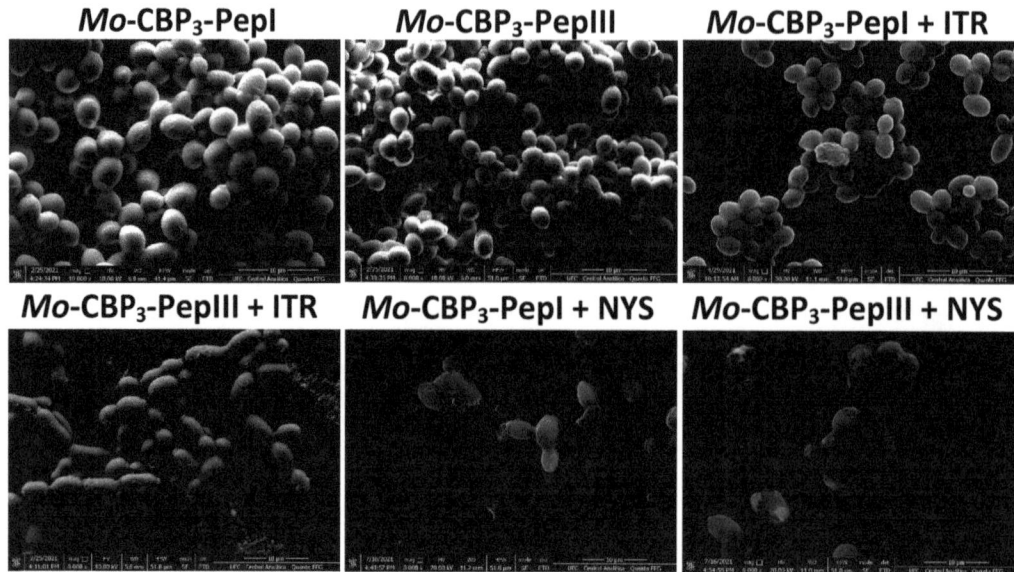

Figure 2. SEM images showing *C. albicans* biofilms after treatment with ITR, NYS, *Mo*-CBP$_3$-PepI, *Mo*-CBP$_3$-PepIII, and their combinations. Control: DMSO-NaCl solution.

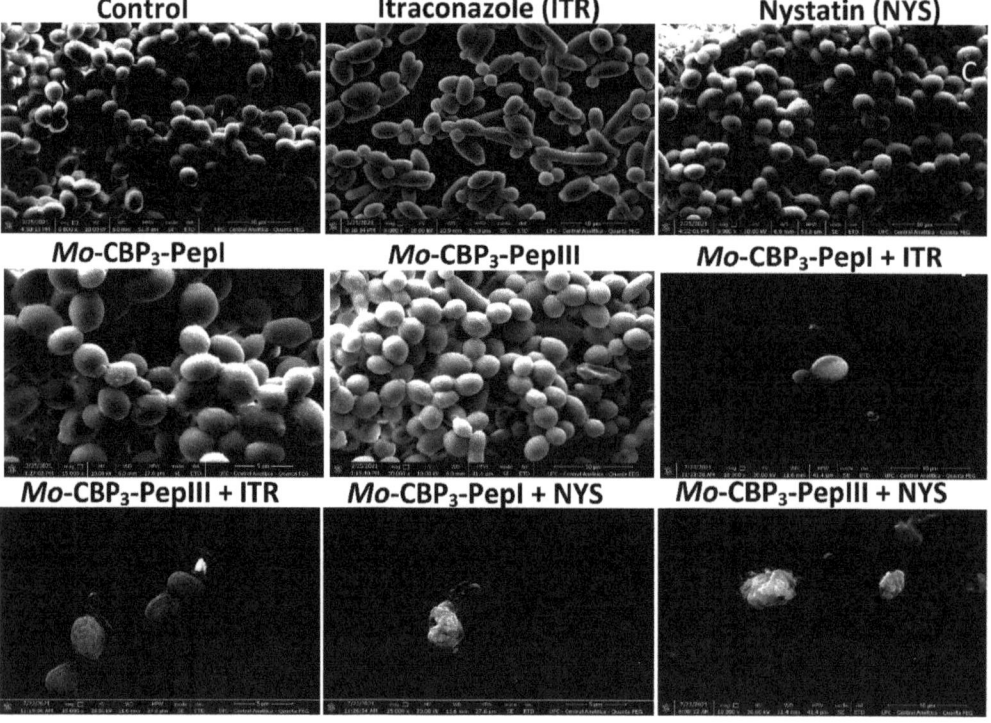

Figure 3. SEM images showing *C. parapsilosis* biofilms after treatment with ITR, NYS, *Mo*-CBP$_3$-PepI, *Mo*-CBP$_3$-PepIII, and their combinations. Control: DMSO-NaCl solution.

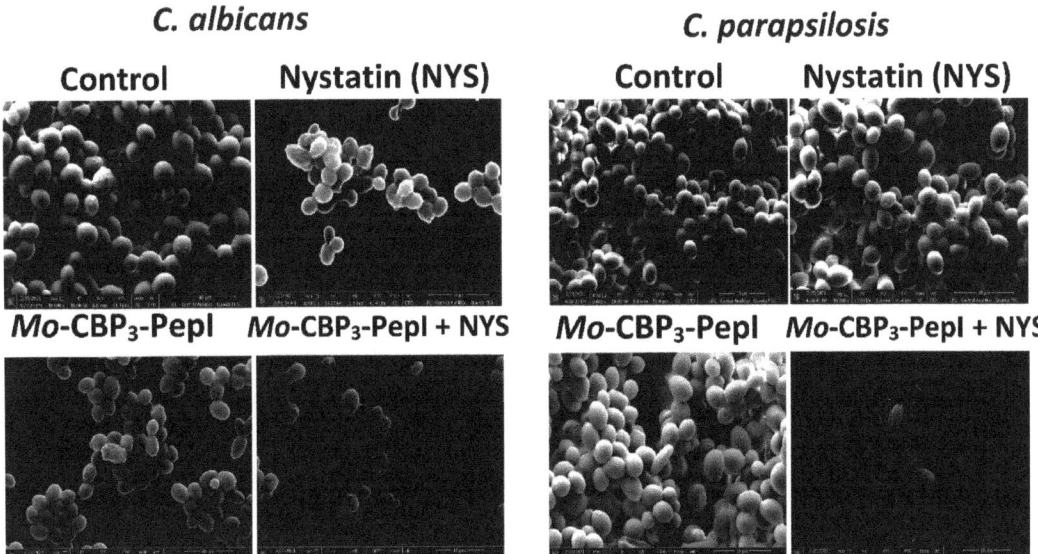

Figure 4. SEM images showing alterations of mature biofilm of *C. albicans* and *C. parapsilosis* after treatment with *Mo*-CBP$_3$-PepI, NYS and *Mo*-CBP$_3$-PepI + NYS. Control: DMSO-NaCl solution.

2.3. Membrane Pore Formation

The propidium iodide (PI) uptake assay was used to evaluate possible damage to the yeast cell membranes. PI interacts with DNA, releasing red fluorescence, but this is only possible when the membrane is damaged, since healthy membranes are impermeable to PI. As expected, the control (DMSO-NaCl solution) did not damage the cell membranes, because no fluorescence was detected. Similarly, cells treated with NYS and ITR did not show any fluorescence. However, *Mo*-CBP$_3$-PepI and *Mo*-CBP$_3$-PepIII, alone or in combination with NYS or ITR, induced red fluorescence in *C. albicans* and *C. parapsilosis* cells, indicating these cells membranes were damaged (Figures 5–9).

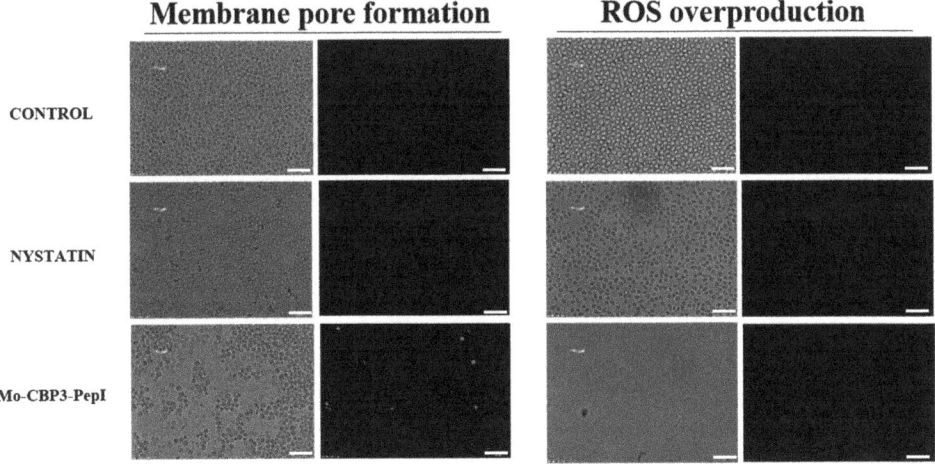

Figure 5. *Cont.*

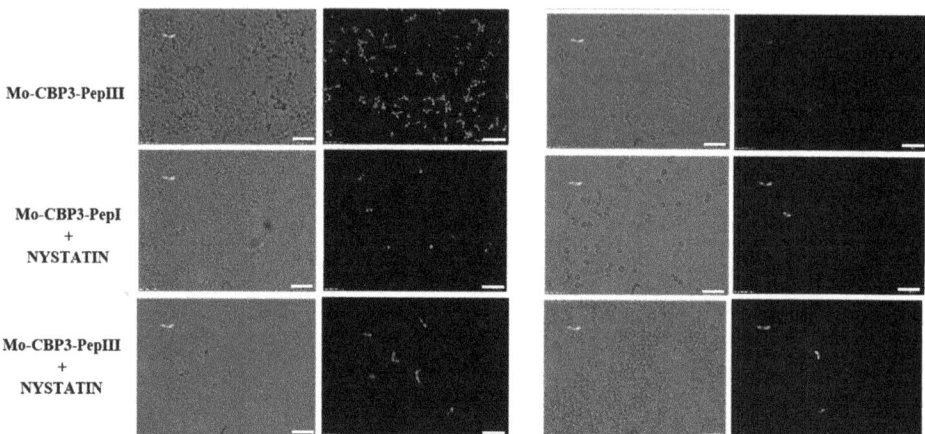

Figure 5. Fluorescence images showing membrane pore formation and ROS overproduction on inhibition of biofilm of *C. albicans* cells. Control solution of DMSO-NaCl, treated with *Mo*-CBP$_3$-PepI and *Mo*-CBP$_3$-PepIII at 50 µg mL^{-1} and synergistic activity of both peptides with NYS. Membrane pore formation was measured by the propidium iodide (PI) uptake assay, and ROS overproduction was detected using 2′, 7′ dichlorofluorescein diacetate (DCFH-DA). Bars: 100 µm.

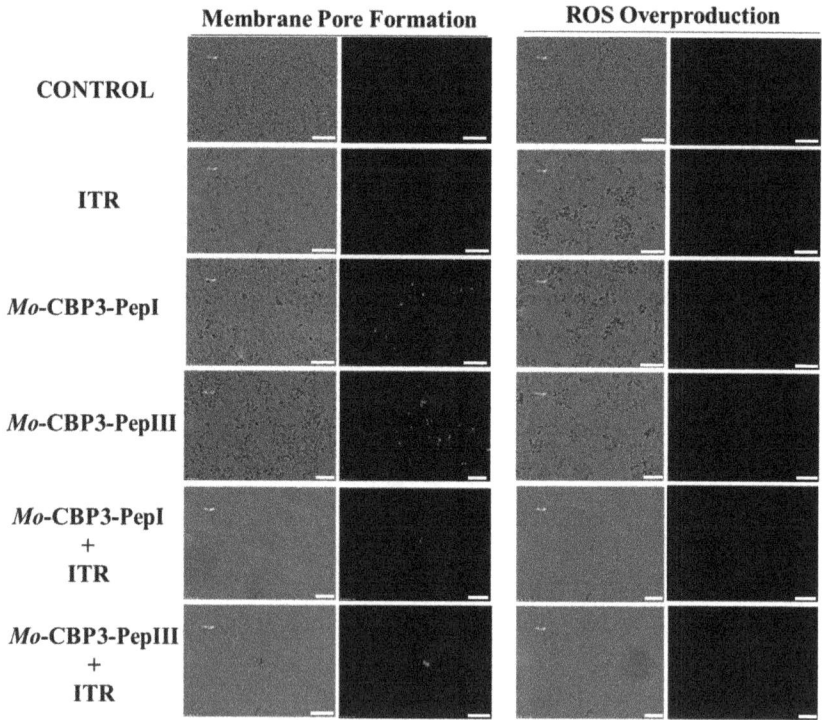

Figure 6. Fluorescence images showing membrane pore formation and ROS overproduction on inhibition of the biofilm of *C. parapsilosis* cells. Control solution of DMSO-NaCl, treated with *Mo*-CBP$_3$-PepI and *Mo*-CBP$_3$-PepIII at 50 µg mL^{-1} and synergistic activity of both peptides with ITR. Membrane pore formation was measured by the PI uptake assay, and ROS overproduction was detected using 2′, 7′ dichlorofluorescein diacetate (DCFH-DA). Bars: 100 µm.

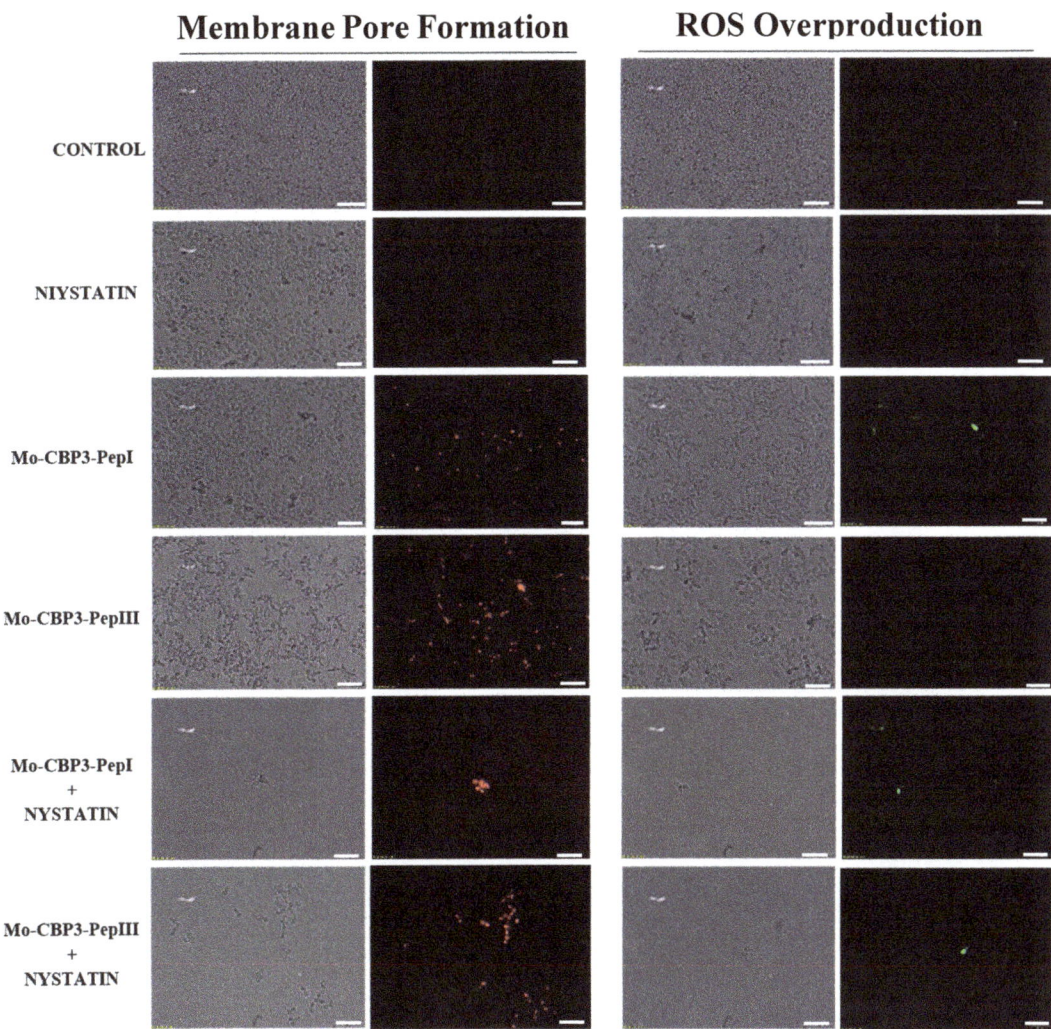

Figure 7. Fluorescence images showing membrane pore formation and ROS overproduction on inhibition of the biofilm of *C. parapsilosis* cells. Control solution of DMSO-NaCl, treated with Mo-CBP3-PepI and Mo-CBP3-PepIII at 50 µg mL^{-1} and synergistic activity of both peptides with NYS. Membrane pore formation was measured by the PI uptake assay, and ROS overproduction was detected using 2', 7' dichlorofluorescein diacetate (DCFH-DA). Bars: 100 µm.

ROS overproduction is another mechanism employed by peptides to inhibit biofilm formation. The results showed that treatment of *C. albicans* cells with NYS or ITR did not induce ROS overproduction, whereas both peptides and their combination with NYS induced a slight production of ROS. None of the treatments induced ROS overproduction by *C. parapsilosis* biofilms (Figures 5–9).

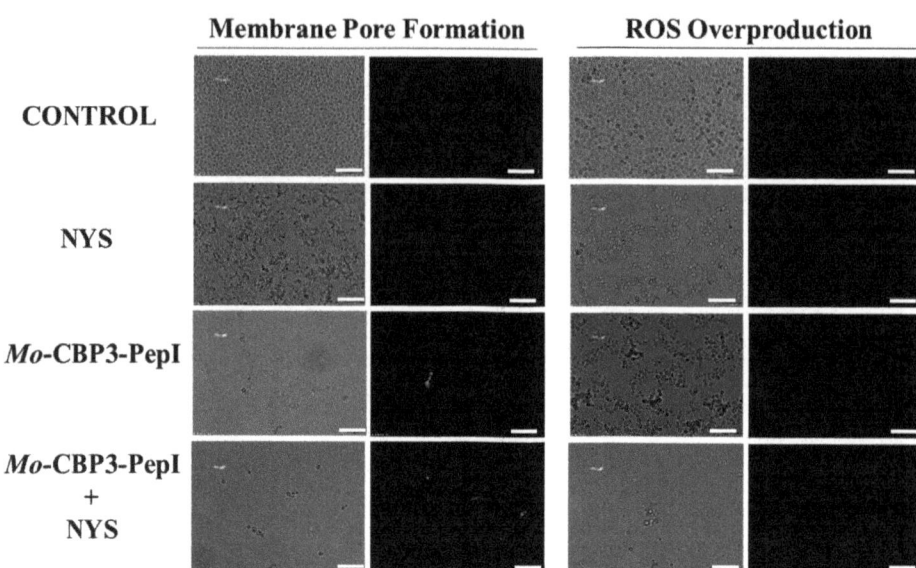

Figure 8. Fluorescence images showing membrane pore formation and ROS overproduction on degradation of the biofilm of C. albicans cells. Control solution of DMSO-NaCl, treated with Mo-CBP3-PepI at 50 µg mL^{-1} and synergistic activity with NYS. Membrane pore formation was measured by the PI uptake assay, and ROS overproduction was detected using 2′, 7′ dichlorofluorescein diacetate (DCFH-DA). Bars: 100 µm.

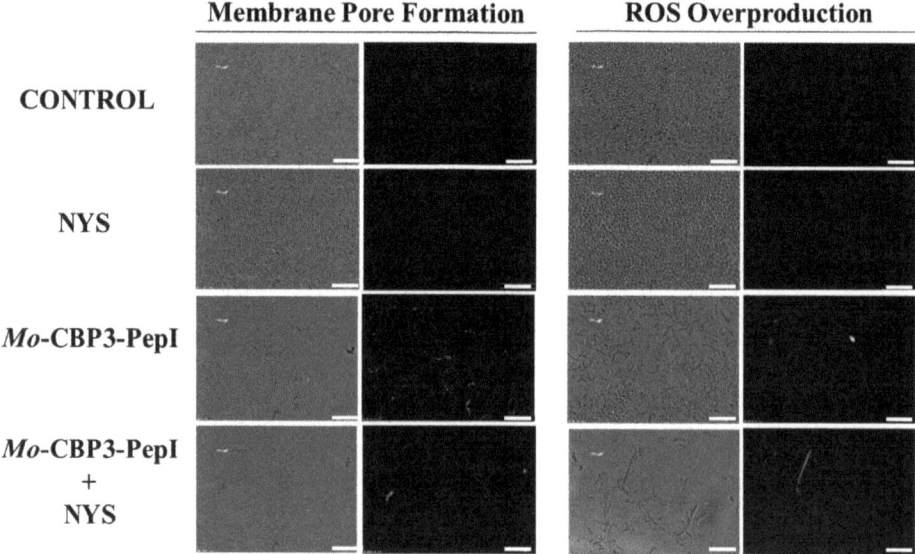

Figure 9. Fluorescence images showing membrane pore formation and ROS overproduction on degradation of the biofilm of C. parapsilosis cells. Control solution of DMSO-NaCl, treated with Mo-CBP$_3$-PepI at 50 µg mL^{-1} and synergistic activity with NYS. Membrane pore formation was measured by the PI uptake assay, and ROS overproduction was detected using 2′, 7′ dichlorofluorescein diacetate (DCFH-DA). Bars: 100 µm.

2.4. Molecular Docking

The molecular docking assays were performed to evaluate the possible interactions of the peptides with NYS and ITR. *Mo*-CBP$_3$-PepI interacted with ITR and NYS with binding interaction energy (LBIE) values of −4.5 and −4.2 kcal.mol^{-1}, respectively (Figure 10A,B). The amino acid residues Pro2 and Ile4 of the Mo-CBP3-PepI peptide showed Pi-Alkyl interactions with the phenyl (4.5 Å), piperazine (4.2 Å), and dichlorophenyl (4.5 Å) groups of ITR. Cys8 had a Pi-Anion (3.4 Å, triazole group) and a Pi-Sulfur (5.1 Å, dichlorophenyl group) interaction with ITR, and Arg6 presented only van der Waals interaction (Figure 10C). *Mo*-CBP$_3$-PepI interacted with NYS by van der Waals forces between Cys8, Gln5, and Cys1. An Alkyl (5.0 Å) interaction with Pro2 and an unfavorable donor-donor (1.3 Å) with Arg6 were also observed (Figure 10D).

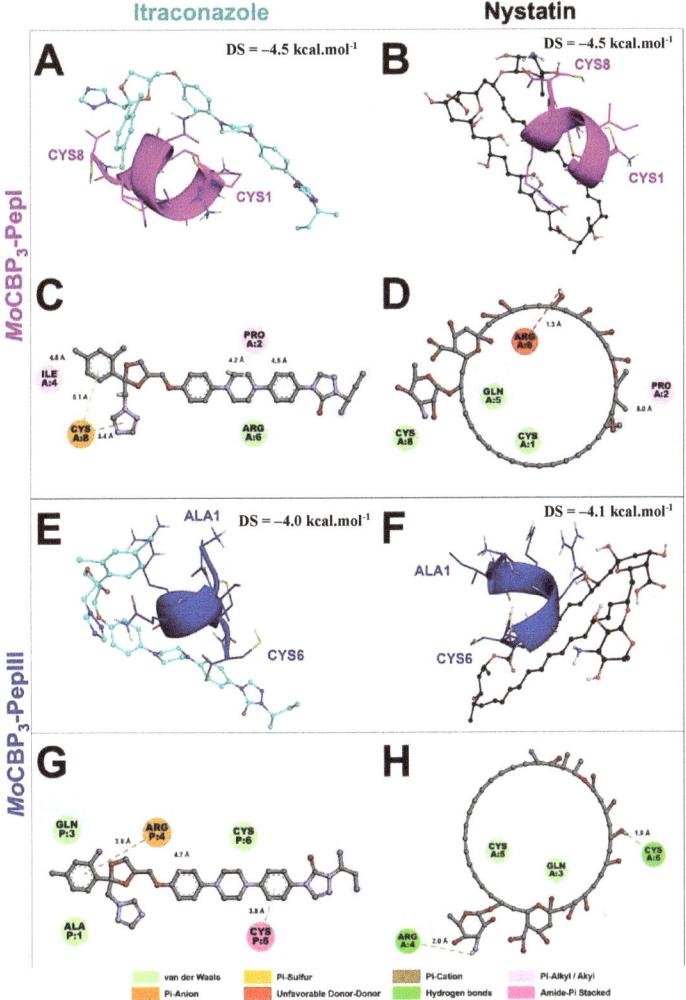

Figure 10. Molecular docking revealed that *Mo*-CBP$_3$-PepI and *Mo*-CBP$_3$-PepIII interact with ITR and NYS. *Mo*-CBP$_3$-PepI is represented in pink (**A**,**B**) and *Mo*-CBP$_3$-PepIII in blue (**E**,**F**). (**C**,**D**,**G**,**H**) show the binding sites of *Mo*-CBP$_3$-PepI and *Mo*-CBP$_3$-PepIII with ITR and NYS.

Mo-CBP$_3$-PepIII presented docking scores of −4.0 and −4.1 kcal.mol^{-1} with ITR and NYS, respectively (Figure 10E,F). *Mo*-CBP$_3$-PepIII interacted through van der Waals forces through residues Ala1, Gln3, and Cys6 with ITR. Cys5 interacted through an Amide-Pi stacked (3.8 Å) with the phenyl group of ITR. The Arg4 of *Mo*-CBP$_3$-PepIII established a Pi-Cation interaction with the dichlorophenyl group (3.8 Å) and a Pi-Alkyl interaction (4.7 Å) with the methoxyphenyl group of itraconazole (Figure 10E,G). The interaction between *Mo*-CBP$_3$-PepIII and NYS was supported by hydrogen bonds between residues Arg4 (2.0 Å) and Cys6 (1.9 Å), as well as through van der Waals interactions through residues Gln3 and Cys5 (Figure 10F,H).

2.5. Hemolytic Assay

As shown in a previous study [16], *Mo*-CBP$_3$-PepI and *Mo*-CBP$_3$-PepIII had no hemolytic activity against any human blood type tested (Table 1), even at 50 µg mL^{-1}. In contrast, NYS (1000 µg mL^{-1}) caused 100% hemolysis in all human blood types, and ITR (1000 µg mL^{-1}) caused 75%, 68%, and 58% hemolysis to Type A, B, and O red blood cells, respectively (Table 1).

Table 1. Hemolytic activity of *Mo*-CBP$_3$-PepI and *Mo*-CBP$_3$-PepIII, antifungal drugs, and combined solutions on human red blood cells.

Peptides/Combinations	% Hemolysis		
	Type A Blood	Type B Blood	Type O Blood
0.1% Triton X-100	100 ± 0.002	100 ± 0.001	100 ± 0.007
DMSO-NaCl Solution	0	0	0
NYS (1000 µg mL^{-1})	100 ± 0.005	100 ± 0.001	100 ± 0.002
ITR (1000 µg mL^{-1})	75 ± 0.007	68 ± 0.004	58 ± 0.003
Mo-CBP$_3$-PepI (50 µg mL^{-1})	0	0	0
Mo-CBP$_3$-PepIII (50 µg mL^{-1})	0	0	0
Mo-CBP$_3$-PepI (50 µg mL^{-1}) + NYS (1000 µg mL^{-1})	14 ± 0.006	23 ± 0.009	2 ± 0.001
Mo-CBP$_3$-PepI (50 µg mL^{-1}) + ITR (1000 µg mL^{-1})	0	4 ± 0.003	8 ± 0.005
Mo-CBP$_3$-PepIII (50 µg mL^{-1}) + NYS (1000 µg mL^{-1})	45 ± 0.001	30 ± 0.001	18 ± 0.007
Mo-CBP$_3$-PepIII (50 µg mL^{-1}) + ITR (1000 µg mL^{-1})	50 ± 0.005	15 ± 0.008	2 ± 0.001

The mean ± standard deviation of three replicates according to ANOVA ($p < 0.05$).

In general, the combination of synthetic peptides decreased the hemolytic effect of both drugs (Table 1). The combination of *Mo*-CBP$_3$-PepI with NYS resulted in hemolytic effects of 14%, 23%, and 2%, and the combination of *Mo*-CBP$_3$-PepI with ITR resulted in 0%, 4%, and 8% hemolysis to Type A, B, and O red blood cells, respectively (Table 1). The combination of *Mo*-CBP$_3$-PepIII with NYS hemolyzed 45%, 30%, and 18%, while the combination of *Mo*-CBP$_3$-PepI with ITR resulted in 50%, 15%, and 2% for Type A, B, and O red blood cells, respectively (Table 1).

3. Discussion

Natural antimicrobial peptides (AMPs) are promising molecules to act as substitutes or adjuvants to treat infections. However, they have some disadvantages, such as toxicity, low resistance to proteolysis, and the high cost of isolation and purification. The development of synthetic antimicrobial peptides (SAMPs) is an alternative solution to overcome these drawbacks, since they have low or no toxicity to mammalian cells, and low chance of developing antimicrobial resistance based on their mechanism of action [1,14].

Bioinspired SAMPs based on natural AMPs can have attributes that are not present in the natural molecule [17,18]. A good example is the synthetic peptide LAH4, designed based on the Magainin 2 sequence, which presented potent activity against *Escherichia coli* and *Staphylococcus aureus* compared with the natural peptide Magainin 2 [17,18]. Recently, our research group designed peptides derived from *Mo*-CBP$_3$ and antifungal chitin-binding protein from *M. oleifera* seeds. *Mo*-CBP$_3$-PepI and *Mo*-CBP$_3$-pepIII inhibited the growth of

C. albicans and *C. parapsilosis* planktonic cells by the stimulation of ROS production, cell wall damage, and membrane pore formation, leading to death [15,16]. It is important to mention that *Mo*-CBP$_3$ did not present anticandidal activity. Based on that, we decided to evaluate the potential of *Mo*-CBP$_3$-PepI and *Mo*-CBP$_3$-pepIII to inhibit biofilm formation and its capacity to promote degradation of mature biofilms of *C. albicans* and *C. parapsilosis*.

Regarding degradation of the mature biofilms of *C. albicans*, *Mo*-CBP$_3$-PepI and *Mo*-CBP$_3$-PepIII had activity of 40% and 70%, respectively (Figure 1). These results corroborate those involving gH625, a peptide analog from gH625-M, which reduced by 61% the biomass of mature biofilms of *C. albicans* [19]. SEM analysis of *C. albicans* and *C. parapsilosis* treated with *Mo*-CBP$_3$-PepI and *Mo*-CBP$_3$-PepIII showed that the biofilms suffered severe structural damage. Furthermore, SEM images suggested that the two peptides induced rupture of the cell wall and membrane pore formation, leading to internal content loss and death. The images also showed the presence of scars, buds, and cracks. These results corroborate those reported by Belmadani and collaborators [20], who observed that Dermaseptin-S1, an antimicrobial peptide from *Phyllomedusa sauvagii*, decreased *C. albicans* biofilm formation by causing changes in the cell wall structure, membrane pore formation, and leakage of internal content. Similar behavior was observed by Sierra et al., where a *C. albicans* biofilm suffered severe damage by the antimicrobial peptide called Histatin-5 [21]. This severe damage observed in the cell wall of both cells via SEM analysis can be explained since *Mo*-CBP$_3$-PepI and *Mo*-CBP$_3$-PepIII are designed based on the sequence of *Mo*-CBP$_3$, which is a chitin-binding protein from *M. oleifera* seeds [16]. Both peptides can interact with the chitin present in the fungal cell wall and cause destabilization of the cell, leading to rupture, electrolyte imbalance, and thus cell death.

Unlike many commercial drugs that have specific targets, SAMPs target the cell membrane and/or the cell wall [14]. The ability of SAMPs to alter the microbial membrane permeability is considered the most common mechanism of action of these molecules, making the development of resistance mechanisms by microorganisms very difficult [1,14]. Fluorescence microscopy analyses were performed to evaluate if our peptides could induce membrane damage. *Mo*-CBP$_3$-PepI and *Mo*-CBP$_3$-PepIII induced PI uptake in *C. albicans* and *C. parapsilosis* biofilms, suggesting pore formation or cell membrane damage, as observed by SEM analysis. Furthermore, the peptides induced ROS overproduction in *C. parapsilosis* and *C. albicans* biofilms. A similar profile was observed using the peptides KP and MCh-AMP1, which are synthetic peptides able to induce ROS overproduction in *C. albicans* biofilm, leading to cell death. ROS are involved in the damage of essential molecules such as proteins, lipids, and DNA [22].

There are some explanations for the synergistic effect of the peptides and antifungal drugs tested here. First, the interactions between both peptides and NYS and ITR (Figure 6) can explain the synergistic activity obtained, where both peptides enhanced the activity of both drugs. Additionally, molecular docking studies were performed to evaluate whether both peptides could interact with NYS and ITR. Similar behavior was detected by Souza et al. [23], where *Mo*-CBP$_3$-PepI and *Mo*-CBP$_3$-PepIII interacted with griseofulvin by weak interactions, such as hydrogen bonds and hydrophobic interactions. The interaction of peptides with griseofulvin enhanced its activity against dermatophytes and reduced the toxicity of the drug, as was also shown in this study.

Two hypotheses can could explain the synergistic action between peptides and NYS. First, peptides target membranes and NYS targets the ergosterol. The interaction between peptides and NYS could result in a coordinated attack on the *Candida* membrane, enhancing the deleterious effect on it. Second, besides targeting the ergosterol in the membrane, NYS also has intracellular targets [24]. Once within the cytoplasm, NYS can attack the vacuole, causing its enlargement and impairing its function. Due to membrane-pore formation, the peptides might facilitate the access of NYS to the cytoplasm. It is known that *Mo*-CBP$_3$-PepI and *Mo*-CBP$_3$-PepIII form pores of 6 and 20 kDa, respectively, in *C. albicans* and *C. parapsilosis* membranes [15,16]. NYS has a molecular weight of 926.1 Da, so it is feasible to suggest that NYS passes through the membrane and attacks the cellular vacuole.

The synergistic effect of peptides with ITR, which has a molecular weight of 705 Da, could be explained by its the passage through the membrane by the pores formed in it as a result of the peptides' action. The facilitated passage of ITR through the pores formed by peptides in the membrane enhances its activity of inhibiting the cholesterol biosynthesis pathways, and thus the ergosterol synthesis [25]. One relevant fact is that both Mo-CBP$_3$-PepI and Mo-CBP$_3$-PepIII improved the activity of NYS and ITR by up to 50% regarding the inhibition of biofilm formation of C. albicans and C. parapsilosis. Moreover, the results showed that Mo-CBP$_3$-PepI enhanced NYS activity up to 60% in degrading the mature biofilms and preformed biofilm of both yeasts. The peptides also enhanced the antifungal activity of NYS and ITR against C. albicans and C. parapsilosis biofilms.

ITR and NYS can cause undesired effects, such as vomiting, nausea, diarrhea, anorexia, abdominal pain, and dizziness. Besides these side effects, cardiotoxicity and hypertension have been attributed to ITR usage. An unexpected and interesting result was that the association of peptides with antifungal drugs reduced their toxicity to human erythrocytes. For example, NYS alone caused hemolysis of 100% in type-A erythrocytes, while Mo-CBP$_3$-PepI + NYS and Mo-CBP$_3$-PepIII + NYS induced hemolysis of 0 and 45%, respectively, for type A blood. All treatments combining peptides with antifungal drugs were able to reduce the drugs' hemolytic effects.

Molecular docking analysis between peptides and drugs revealed a clue about how peptides reduced these hemolytic effects. The membrane of erythrocytes has neutral phospholipids, which means that any interaction with those membranes must be driven by hydrophobic interactions [24]. It is known that NYS and ITR are hydrophobic drugs [25,26]. Thus, hydrophobic interactions with membranes of erythrocytes may drive the hemolytic activity of NYS and ITR. The molecular docking experiments revealed that peptides had hydrophobic interactions with NYS and ITR, suggesting that the hydrophobic interactions between peptides and both drugs prevented the interaction with the erythrocyte membranes, reducing their hemolytic effect.

4. Materials and Methods

4.1. Ethics Statement

Does not apply to this study.

4.2. Biological and Chemical Materials

C. albicans (ATCC 10231) and C. parapsilosis (ATCC 22019) were obtained from the Laboratory of Plant Toxins of the Department of Biochemistry and Molecular Biology of Federal University of Ceará, Brazil. All chemicals were purchased from Sigma-Aldrich Co. (St. Louis, MO, USA).

4.3. Peptide Synthesis

The synthetic peptides Mo-CBP$_3$-PepI (CPIAQRCC) and Mo-CBP$_3$-PepIII (AIQRCC) were chemically synthesized by the company GenOne (São Paulo, Brazil), and the quality and purity ($\geq$95%) were analyzed by reverse-phase high-performance liquid chromatography (RP-HPLC, Jasco, Easton, MD, USA) and mass spectrometry (Waltham, MA, USA).

4.4. Biological Activity

Antibiofilm Assay

The assays against C. albicans and C. parapsilosis biofilms were performed following the method described by [27–29], with some modifications. To evaluate the inhibition of the biofilm formation, 100 µL of C. albicans or C. parapsilosis suspension (2.5×10^3 CFU/mL in Sabouraud liquid medium) was incubated in 96-well plates with 100 µL of Mo-CBP$_3$-PepI, Mo-CBP$_3$-PepII or Mo-CBP$_3$-PepIII (50 µg mL^{-1}, as defined by [14–16,23]), at 37 °C for 48 h. The supernatant was removed and the wells were washed three times with sterile 0.15 M NaCl. Next, the cells were fixed with 100 µL of 100% methanol for 15 min at 37 °C and the plates were air-dried under the same conditions. Then, 200 µL of an aqueous solution of 0.1% crystal violet was added and incubated for 30 min at 24 °C. To remove the excess crystal violet, the plates were washed three times with distilled water and finally 100 µL of 33% acetic acid to solubilize the dye bound in the biofilm. After 15 min, the absorbance was measured at 600 nm using an automated microplate reader (Epoch, Biotek, Santa Clara, CA, USA).

To evaluate the degradation of mature biofilm, the cell suspensions of both yeasts (100 µL, 2.5×10^3 CFU/mL in Sabouraud liquid medium) were first incubated at 37 °C for 24 h in 96-well plates. Then, the supernatant was removed, and 100 µL of the Sabouraud liquid medium and 100 µL of each peptide (50 µg mL^{-1}) were added and incubated again for 24 h. The culture medium was again discarded, and the same procedure that used 0.1% crystal violet was employed to quantify the biofilm mass. In both experiments, a solution of 5% DMSO in 0.9% NaCl was used as a negative control. NYS (1000 µg mL^{-1}) and ITR (1000 µg mL^{-1}) were used as positive controls. The synergism assays were carried out by combining the peptides (50 µg mL^{-1}) with NYS or ITR (1000 µg mL^{-1}) and the effectiveness was compared with the activity of the peptides and drugs alone.

4.5. Overproduction of Reactive Oxygen Species (ROS)

The ROS overproduction was determined following the method described by Dias et al. [29], with some modifications. C. albicans and C. parapsilosis were incubated with the three peptides under the same conditions as described above. Then, 50 µL of cell suspension (2.5×10^3 CFU/mL) was incubated with 50 µL of each peptide (50 µg mL^{-1}) for 24 h and the formed biofilm was washed with 0.15 M NaCl three times to remove the Sabouraud liquid medium. Next, 20 µL of 2',7' dichlorofluorescein diacetate (DCFH-DA, Sigma, St. Louis, MI, USA) was added and incubated in the dark for 30 min at 24 °C. Finally, the biofilms were washed with 0.15 M NaCl and observed under a fluorescence microscope (Olympus System BX 41, Tokyo, Japan) with an excitation wavelength of 488 nm and emission wavelength of 525 nm.

4.6. Cell Membrane Integrity Assay

The cell membrane integrity of C. albicans and C. parapsilosis was tested as described by Dias et al. [29], with some modifications. The biofilms were treated as described for ROS overproduction analysis. Thus, 20 µL of propidium iodide (PI, Sigma, St. Louis, MI, USA) was added and incubated in the dark for 30 min at 24 °C. Then the samples were washed three times with 0.15 M NaCl to remove the excess of PI and observed with a fluorescence microscope (Olympus System BX 41, Tokyo, Japan) with an excitation wavelength of 535 nm and emission wavelength of 617 nm.

4.7. Scanning Electron Microscopy (SEM) Analysis

The morphological changes in the cells of C. albicans and C. parapsilosis were evaluated by SEM (Billerica, MA, USA), using the method described by Staniszewska et al. [30]. Biofilms were fixed with 1% (v/v) glutaraldehyde in 0.15 M sodium phosphate buffer at pH 7.0 for 16 h. Then the biofilms were washed with 0.15 M sodium phosphate buffer (pH 7.0) three times. Next, 0.2% (v/v) osmium tetroxide was added to the samples and incubated for 30 min at 37 °C and washed again under the same conditions described above. Samples were successively dehydrated with increased ethanol concentrations (30%, 50%, 70% 100% and 100% [v/v]) for 10 min each at 24 °C. Last, the final dehydration was realized with 50% hexamethyldisilane (HMDS, Sigma, St. Louis, MI, USA) diluted in ethanol for 10 min and then 100% HDMS. The biofilms were placed on stubs and coated with a 20 nm gold layer using a positron-emission tomography (PET) coating machine (Emitech-Q150TES, Quorum Technologies, Lewes, England). The images were obtained with an FEI inspectTM50 scanning electron microscope, equipped with a low energy detector (Everhart-Thornley), and the acceleration used was 20,000 kV and 20,000× detector magnification.

4.8. Obtainment, File Preparation, and Molecular Docking

The three-dimensional (3D) structures of *Mo*-CBP$_3$-PepI and *Mo*-CBP$_3$-PepIII were predicted using the PepFold server 3 (https://bioserv.rpbs.univ-paris-diderot.fr/services/PEP-FOLD/ accessed on 15 February 2022) [31]. The amino acid protonation of the peptides was adjusted to pH 7.4 using Protein Prepare [32]. NYS (accession number CID 16219709) and ITR (accession number CID 55283) 3D structures were obtained from the database of PubChem (https://pubchem.ncbi.nlm.nih.gov/ accessed on 15 February 2022) [33]. The protonation of the ligands was adjusted using the Marvin Sketch software version 15.6.15. The energy minimization of the peptide hydrogens and the ligand was conducted using Discovery Studio v. 20.1 (https://discover.3ds.com/discovery-studio-visualizer-download accessed on 15 March 2022) and Open Babel version 2.4.0 (https://osdn.net/projects/sfnet_openbabel/downloads/openbabel/2.4.0/OpenBabel-2.4.0.exe/ accessed on 5 March 2022).

Molecular docking assays were carried out using Autodock Vina, version 1.1.2 [34]. Additionally, the Autodock graphical interface version 1.5.6 was used to maintain polar hydrogens and provide charges to peptides and drugs using Kollman united charges [35]. The *Mo*-CBP$_3$-PepI and *Mo*-CBP$_3$-PepIII were considered rigid molecules, and NYS and ITR were docked as flexible molecules. The grid box was defined as a 24 Å × 24 Å × 24 Å cube with the peptides in the center. The exhaustiveness was set to 16, and all other parameters were used as default. The software Discovery Studio v. 20.1 and the 3D interaction representations were realized using the Pymol program (https://pymol.org/2/ accessed on 8 March 2022).

4.9. Hemolytic Assay

The hemolytic activities of *Mo*-CBP$_3$-PepI, *Mo*-CBP$_3$-PepIII, NYS, and ITR, alone and in their different combinations, were assessed using A, B, and O types of human erythrocytes as described by Souza et al. [14]. The concentrations of all solutions were the same as used in the synergism assays. The blood types were provided by the Hematology and Hemotherapy Center of Ceará (Fortaleza, Brazil).

The blood was collected in a tube with heparin (5 IU mL^{-1}, Sigma Aldrich, São Paulo, Brazil), centrifuged at 300× g for 5 min at 4 °C, washed with sterile 0.15 M NaCl, and diluted to a concentration of 2.5%. Each blood type was incubated (100 µL) with solutions of Mo-CBP3-PepI, Mo-CBP3-PepIII (50 µg mL^{-1}), NYS (1000 µg mL^{-1}), or ITR (1000 µg mL^{-1}) for 30 min at 37 °C, followed by centrifugation (300× g for 5 min at 4 °C, centrifuge Eppendorf 5810, Hannover, Germany). Supernatants were collected and transferred to 96-well microtiter plates and the hemolysis (%) was calculated by reading the absorbance at 414 nm using an automated absorbance microplate reader using DMSO-NaCl solution (0%) and 0.1% Triton X-100 (100%) as negative and positive controls for hemolysis, respectively. The hemolysis was calculated by the equation: [(Abs$_{414nm}$ of sample treated with peptides or drugs-Abs$_{414nm}$ of samples treated with DMSO-NaCl)/[(Abs$_{414nm}$ of samples treated with 0.1% TritonX-100-Abs$_{414nm}$ of samples treated with DMSO-NaCl] × 100.

4.10. Statistical Analysis

All the assays were performed individually three times and the values are expressed as the mean ± standard error. The data were submitted to ANOVA followed by the Tukey test. GraphPad Prism version 5.01 (GraphPad Software company, Santa Clara, CA, USA) was used to generate all graphics, with a significance of $p < 0.05$.

5. Conclusions

The antibiofilm activity, absence of toxicity, and synergistic effect enhancing the activity of NYS and ITR, strongly indicated that *Mo*-CBP$_3$-PepI and *Mo*-CBP$_3$-PepIII are promising antibiofilm peptides which could act as new antimicrobial agents. We also highlight their use for clinical application or adjuvants to conventional drugs to overcome resistance developed by *Candida* species.

Author Contributions: All authors made substantial contributions. The conception and design of the study and acquisition of data, analysis, docking analysis, and interpretation were performed by L.P.B., C.D.T.F., A.F.B.S., N.A.S.N., J.L.A., A.L.C.P., J.T.A.O. and P.F.N.S. Microscopic analyses were carried out by R.G.G.S. and A.F.B.S. Writing or revising the article was done by L.P.B., A.L.C.P., G.H.G., F.P.M. and P.F.N.S. P.F.N.S. gave final approval of the version to be submitted. All authors have read and agreed to the published version of the manuscript.

Funding: This work was supported by grants from the following Brazilian agencies: Conselho Nacional de Desenvolvimento Científico e Tecnológico (CNPq) (process numbers 308107/2013-6 and 306202/2017-4); Coordenação de Aperfeiçoamento de Pessoal de Nível Superior (CAPES); Instituto Nacional de Ciências e Tecnologia de Bioinspiração (Process Number: 465507/2014-0) and Fundação Cearense de Apoio ao Desenvolvimento Científico e Tecnológico (FUNCAP). CAPES provided the postdoctoral grant to Pedro F. N. Souza (grant number 88887.318820/2019-00). We are also grateful to the staff of the central analytical facilities of UFC, Brazil.

Institutional Review Board Statement: Not applicable.

Informed Consent Statement: Not applicable.

Data Availability Statement: The data that support the findings of this study are available on request from the corresponding author.

Acknowledgments: Special thanks to CAPES for providing the postdoctoral grant to Pedro F. N. Souza. We are also grateful to the staff of the central analytical facilities of UFC, Brazil.

Conflicts of Interest: The authors report no conflict of interest. The authors alone are responsible for the content and the writing of the paper.

References

1. Lima, P.G.; Oliveira, J.T.A.; Amaral, J.L.; Freitas, C.D.T.; Souza, P.F.N. Synthetic antimicrobial peptides: Characteristics, design, and potential as alternative molecules to overcome microbial resistance. *Life Sci.* **2021**, *278*, 119647–119660. [CrossRef] [PubMed]
2. Kumar, A.; Alam, A.; Rani, M.; Ehtesham, N.Z.; Hasnain, S.E. Biofilms: Survival and defense strategy for pathogens. *Int. J. Med. Microbiol.* **2017**, *307*, 481–489. [CrossRef] [PubMed]
3. Kovács, R.; Majoros, L. Fungal quorum-sensing molecules: A review of their antifungal effect against *Candida* biofilms. *J. Fungi* **2020**, *6*, 99. [CrossRef] [PubMed]
4. Zarnowski, R.; Westler, W.M.; Lacmbouh, G.A.; Marita, J.M.; Bothe, J.R.; Bernhardt, J.; Lounes-Hadj Sahraoui, A.; Fontaine, J.; Sanchez, H.; Hatfield, R.D.; et al. Novel entries in a fungal biofilm matrix encyclopedia. *MBio* **2014**, *5*, e01333-14. [CrossRef]
5. Fox, E.P.; Nobile, C.J. A sticky situation. *Transcription* **2012**, *3*, 315–322. [CrossRef] [PubMed]
6. Kullberg, B.J.; Oude Lashof, A.M.L. Epidemiology of opportunistic invasive mycoses. *Eur. J. Med. Res.* **2002**, *7*, 183–191. [PubMed]
7. Weig, M. Clinical aspects and pathogenesis of *Candida* Infection. *Trends Microbiol.* **1998**, *6*, 468–470. [CrossRef]
8. Baillie, G.S. Matrix polymers of *Candida* biofilms and their possible role in biofilm resistance to antifungal agents. *J. Antimicrob. Chemother.* **2000**, *46*, 397–403. [CrossRef]
9. Sasso, M.; Roger, C.; Sasso, M.; Poujol, H.; Barbar, S.; Lefrant, J.-Y.; Lachaud, L. Changes in the distribution of colonising and infecting *Candida* Spp. isolates, antifungal drug consumption and susceptibility in a french intensive care unit: A 10-year study. *Mycoses* **2017**, *60*, 770–780. [CrossRef]
10. LaFleur, M.D.; Kumamoto, C.A.; Lewis, K. *Candida albicans* biofilms produce antifungal-tolerant persister cells. *Antimicrob. Agents Chemother.* **2006**, *50*, 3839–3846. [CrossRef]
11. Ramage, G. Investigation of multidrug efflux pumps in relation to fluconazole resistance in *Candida albicans* biofilms. *J. Antimicrob. Chemother.* **2002**, *49*, 973–980. [CrossRef] [PubMed]
12. Arendrup, M.C.; Patterson, T.F. Multidrug-resistant *Candida*: Epidemiology, molecular mechanisms, and treatment. *J. Infect. Dis.* **2017**, *216*, S445–S451. [CrossRef] [PubMed]
13. Katiyar, S.; Pfaller, M.; Edlind, T. *Candida albicans* and *Candida glabrata* clinical isolates exhibiting reduced echinocandin susceptibility. *Antimicrob. Agents Chemother.* **2006**, *50*, 2892–2894. [CrossRef] [PubMed]
14. Souza, P.F.N.; Marques, L.S.M.; Oliveira, J.T.A.; Lima, P.G.; Dias, L.P.; Neto, N.A.S.; Lopes, F.E.S.; Sousa, J.S.; Silva, A.F.B.; Caneiro, R.F.; et al. Synthetic antimicrobial peptides: From choice of the best sequences to action mechanisms. *Biochimie* **2020**, *175*, 132–145. [CrossRef]
15. Lima, P.G.; Souza, P.F.N.; Freitas, C.D.T.; Oliveira, J.T.A.; Dias, L.P.; Neto, J.X.S.; Vasconcelos, I.M.; Lopes, J.L.S.; Sousa, D.O.B. Anticandidal activity of synthetic peptides: Mechanism of action revealed by scanning electron and fluorescence microscopies and synergism effect with nystatin. *J. Pept. Sci.* **2020**, *26*, e3249. [CrossRef]
16. Oliveira, J.T.A.; Souza, P.F.N.; Vasconcelos, I.M.; Dias, L.P.; Martins, T.F.; Van Tilburg, M.F.; Guedes, M.I.F.; Sousa, D.O.B. Mo-CBP$_3$-PepI, Mo-CBP$_3$-PepII, and Mo-CBP$_3$-PepIII are synthetic antimicrobial peptides active against human pathogens by stimulating ROS generation and increasing plasma membrane permeability. *Biochimie* **2019**, *157*, 10–21. [CrossRef]

17. Mason, A.J.; Moussaoui, W.; Abdelrahman, T.; Boukhari, A.; Bertani, P.; Marquette, A.; Shooshtarizaheh, P.; Moulay, G.; Boehm, N.; Guerold, B. Structural determinants of antimicrobial and antiplasmodial activity and selectivity in histidine-rich amphipathic cationic peptides. *J. Biol. Chem.* **2009**, *284*, 119–133. [CrossRef]
18. Mason, A.J.; Gasnier, C.; Kichler, A.; Prévost, G.; Aunis, D.; Metz-Boutigue, M.H.; Bechinger, B. Enhanced membrane disruption and antibiotic action against pathogenic bacteria by designed histidine-rich peptides at acidic PH. *Antimicrob. Agents Chemother.* **2006**, *50*, 3305–3311. [CrossRef]
19. Galdiero, E.; de Alteriis, E.; De Natale, A.; D'Alterio, A.; Siciliano, A.; Guida, M.; Lombardi, L.; Falanga, A.; Galdiero, S. Eradication of *Candida albicans* persister cell biofilm by the membranotropic peptide GH625. *Sci. Rep.* **2020**, *10*, 5780–5791. [CrossRef]
20. Belmadani, A.; Semlali, A.; Rouabhia, M. Dermaseptin-S1 decreases *Candida albicans* growth, biofilm formation and the expression of hyphal wall protein 1 and aspartic protease genes. *J. Appl. Microbiol.* **2018**, *125*, 72–83. [CrossRef]
21. Sierra, J.M.; Fusté, E.; Rabanal, F.; Vinuesa, T.; Viñas, M. An overview of antimicrobial peptides and the latest advances in their development. *Expert Opin. Biol. Ther.* **2017**, *17*, 663–676. [CrossRef] [PubMed]
22. Seyedjavadi, S.S.; Khani, S.; Eslamifar, A.; Ajdary, S.; Goudarzi, M.; Halabian, R.; Akbari, R.; Zare-Zardini, H.; Imani Fooladi, A.A.; Amani, J.; et al. The antifungal peptide MCh-AMP1 derived from *Matricaria chamomilla* inhibits *Candida albicans* growth via inducing ROS generation and altering fungal cell membrane permeability. *Front. Microbiol.* **2020**, *10*, 3150. [CrossRef] [PubMed]
23. Souza, P.F.N.; Lima, P.G.; Freitas, C.D.T.; Sousa, D.O.B.; Neto, N.A.S.; Dias, L.P.; Vasconcelos, I.M.; Freitas, L.B.N.; Silva, R.G.G.; Sousa, J.S.; et al. Antidermatophytic activity of synthetic peptides: Action mechanisms and clinical application as adjuvants to enhance the activity and decrease the toxicity of griseofulvin. *Mycoses* **2020**, *63*, 979–992. [CrossRef] [PubMed]
24. Bhuiyan, M.S.A.; Ito, Y.; Nakamura, A.; Tanaka, N.; Fujita, K.; Fukui, H.; Takegawa, K. Nystatin effects on vacuolar function in *Saccharomyce*. *Biosci. Biotechnol. Biochem.* **1999**, *63*, 1075–1082. [CrossRef] [PubMed]
25. Borgers, M.; Van de Ven, M.-A. Mode of action of itraconazole: Morphological aspects. *Mycoses* **1989**, *32* (Suppl. 1), 53–59. [CrossRef] [PubMed]
26. Huang, Y.; Huang, J.; Chen, Y. Alpha-helical cationic antimicrobial peptides: Relationships of structure and function. *Protein Cell* **2010**, *1*, 143–152. [CrossRef]
27. Benavent, C.; García-Herrero, V.; Torrado, C.; Torrado-Santiago, S. Nystatin antifungal micellar systems on endotracheal tubes: Development, characterization and in vitro evaluation. *Pharmazie* **2019**, *74*, 34–38. [CrossRef]
28. Lang, B.; Liu, S.; McGinity, J.W.; Williams, R.O. Effect of hydrophilic additives on the dissolution and pharmacokinetic properties of itraconazole-enteric polymer hot-melt extruded amorphous solid dispersions. *Drug Dev. Ind. Pharm.* **2016**, *42*, 429–445. [CrossRef]
29. Dias, L.P.; Souza, P.F.N.; Oliveira, J.T.A.; Vasconcelos, I.M.; Araújo, N.M.S.; Tilburg, M.F.V.; Guedes, M.I.F.; Carneiro, R.F.; Lopes, J.L.S.; Sousa, D.O.B. RcAlb-PepII, a synthetic small peptide bioinspired in the 2S albumin from the seed cake of *Ricinus communis*, is a potent antimicrobial agent against *Klebsiella pneumoniae* and *Candida parapsilosis*. *Biochim. Biophys. Acta-Biomembr.* **2020**, *1862*, 183092–183102. [CrossRef]
30. Staniszewska, M.; Bondaryk, M.; Swoboda-Kopec, E.; Siennicka, K.; Sygitowicz, G.; Kurzatkowski, W. *Candida albicans* morphologies revealed by scanning electron microscopy analysis. *Braz. J. Microbiol.* **2013**, *44*, 813–821. [CrossRef]
31. Lamiable, A.; Thévenet, P.; Rey, J.; Vavrusa, M.; Derreumaux, P.; Tufféry, P. PEP-FOLD3: Faster de novo structure prediction for linear peptides in solution and in complex. *Nucleic Acids Res.* **2016**, *44*, W449–W454. [CrossRef] [PubMed]
32. Martínez-Rosell, G.; Giorgino, T.; De Fabritiis, G. PlayMolecule ProteinPrepare: A web application for protein preparation for molecular dynamics simulations. *J. Chem. Inf. Model.* **2017**, *57*, 1511–1516. [CrossRef] [PubMed]
33. Kim, S.; Chen, J.; Cheng, T.; Gindulyte, A.; He, J.; He, S.; Li, Q.; Shoemaker, B.A.; Thiessen, P.A.; Yu, B.; et al. PubChem 2019 update: Improved access to chemical data. *Nucleic Acids Res.* **2019**, *47*, D1102–D1109. [CrossRef]
34. Trott, O.; Olson, A.J. AutoDock Vina: Improving the speed and accuracy of docking with a new scoring function, efficient optimization, and multithreading. *J. Comput. Chem.* **2009**, *31*, 455–461. [CrossRef]
35. Morris, G.M.; Huey, R.; Lindstrom, W.; Sanner, M.F.; Belew, R.K.; Goodsell, D.S.; Olson, A.J. AutoDock4 and autodocktools4: Automated docking with selective receptor flexibility. *J. Comput. Chem.* **2009**, *30*, 2785–2791. [CrossRef] [PubMed]

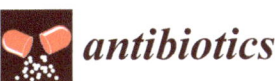

Review

Antisense and Functional Nucleic Acids in Rational Drug Development

Robert Penchovsky *, Antoniya V. Georgieva, Vanya Dyakova, Martina Traykovska and Nikolet Pavlova

Laboratory of Synthetic Biology and Bioinformatics, Faculty of Biology, Sofia University, "St. Kliment Ohridski", 8 Dragan Tzankov Blvd., 1164 Sofia, Bulgaria
* Correspondence: robert.penchovsky@hotmail.com; Tel./Fax: +359-28167340

Abstract: This review is focused on antisense and functional nucleic acid used for completely rational drug design and drug target assessment, aiming to reduce the time and money spent and increase the successful rate of drug development. Nucleic acids have unique properties that play two essential roles in drug development as drug targets and as drugs. Drug targets can be messenger, ribosomal, non-coding RNAs, ribozymes, riboswitches, and other RNAs. Furthermore, various antisense and functional nucleic acids can be valuable tools in drug discovery. Many mechanisms for RNA-based control of gene expression in both pro-and-eukaryotes and engineering approaches open new avenues for drug discovery with a critical role. This review discusses the design principles, applications, and prospects of antisense and functional nucleic acids in drug delivery and design. Such nucleic acids include antisense oligonucleotides, synthetic ribozymes, and siRNAs, which can be employed for rational antibacterial drug development that can be very efficient. An important feature of antisense and functional nucleic acids is the possibility of using rational design methods for drug development. This review aims to popularize these novel approaches to benefit the drug industry and patients.

Keywords: antisense oligonucleotides; antisense therapies; drug delivery; drug discovery; nucleic acid engineering; ribozymes; riboswitches

1. Introduction

Nucleic acids have been suitable tools for engineering biosensors for various in vitro and in vivo applications over the last two decades. At the same time, new natural mechanisms for the control of gene expression have been discovered based on various types of RNAs, including micro(mi)RNAs, small interfering(si)RNAs, riboswitches [1], and ribozymes. There are currently four different nucleic acid engineering strategies to inhibit the expression of specific RNAs in the cell, such as siRNAs [2], antisense oligonucleotides (ASOs) [3], ribozymes [4,5], and CRISPR-Cas9 systems [6]. All tools used for nucleic acid-based drug development are inherited based on rational design methods, being novel and the main point of this review.

This review discusses all distinct strategies for RNA inhibition and the engineering methods that make them possible. We also describe the applications of the mRNA inhibition approaches in drug development [7,8], providing validated, proven examples.

Nucleic acids have unique properties that play two essential roles in drug discovery, including drug targets and drugs. Various RNAs can be employed as drug targets, including messenger, ribosomal, non-coding RNAs, ribozymes, riboswitches, etc. Various antisense and functional nucleic acids can be employed as RNA targeting tools. Thus, nucleic acids can be drug targets and drugs themselves.

RNA has the most diverse roles of all biomacromolecules in the cell. The most important roles of RNA are the transcription and translation of genetic instructions involving messenger (m), transfer (t), and ribosomal (r) RNAs. RNAs can also have a catalytic function through the ribozymes and gene regulatory roles through the non-coding (nc) RNAs and the riboswitches. The new high-throughput sequencing and many bioinformatics and biochemical methods are new insights into the role of RNA in biological systems [9].

RNA can exhibit a catalytic function when it works as a ribozyme and a biosensing function as a riboswitch. Naturally occurring RNAs, such as the glmS gene control element, have biosensing and catalytic functions [10]. The proteins are usually responsible for the catalytic and biosensing functions in the cell.

RNA executes essential and complex biochemical functions in the cell and uniquely combines different biochemical properties. Functional RNAs like riboswitches can form complex tertiary structures similar to proteins. For instance, riboswitches can precisely sense the presence of small molecules in the cell, such as guanine, adenine, thiamine pyrophosphate (TPP), and many others, as proteins can. RNA can also specifically hybridize with other nucleic acids [10]. Thus, some RNAs work via Watson-Crick base-pairing while others operate via their 3D structures. These unique biochemical properties make functional RNA molecules very promising targets for drug discovery.

RNA is less chemically stable than DNA due to a 2'-hydroxyl group of the ribose, which, in inline conformation, leads to transesterification of the phosphodiester bond of RNA [11]. Many catalytic RNAs, such as hammerhead ribozymes, can speed up the transesterification reaction up to a million times [11].

The mRNA destabilization is an essential mechanism in regulating gene expression in eukaryotic and prokaryotic organisms. However, for eukaryotic organisms that possess RNA-interfering pathways for sequence-specific mRNA decay [12], the non-coding RNAs (ncRNAs) are classified into three groups such as long non-coding RNA (lncRNA), short non-coding RNA (sncRNA), and translational/structural RNA, which possess diverse functions [13]. Their regulation can enhance treatments against different diseases by chromatin modification, inducing immunity via RNA-based vaccination, targeting mRNA for its cleavage via antisense oligonucleotides (ASOs), RNA alternative splicing, RNA masking, shRNA or miRNA-based gene silencing, and transcriptional or translational interference [14,15]. The discovery of gene silencing by ncRNAs in many different organisms, from plants to mammalians, including humans, has extended our understanding of the role of RNA in the cell and given us the opportunities to use non-coding RNA molecules as new targets for drug discovery and drug development.

Understanding RNA interference (RNAi) mechanisms for controlling gene expression has provided us with novel molecular tools that can be used to develop novel drugs. The RNAi pathway regulates mRNA stability and translation in human cells. siRNAs could trigger the RNA silencing of specific genes [16].

Rational design approaches of functional and ASOs can significantly reduce the time and overall cost and increase the rate of successful drug development.

2. ASO-Based Strategies for Drug Development

mRNAs are universally present in all forms of life. Therefore, they are more often becoming targets for treating various RNA-associated diseases such as cancer, neurodegenerative diseases, and many others. One promising method that has attracted more attention in the past decade is antisense oligonucleotide technology (ASOT), which has various applications in drug development, including specific gene silencing [17]. ASOs are single-stranded synthetic oligonucleotides that hybridize to a particular mRNA or other type of RNA and inhibit gene expression [18]. Typically, the length of an ASO is between 15 and 25 nucleotides, which, via Watson-Crick base-pairing, binds complementarily to the target RNA to form a duplex. The ASO-based inhibition is achieved by steric blocking of translation or splicing or by cleavage of the target RNA in the duplex via the RNase H or RNase P enzymes, exon skipping [19], and exon inclusion (Figure 1). Apart from that, ASO can be employed to block the transcription by targeting the genome DNA (Figure 1A).

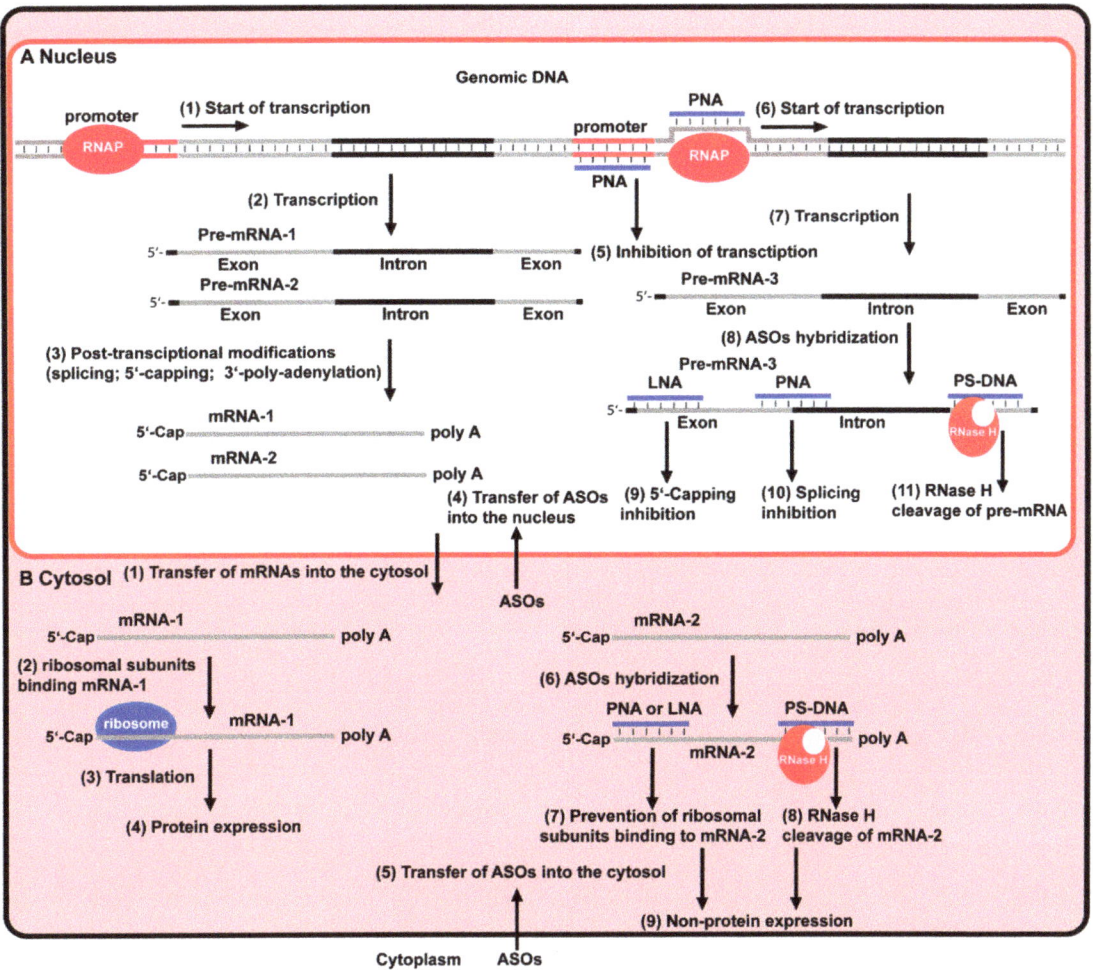

Figure 1. Control of gene expression in eukaryotes by ASOs. (**A**) In the nucleus, genomic DNA has promoter sites. The binding of RNAP to the promoter site (1) triggers pre-mRNA-1 and pre-mRNA-2 (2). These pre-mRNAs undergo post-transcriptional modifications and become mRNA-1 and mRNA-2 (3). ASOs can be transferred into the nucleus (4). One of these ASOs, PNA, can bind to the promoter and inhibit transcription (5). PNA can bind to one of the DNA strands (6) and induce the transcription of pre-mRNA-3 (7). ASOs present in the nucleus can hybridize to complementary sequences of pre-mNA-3 (8); hybridizing of LNA leads to 5′-capping inhibition (9); hybridizing of PNA leads to splicing inhibition of mRNA-3 (10); hybridizing of PS-DNA leads to the formation of a chimeric structure that is a substrate for RNase H, which recognizes, binds and cleaves mRNA-3 (11). (**B**) The spliced mRNAs are transferred from the nucleus (1). Ribosomal subunits recognize RBS and bind (2). The ribozyme binding triggers translation (3) and protein expression (4). When ASOs are transferred from the cytoplasm into the cytosol (5), they hybridize with complementary sequences of mRNA-2 (6); hybridizing of LNA leads to the prevention of ribosomal binding to mRNA-2 (7); hybridizing of PS-DNA leads to the formation of a chimeric structure (duplex) which is a substrate for RNase H, which recognizes, binds and cleaves mRNA-2 (8) leading to non-protein expression (9).

The unmodified *ASOs* quickly degrade due to the circulating nucleases and are rapidly excreted by the kidneys. This makes them unsuitable for creating therapeutic drugs. Hence, chemical modifications play a crucial role in increasing the stability of ASOs in vivo and the success of an antisense strategy [20]. According to their modifications, there are three generations of antisense oligonucleotides.

2.1. First-Generation ASOs

The first-generation ASO (Figure 2A) has a sulfur atom instead of one of the non-bridging oxygen atoms in the phosphodiester bond (i.e., PS modification). Another substitute for the same oxygen atom can be methyl or amine. This modification makes the ASO more resistant to nucleases and prolongs its half-life in vivo compared with non-modified DNA. The PS-modified ASOs activate RNase H, and, as a result, the target RNA is cleaved right after the hybridization with the ASO under multiple-turnover conditions. However, this generation of ASOs has a few shortcomings, such as the possibility of non-specific binding with proteins by forming S-S bonds and slightly reduced affinity to the target RNAs. The first-generation ASOs have a reduced affinity for mRNA hybridization by approximately 0.5 °C per nucleotide. First-generation ASOs are still widely used in vitro and in vivo, particularly in combination with second-generation ASOs. This combination decreases the shortcomings of first-generation ASOs by reducing the number of PS-modified bases.

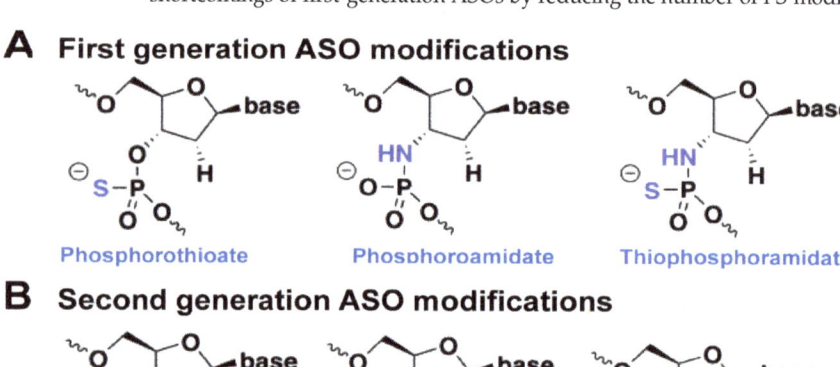

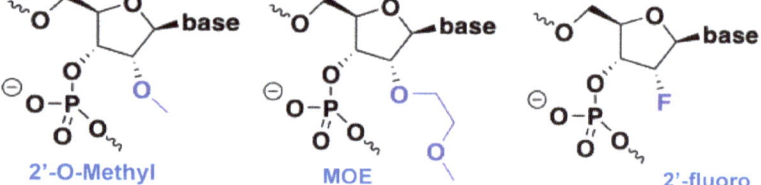

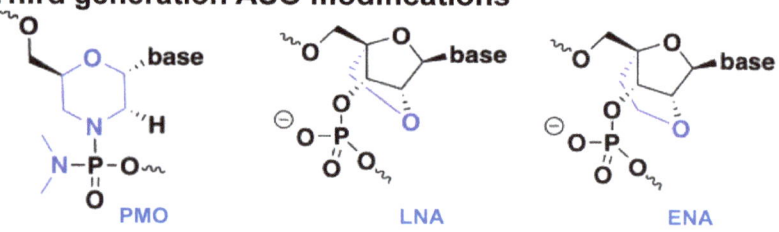

Figure 2. Chemical modifications of various ASOs. (**A**) First-generation ASOs: phosphorothioate, phoshoroamidate, and thiophosphoramidate. They contain phosphodiester bonds in which one of the non-bridging oxygen is replaced by a sulfur atom, an amide group, and a sulfur and amide group. (**B**) In the second-generation ASOs, the nuclease resistance is increased by 2′-alkyl modifications of the ribose and fluorine. (**C**) Third generation ASOs: phosphoramidite morpholino oligomer (PMO), locked nucleic acid (LNA), and ethylene-bridged nucleic acid (ENA).

2.2. Second-Generation ASOs

The second-generation ASO is characterized mainly by 2′-O-methyl and 2′-O-methoxyethyl (i.e., 2′-alkyl) modifications of the ribose (Figure 2B). These modifications correct the flaws of the previous generation by increasing the specific binding affinity and the hybridization stability of the formed duplex. However, on the other hand, a new disadvantage occurs since the 2′-alkyl modification prevents the cleavage of the target RNA because RNase H cannot be activated and, thus, works under single-turnover conditions. Thus, a chimeric design that combines the first and second generation of modifications is often employed. The ASO has a central part built of a PS-modified 2′-deoxynucleotide and flanking regions on both sides made of 2′-alkyl-modified nucleotides. The main feature is typically between 8 and 16 nt long [21], whereas the flanking wings are between 5 and 10 nt long. Such chimeric ASOs activate RNase H-mediated cleavage while the flanking wings had better protect the ASO from nuclease degradation [22].

2.3. Third-Generation ASOs

Third-generation ASO modifications (Figure 2C) mainly involve the furanose ring of the nucleotides. They are primarily electric neutral, unlike the previous two generations, and therefore, they can easily pass the phospholipid bilayer of the cells [23]. Moreover, third-generation ASOs have improved nuclease resistance, target affinity, and pharmacokinetics [24]. Frequently used ASOs from this generation are locked nucleic acid (LNA), peptide nucleic acid (PNA), 2′-O,4′-C-ethylene-bridged nucleic acid (ENA), and phosphorodiamidate morpholino oligomer (PMO) (Figure 2C). However, these ASOs cannot induce an RNA cleavage via RNase H and inhibit RNA by blocking translation under single-turnover conditions [22,25].

2.3.1. LNA

LNA follows the Watson–Crick base-pairing rules and forms duplexes with complementary DNA or RNA with increased stabilities and selectivities [26]. Imanishi's collective presents bicyclic nucleoside analogs—2′-O,4′-C-methylene uridine, and -cytidine, with fixed N-type conformation incorporated into oligonucleotides. Typically, 2′-O,4′-C-methylene uridine, and -cytidine analogs have a C3′-*endo* sugar puckering, synthesized from uridine [27]. LNA has a modified ribose with an extra bridge connecting the 2′-oxygen and 4′-carbon (Figure 2C). As a result, the ribose is locked in the 3′-end (north) conformation, often found in A-form duplexes, which significantly increases the melting temperature and specificity of hybridization. For instance, LNA/DNA hybrids possess increased T_m from 2 °C to 6 °C per monomer compared with DNA/DNA hybrids with the same sequence. LNA/RNA hybrids have even higher T_m, rising from 3 °C to 8 °C per monomer. LNA oligomers can be synthesized by conventional phosphoramide chemistry, allowing automated synthesis that will be inexpensive when its intellectual property rights expire. Furthermore, LNA oligomers can be easily synthesized as chimeras having DNA, RNA, and other modified bases or labels. For example, two sets of iso-LNA-modified gapmers were tested in HeLa cells for target knockdown activity, systematically changing the number and positions of the long nucleic acid modifications. Based on the structure specifications, the results showed 768 different gapmers targeting the HeLa cells for target knockdown activity and cytotoxic potential because of the binding affinity between the ASOs and the mRNA target [28]. When the accessible regions in the specific target are chosen or identified, it is possible to optimize the LNA gapmers with improved pharmacological profiles to target them.

Usually, the chimeric ASOs, like phosphorothioate DNA, are flanked by stability-enhancing modified nucleotides such as D-2-O-methylribose modifications [29]. Nucleotide modifications of D-2-O-methylribose in the central DNA gap could disturb the RNase H function [29]. LNA gapmers can activate RNase H. One of the first experiments conducted with LNA/DNA gapmers was performed on the central nervous system of rats, targeting their delta-opioid receptor mRNA [28]. It was designed superior to dose-dependent and sequence-specific inhibition by an iso-sequential DNA antisense oligonucleotide [30]. Subsequent experiments based on receptor binding showed that LNA, DNA, and PS ASOs reduce the delta-opioid receptor density by 35% to 55%. In another experiment, LNAs/DNAs were tested targeting the 3′-UTR of intercellular adhesion molecule-1 mRNA [31]. Results showed that an LNA/DNA/LNA gapmer with nine consecutive DNA nucleotides in the gap is a dose-dependent and sequence-specific inhibitor of the intercellular adhesion molecule-1 expression in the primary human umbilical vein endothelial cells [31]. In other experiments, LNA/DNA/LNA gapmers showed results as activators of RNase H-mediated RNA degradation and the known iso-sequential 2′-O-methyl gapmers [32].

2.3.2. PNA

Peptide nucleic acid (PNA) was first synthesized by Danish scientists in 1991 [33]. PNA is a misnomer because it is not an acid. Unlike the phosphodiester backbone of DNA, RNA, and LNA, PNA has a peptide backbone usually built of N-(2-amino-ethyl)-glycine repeats. As a result, PNA possesses a unique combination of chemical, physical, and biological properties used in various antisense therapies. PNA can hybridize with RNA or DNA via Watson-Crick and also via Hoogsteen base pairing [34]. It is much more chemically stable and resistant to enzymatic decay than DNA and RNA. Due to the lack of electrostatic repulsion, PNA hybridizes with single-stranded RNAs and DNA molecules much more robustly and faster than the complementary DNA and RNA strands.

Moreover, PNA binds to nucleic acid target molecules both in vitro and in vivo. One PNA antisense nucleic compound, conjugated to the $(RXR)_4XB$ (cell-penetrating peptide), was targeted to *carA*, an essential gene for the MDR human pathogen *Acinetobacter baumannii*. The minimal medium in vitro experiments demonstrated that the PNA inhibited four strains at 1.25 µM concentration. The tested PNA compound did not affect the bacteria in lower concentrations [35].

2.3.3. PMO

Morpholino oligonucleotides (PMOs) are neutrally charged DNA analogs with morpholino rings instead of ribose ones. Their syntheses are inexpensive and combined with characteristics such as solid nuclease resistance, binding affinity, and stability in serum and plasma, making PMOs a preferred object for pharmaceutical research. However, they have a lower melting temperature than DNA, therefore, higher concentrations are needed for successful inhibition. Also, their cellular uptake is inferior, but that can be significantly improved by attaching arginine-rich CPP to the PMO [36]. Other techniques to deliver PMO into the target cells are microinjection and scraping (electroporation or endosomal escape reagents). One designed and tested PMO reduces the neurofilament synthesis and inhibits axon regeneration in lamprey reticulospinal neurons [37]. Another two PMOs—peptide-conjugated PMO (PPMO) and non-conjugated PMO have been tested against Ebola virus infection in vitro and in vivo. The PPMO oligomers with a length of 22 nt targeted the translation start site region of EBOV VP35 positive-sense RNA and showed inhibitor effects in vitro. The in vivo experiments showed that PMO plus is an effective antisense oligonucleotide agent against Ebola infection in monkeys [38].

2.4. ASOs as Drugs

ASO-based technologies have certain advantages when applied to drug development for two main reasons. The mRNA is a universal target for drug development, which is present in every organism. Therefore, the antisense approach can be considered a versatile and universal drug development strategy. Also, we can easily design ASOs, which target predefined mRNA(s) using rational methods based on nucleic acid hybridization. Therefore, we can promptly engineer the ASOs that will down-regulate the expression of the desired gene.

Most medicines developed now are small molecules that specifically bind to a target molecule in the cell. Most of the target molecules for these drugs are proteins and some functional RNAs with complex 3D structures and form binding pockets where small molecules can specifically bind. Unfortunately, finding such small molecules that specifically bind their molecular targets in the cell is a time-consuming and costly process with no guarantee of success. Much more effort will be needed to find a small molecule that specifically binds a protein of interest and inhibits its function, a general and universal approach in drug discovery compared with the design of ASOs.

Half of the approved ASOs as therapeutic agents are splice-switching oligonucleotides (SSOs). They are short, modified synthetic antisense oligonucleotides complementary to pre-mRNA, disturbing the regular splicing repertoire of the transcript, causing a block of the RNA–RNA base-pairing or protein–RNA binding interactions [39]. The splicing of pre-mRNA is required to express most protein-coding genes, regulating gene expression and protein production. Splice-switching oligonucleotides target and alter the splicing in a therapeutic healing effect. In 2016, the U.S. Food and Drug Administration (FDA) approved another antisense drug called Eteplirsen (Exondys 51), a 30 nt neutrally charged PMO. Eteplirsen alters the splicing of the Duchenne muscular dystrophy pre-mRNA by hybridizing to exon 51 of the DMD gene, which leads to the correction of the translational reading frame and the production of shortened but functional dystrophin proteins. Duchenne muscular dystrophy is an X-linked recessive disease that affects one in 3500–5000 males, leading to progressive muscular deterioration that until now was untreatable [40]. Fortunately, with the approval of Eteplirsen, 14% of all DMD patients can be treated to slow down the progression of the disease. However, there has been controversy about the drug's efficiency because of insufficient patients and inconsistent results [41,42]. That is why there are currently four additional trials to confirm its therapeutic effect: NCT01540409, NCT02255552, NCT02286947, and NCT02420379.

Three more nucleic acid-based drugs have been accepted and used to treat Duchenne muscular dystrophy. The first is Vyondys, also known as Dolodirsen injection, approved by the FDA in 2019. Vyondys also treats patients with DMD with a confirmed mutation in the dystrophin gene that can be treated by skipping exon. As a result, dystrophin production in skeletal muscle is increased. Viltepso, also known as Viltolarsen, is an approved therapy developed by NS Pharma, with its parent company Nippon Shinyaku (Kyoto, Japan), treating DMD resulting from mutations amenable to exon skipping. It is administered as an infusion into the bloodstream. Its application is possible at home as well as in the hospital. The FDA approved it in 2020. The third Amondys, known as Casimersen, was approved by FDA in 2021 as the first treatment for patients with DMD with a mutation amenable to skipping exon. That is the third Sarepta-approved RNA exon-skipping therapy for DMD after Exondys and Vyondys.

The FDA accepted one more ASO-based drug in December 2016 called Nusinersen (Spinraza). It is meant to treat spinal muscular atrophy (SMA), an autosomal recessive neurodegenerative disease affecting 1 in 10,000 live births and leading to motor neuron degeneration in the spinal cord and brainstem, concluding with muscle atrophy and general weakness [43,44]. Nusinersen is a second-generation modified ASO (2′-O-2-methoxyethyl phosphorothioate) administered mainly intrathecally into the CSF and modulates the splicing of SMN2 mRNA. This increases levels of the otherwise insufficient full-length SMN protein and helps patients with all three types of SMA. Moreover, it averts the manifestation of spinal muscular atrophy when treated earlier.

3. Synthetic Non-Coding RNAs as Therapeutic Agents

3.1. RNAi

RNAi is found in a broad spectrum of eukaryotic organisms. Small interfering RNAs (siRNAs) are approximately 21–22 bp double-stranded molecules with two nucleotides overhanging at the 3′-end specific sequences and direct mRNA cleavage [45], which leads to inhibition of the translation of the targeted RNA due to its degradation. Therefore, synthetic siRNAs can be used in mammalian cells to tackle disease-causing genes (Figure 3). Synthetic non-coding RNAs can also specifically inhibit a target RNA via its microRNA (miRNA) function. For instance, short hairpin RNA (shRNA) and bifunctional short hairpin RNA (bi-shRNA) can inhibit target wild mRNAs or mutate mRNAs [46].

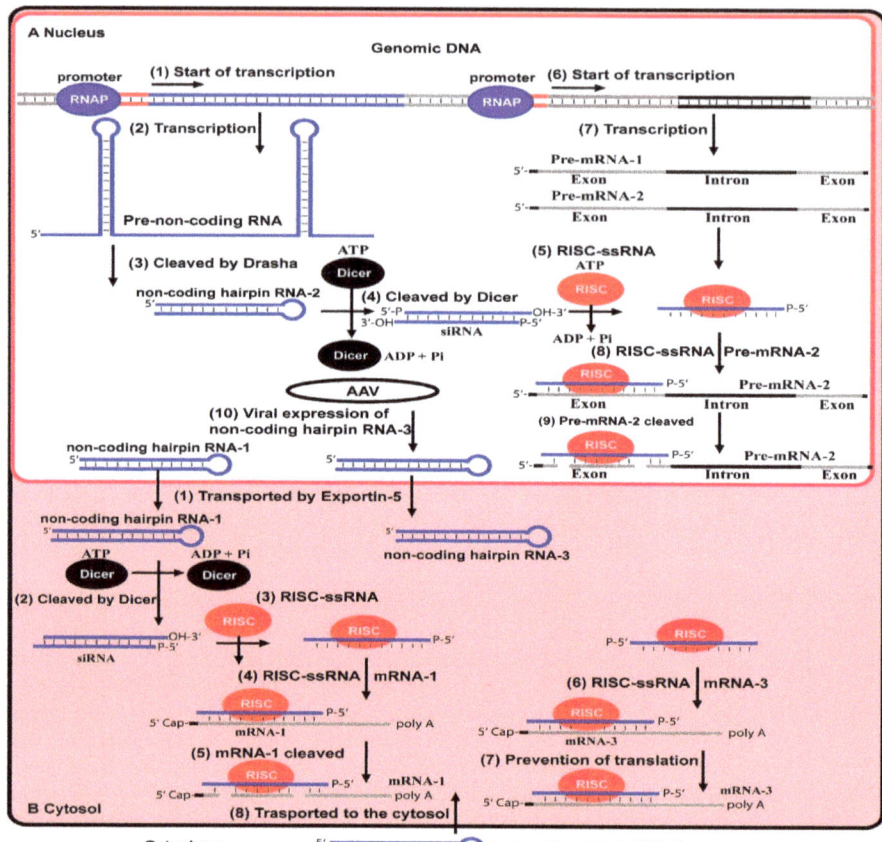

Figure 3. Control of gene expression in eukaryotes via the RNA interference pathway. (**A**) The genomic DNA in the nucleus has promoter sites responsible for pre-mRNA transcription. The binding of RNAP to the promoter sites triggers transcription (1) of DNA in pre-non-coding mRNA containing hairpin structures (2). Through the action of the Dicer enzyme, which is part of the RNA interference complex, the non-coding hairpin RNA-2 and hairpin RNA-1 are formed (3). The siRNA molecules are created by the action of the Dicer enzyme, which cleaves the dsRNAs into short dsRNA fragments—siRNAs (4). Due to the use of ATP by the Dicer enzyme, ADP and Pi are released in the reaction. siRNA is used as a template for recognizing complementary mRNA by RISC. The formation of the RISC-ssRNA complex requires ATP, so ADP and Pi are released (5). The binding of RNAP to the other promoter site (6) triggers the transcription of two pre-mRNAs, pre-mRNA-1 and pre-mRNA-2 (7). Pre-mRNA-2 is complementary to ssRNA from the RISC-ssRNA complex (8). By binding pre-mRNA-2, RISC is activated and induces cleavage. (**B**) The non-coding hairpin-RNA-1 produced from the Dicer enzyme and non-coding hairpin RNA-3 expressed from the viral vector AAV are transported from the nucleus into the cytosol via Exportin-5 (1). In the cytosol, the non-coding hairpin-RNA-1 is cleaved into siRNA molecules by the Dicer enzyme in an ATP-depended reaction (2). The formed RISC-ssRNA complex (3) binds to the complementary sequence mRNA-1 (4). The binding activates RISC and induces cleavage of mRNA-1 (5). RISC-ssRNA complex can also bind to non-coding mRNA-3 (6), which leads to the prevention of translation (7). RNA interference can be affected by incorporating a non-coding mRNA-4 from the cytoplasm inside the cytosol (8).

RNAi is also used to develop novel approaches for viral infections, cancer, and autoimmune diseases [47]. Approximately 20 clinical trials have been initiated using micro(mi)RNA and siRNA, and 19 ongoing trials are with siRNA only [48,49]. The first RNAi-based drug accepted and approved by the FDA (the U.S. Food and Drug Administration) is Patisiran (ONPATTRO™) [48,50–52]. Patisiran, a siRNA drug administered by IV infusion to treat hereditary TTR amyloidosis (hATTR), was accepted by the US FDA. hATTR is a medication for treating polyneuropathy caused by the rare lethal disease hereditary transthyretin-mediated amyloidosis. It is an effective gene-silencing drug. In the same month, another drug treating hTTR applied for NDA called Inotersen (ASO-based) by Ionis Pharmaceuticals (Carlsbad, CA, USA). As a result, the production of an abnormal form of transthyretin is inhibited (a genetic autosomal dominant disease caused by a mutation in the TTR gene, rapidly progressive, and affecting approximately 50,000 people worldwide). In November 2017, Alnylam Pharmaceuticals announced positive results from the APPOLO Phase 3 study and submitted an enrollment to the FDA for new drug discovery. In addition to their precise mechanism of action, siRNAs have higher specificity, higher potency, and greater reduced toxicity than protein-based drugs or other small molecules, making them apposite for cancer researchers [53,54].

Moreover, multiple genes (oncogenes, mutated tumor suppressors) can be targeted. More modifications are being constantly made to improve their biological safety, serum stability, off-target effects, and appropriate in vivo delivery [55]. For example, adding a 2'-modification of the ribose ring increases the endonuclease resistance of the siRNA.

Silenseed's drug, siG12D-LODER, targets pancreatic cancer and, combined with chemotherapy, shows improvement in Phase I clinical trials [56]. In 2017, the company announced that they would continue with Phase II trials with clinical trials gov. identifier: NCT01676259. Another up-and-coming drug is RXI-109 by RXi Pharmaceuticals. It is a self-delivering siRNA that decreases the expression of connective tissue growth factor (CTGF) and improves the visual appearance of fibrosis and post-surgical scars. In August 2018, positive results were announced by Rxi Pharmaceuticals in Phase 1/2 clinical trial with RXI-109 for retinal scarring.

3.2. Guide RNA

CRISPR (clustered, regularly interspaced short palindromic repeats) is the name attributed to a family of DNA segments containing short repeated sequences from viruses, bacteriophages, or plasmids that have infected the bacterium in the past. CRISPRs are present in the locus CRISPR and other gene elements in bacteria and archaea. The bacterium uses short repeats to recognize and destroy the genomes of viruses similar to those that originated CRISPRs, thus constituting a form of acquired immunity system of prokaryotes [57]. CRISPRs are one of the essential elements of the CRISPR/Cas system, which is also involved in the acquired immunity of prokaryotes. The specificity of action of the CRISPR/Cas9 system is performed by a guide (g) RNA, which has specific primary and secondary structures.

A simplified version of this system has been created to provide a robust and precise genetic editing tool, which is much easier to use and, at the same time, cheaper than previous technologies. The new CRISPR-based strategies expand the possibilities, resulting in better diagnostics and environmental monitoring [58]. Thanks to the CRISPR/Cas9 system, it has been possible to modify the genes of multiple organisms permanently.

Recently, a technique was used to inhibit the urothelial cancer-associated 1 (UCA1) long non-protein-coding RNA by CRISPR/Cas9 to prove that the target has a role in the progression of bladder cancer [59]. UCA1 regulates embryonic development and bladder cancer invasion and advances as a regulator of the expression of different genes involved in tumorigenesis and embryonic development [60]. Several studies show that UCA1 is pivotal in anti-cancer drug resistance [61]. Its overexpression correlates with chemotherapeutic resistance (cisplatin, gemcitabine, EGFR-TKIs, imatinib, tamoxifen, and 5-FU). In that case, UCA1's knockdown results in a drug sensitivity restoration and is expected to be a suitable diagnostic marker [61]. UCA1's knockdown was revealed to restrain cell proliferation, migration, and invasion in large B-cell lymphoma by suppressing miR-331-3p expression [62]. It was also suggested as a possible medicinal target and biomarker for large B-cell lymphoma.

4. Functional Synthetic Nucleic Acids as Tools for Drug Discovery

Synthetic Hammerhead Ribozymes as Therapeutics

Ribozymes are RNA enzymes that catalyze a chemical reaction like any other protein enzyme. They are highly applicable to manipulating various biological systems [63]. Since the identification of the first ribozyme in 1980 by Thomas R. Chech, applications of new synthetic ribozymes have been of great interest. The hammerhead ribozyme (HHRz) is one of the most frequently used types of catalytic RNA in drug discovery and development (Figure 4). Allosteric HHRz can be engineered as a biosensor by computational [64] and in vitro selection methods [65]. HHRz is a small ribozyme well-known for its capability of catalyzing the site-specific cleavage of a phosphodiester bond by hydrolyzes. HHRz consists of approximately 30 nucleotides that form 3 base-paired stems and a core of non-complementary nucleotides responsible for catalysis. The great interest in research in hammerhead ribozymes is due to their ability to block gene expression; therefore, they take place in developing new therapeutic agents [66].

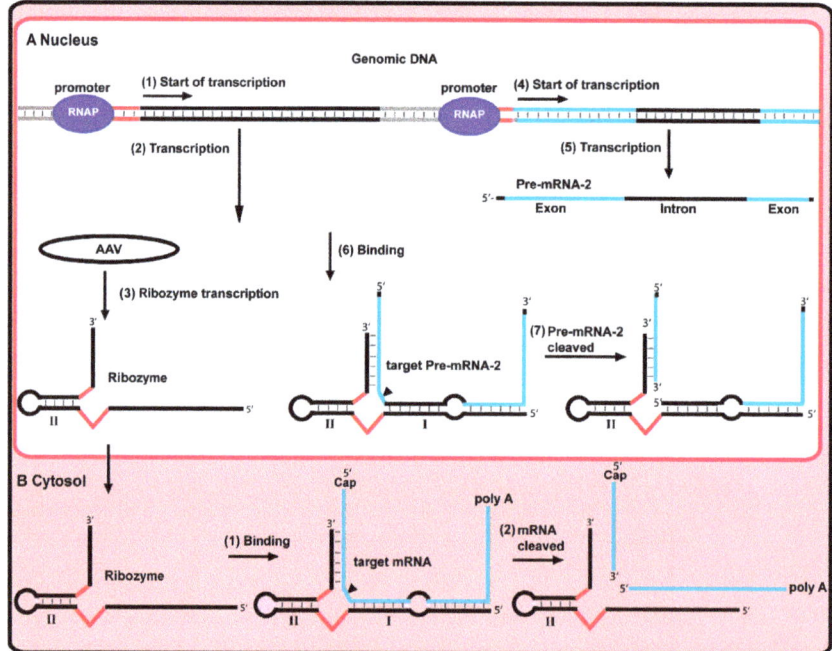

Figure 4. Control of gene expression by synthetic ribozymes. (**A**) Inside the nucleus, genomic DNA has promoter sites. The binding of RNAP to the first promoter site (1) triggers ribozyme transcription (2). A viral vector AAV in the nucleus (3) can also express the ribozyme. The binding of RNAP to the other promoter site triggers (4) the transcription of pre-mRNA-2 (5). The synthesized pre-mRNA-2 complement the ribozyme sequence and binds it (6). When bound to the pre-mRNA-2, the ribozyme is activated and cleaved at the cleavage site (black arrow). Along with that, the pre-mRNA-2 is also cleaved (7). (**B**) The ribozyme can also bind to the target mRNA inside the cytosol via complementary sequences (1). The ribozyme is activated and cleaves at the cleavage site (black arrow). Along with that, the mRNA is also cleaved (2), which leads to no translation of the mRNA.

Hammerhead ribozymes cleave the HIV-1 sequences in a cell-free environment in research. This has led to the development of human cells expressing the hammerhead ribozyme that, once treated with HIV-1, decreases the levels of HIV-1 gag RNA, which has been observed [67].

In gene therapy research, a HHRz was introduced to gastric carcinoma cells overexpressing a carrier protein responsible for multidrug resistance (MDR) in breast cancer cells (BPCR). The hammerhead ribozyme in question is an anti-BPCR agent that targets the BPCR-mRNA. By this method, the expression of the BPCR decreased dramatically (Figure 4) [68].

Investigations in trans-activating ribozymes showed that HHRz can be developed to attack the desired RNA and consequently block its gene expression. This represents a powerful tool in gene therapy against pathogens or genetic diseases [69]. There are results for the pseudoknot-type hammerhead ribozyme PK-HHRz, activated by a pseudoknot interaction between loops I and II, with higher cleavage activity than the wild-type sequence [70]. The increased activity of the pseudoknot-type hammerhead ribozyme PK-HHRz is achieved by elongating loop II. PK-HHRz could be used as a fundament for designing new variants of gene-regulating drugs. Recently, M1 ribozymes have been successfully used to target various RNA viruses in vitro and in vivo. This ribozyme is based on the RNA part of the RNase P of *E. coli* [71].

5. Factors Affecting Therapeutic Potency

Several essential factors generally affect the therapeutic potency of functional nucleic acids and ASOs, such as delivery in vivo, nuclease resistance, renal filtration, and toxicology.

5.1. Delivery

Although in the last 20 years, a lot of progress has been made in ASOs, one of the biggest challenges is still the successful delivery of the drug to its target in vivo [72]. The delivery of ASO in the human body depends on its generation. ASOs have different modifications and varying physical and chemical properties. Thus, they must be considered when choosing the methods for ASO delivery. Highly charged ASOs (PS-ASO) cannot passively diffuse across the lipid bilayer [23]. Examples of specific uptake of various charged and uncharged ASOs by different cultured cells and mouse models, known as gymnotic uptake, are exceptions to the rule. There are also results showing the uptake of uncomplexed ASOs, which occur in vivo in lung tissues [73].

There are different ways of administering ASOs, such as systematic applications that include subcutaneous, intradermal, intravenous, intrathecal, and topical applications. ASOs can be directly administered to cerebrospinal fluid (CSF) by intracerebroventricular or intrathecal infusion and via intranasal administration for delivery to brain cells. Once ASOs are in the organism, there are two main barriers to delivering them to their target. The first is the tissue barrier that the therapeutic ASO has to reach. Whether ASOs can successfully pass the vascular endothelial barrier, reticuloendothelial system (RES), blood-brain barrier, or renal excretion depends significantly on their size. Molecules transported between the blood and the parenchymal space are of limited size, up to 70 nm. Even if individual ASOs fit this criterion, they can still be removed by phagocytes or ultrafiltered by the kidneys. Different methods exist to avoid it, such as applying modified surfaces with polyethylene glycol or PS-ASOs that bind to specific plasma proteins [74]. The other main barrier is the permeation into the cells (cellular uptake), intracellular transport, and endosome escape. Generally, ASOs are taken into the cells by endocytosis, caveolar potocytosis, or pinocytosis.

There is an additional difference in the delivery of the ASO to its target cell depending on whether it is only the ASO or ASO attached to a carrier to facilitate the transportation. These carriers can be liposomes, lipids, nanoparticles, polymers, cell-penetrating peptides (CPPs), antibody conjugates, etc.

Liposomes and charged lipids are often used for ASO and siRNA delivery. Liposomes are spherical vesicles with at least one phospholipid bilayer [75]. On their inside, they are aqueous and can contain polar therapeutic molecules, including first and second-generation ASOs. On the other hand, cationic lipids are effective at transportation because they form strong complexes with ASOs due to their opposite charges. Liposomes are taken into the cells by membrane fusion, while the cationic lipids are via endocytosis.

CPPs have shown promising results as carriers of therapeutic molecules for different diseases. They are oligopeptides (6–30 residues) and can move through the cell membrane at low concentrations in vitro and in vivo [76]. They can be covalent or noncovalent to their cargo, but the covalent bond provides more stable conjugates [77]. It can be considered that negatively charged ASOs coupled with conjugated cationic CPPs could interact and lose their antisense or delivery properties. However, this does not affect neutrally charged ASOs such as LNA, PMO, and chimeric first and second-generation ASOs. Another occurrence is that the bond position matters, too, as CPP coupled at the 5′-end of the PMO is more active than at the 3′-end. CPP-PMO is an example of successful ASO transportation and general therapeutic effects, which passes the blood-brain barrier (BBB) and corrects aberrant splicing in ataxia-telangiectasia [78].

Antibodies have proven pharmaceutical significance as therapeutic agents. Specifically, monoclonal antibodies (mAbs) come from a single clone of cells designed to target specific antigens available in particular cells or tissues [79]. They can be used for conjugation with ASOs, and once administered, they are recognized by specific receptors, which will help them with cellular uptake by endocytosis. For instance, radioactively labeled anti-luciferase PNA conjuring to OX26 mAb successfully passes the blood-brain barrier and shows the luciferase-expressing brain tumors in rats in vivo [80].

N-acetylgalactosamine (GalNAc) is an amide derivative of the monosaccharide galactose. It involves intercellular communication and can be a targeting ligand of specific ASOs and siRNA. It binds to the asialoglycoprotein receptors on hepatocytes and ensures the introduction of the drug into the liver. Most of the recently approved siRNAs are conjugated with GalNAc. For example, GalNAC-siRNA conjugates have been used for delivery to the liver and eliminate the siRNA delivery problem for liver hepatocytes [81].

As many tissues can be reached only by systemic administration in vivo, the small RNAi therapeutic molecules must be conjugated with bigger carriers for filtration resistance and successful delivery to their target [82]. Such carriers are often non-viral vectors, such as nanotechnology-based ones. Among the frequently used are lipid-based—liposomes and lipoplexes. A cholesterol conjugate is another transporter that can carry inside the designed RNAi. As cholesterol is a component of the cell membranes, the conjugate passes quickly through the membrane and releases the RNAi inside the cell [83].

5.2. Stability

The drug's half-life depends directly on its volume of distribution or on how widely it is distributed in the body. As much as the drug is widespread in the patient's body, its half-life is longer. In addition, the half-life of this same drug is inversely dependent on its release from the body, which means the half-life is shorter when the drug release rate from the body is higher.

One of the most significant limitations in achieving the required effective dose of antisense oligonucleotide without reaching toxic therapy levels is that ASOs have a short cell half-life. That means the amount of drug needed to reach the effective dose will be achieved with a daily intake of common medications with a supporting role. Because the drug will be taken on a schedule, the half-life in the body plays a role to the extent that it determines the frequency of taking medicine. If we talk about drugs taken sporadically and at longer intervals than their half-life, the drug will not stay in the body long enough, and its short half-life will negatively affect its effectiveness.

DNA and RNA have phosphodiester backbones, which are susceptible to nuclease degradation. This limits the application of antisense oligonucleotides as therapeutic agents if they are not modified. The chemical modification of the ASO could enhance metabolic stability. The phosphorothioate modification (PS modification) is the most widely used modification, which replaces a single oxygen atom from the backbone with a sulfur atom. This chance increases the stability of the antisense oligonucleotides and enhances their binding affinity to their target [84]. Unmodified ASOs have a short half-life in vivo—around one hour in human serum. First-generation ASOs have half-lives of 9–10 h in human serum and 19 h in the cerebrospinal fluid of rats due to their PS modification and ability to attach to plasma proteins (thus, be safe from filtration). The LNA antisense oligonucleotide lifespan depends on the design of the chemical structure and could be up to 5–8 days. Laboratory tests showed that unmodified oligodeoxynucleotides had a half-life of 1.5 h. Another four LNA have been tested, increasing human serum lifespan ~10-fold to ~15 h. The main conclusion from the monitored results is that the stability of chimeric LNA/DNA oligonucleotides is much higher compared with 2'-O-methyl and phosphorothioate gapmers with half-lives of 12 and 10 h, respectively [32]. The half-life of the PMO-based Eteplirsen is 2 to 6 h in plasma.

Regarding RNA interference, unmodified siRNA has a shorter half-live in serum than the modified [83]. For example, it is proven that cholesterol conjugates added to siRNA increase their half-life in human serum and protect it from renal clearance. There are statistical analyses of PS-ASO experiments with enhanced antisense efficiency, which found motifs like: "CCAC", "TCCC", "ACTC", "GCCA", and "CTCT". When the PS-ASO shows diminished antisense efficiency, found in motifs like "GGGG", "ACTG", "AAA", and "TAA" [85].

5.3. Toxicity of ASOs

In contrast to many synthetic proteins, ASOs rarely induce or induce an immune response in humans, which is a significant advantage for their clinical usage. ASOs tend to produce transient toxicities in rodents, primates, and humans. Sometimes, however, the toxicities can have mild to moderate effects. The toxicities of ASOs can be sequence-independent or sequence-dependent. The sequence-independent toxicity is caused by backbone chemical modifications that may lead to unwanted non-specific protein binding. For instance, PS-ASOs may form disulfide bonds with peptides. A vigorous bioinformatics search can avoid the sequence-independent toxicities that can reduce off-target hybridization to a minimum during the designer stage of ASOs. The most common types of acute toxicity are high serum transaminase levels, partial thromboplastin prolongation, and transient activation of complement cascades. ASO toxicity can lead mainly to proinflammation, nephrotoxicity, hepatotoxicity unrelated to lysosomal accumulation, and thrombocytopenia [86]. There is a clear dependency between the accuracy and the thermodynamic stability of ASO/mRNA hybridization and ASO's cytotoxicity published by us this year in Antibiotics [65]. These findings can be used by the design of the ASOs to reduce their non-specific cytotoxicity.

For example, the CpG-motif ASOs trigger a proinflammatory response, causing activation of Toll-like receptor 9, also known as TLR9. CpG motif ASO's properties have been tested for therapeutics for cancer therapies. However, antisense oligonucleotides have a specific design and minimize the proinflammatory responses by avoiding CpG motifs. They can elicit a proinflammatory reaction if their dose level is high in the body and weaker than the CpG-motifs [87].

The human immune system possesses a specific innate immune pathway that senses cytosolic DNA [88]. It is known as the STING pathway and is responsible for activating downstream signaling events such as interferon regulatory factor 3 (IRF3) activation and human interferon-beta protein (IFN-β) gene expression [88]. IFR3 is an analog of the interferon regulatory factors 1 and 2, with functional domains like a nuclear export signal, a DNA-binding domain, a C-terminal IRF association domain, and regulatory phosphorylation sites. It is part of the interferon transcription factors family. In the cytoplasm, it is inactive. After phosphorylation with serine or threonine, it forms a complex, which translocates to the nucleus. It manifests its transcriptional activity role affecting the interferons alpha and beta genes [89]. The fibroblasts' antiviral activity mainly involves the innate immune response by producing IFN-β proteins. Multiple post-translational modifications regulate different steps of the STING pathway. The STING pathway detects sequence-nonspecific cytosolic DNA species with more than ~70 bp in human cells [90]. It also senses different RNAs, cyclic-di-GMP, and cyclic-di-AMP generated by numerous intracellular bacteria, such as *Listeria monocytogenes*, essential in microbial pathogenesis mechanisms of host defense causes of inflammatory disease and cancer.

6. Riboswitches as a Target for Antibacterial Drug Discovery

Riboswitches are strongly conservative gene control elements, primarily found in the 5′-UTR region of mRNA, where they control the gene expression of some vitamin precursors like riboflavin, thiamin, and cobalamin, amino acids like methionine and lysine, the synthesis of some nucleotides like adenine, and guanine, and other essential metabolites by two main regulatory mechanisms such as termination of transcription, and prevention of translation [91,92]. Some riboswitches regulate gene expression by trans-acting regulatory mechanisms and self-cleavage. As biosensors, they sense the presence of small molecules and bind to specific essential ligands that trigger conformational changes or have an essential role in biofilm formation [93]. The riboswitches are found in many bacteria, archaea, plants, and fungi but are still not in the human genome. There are criteria to classify the suitability of each riboswitch class for targeting antibacterial drugs [10,94]. The first one is the riboswitch found in human bacterial pathogen bacteria. The second is the riboswitch to control the biochemical pathway(s) to synthesize essential metabolites in the bacterium, which does not have an alternative biosynthetic pathway without riboswitch control.

The third criterion is the synthesis of transporter protein for the essential metabolite to be under riboswitch control. It must fulfill all requirements to be classified as a promising riboswitch class for an antibacterial target. The design of therapeutic molecules, such as ASOs, which can bind in vivo to the aptamer domain, might be the answer to successfully creating entirely new classes of antibiotics [64]. Recent studies prove the inhibition effect of chimeric ASOs on the bacterial growth of *S. aureus* targeting SAM-I riboswitch [95]. The combined application of the first two ASOs, which target the glucosamine-6-phosphate (*glmS*) riboswitch and the *nagA* mRNA, block the synthesis of glucosamine-6-phosphate entirely and inhibits the bacterial growth of *S. aureus* [3]. Other engineered ASOs have been tested as antibacterial agents that target the flavine mononucleotide (FMN) riboswitch and inhibit the growth of *E. coli*, *L. monocytogenes*, and *S. aureus* [96]. Moreover, we have successfully targeted thiamine pyrophosphate (TPP) riboswitch in *S. aureus* for antibacterial drug development [97]. The compounds with proven antibiotic effects include Roseoflavin (RoF) and 8-dimethyl-8-amino-riboflavin (AF), where the latter has lower toxicity [98].

7. Prospective of Applying Antisense Nucleic Acid-Based Strategies for Drug Development

Antisense nucleic acid-based therapies can offer suitable treatment for genetic disorders or infectious diseases. The antisense therapies must be adaptable, precisely created, and selectively target the specific gene(s). ASOs are stable single-stranded molecules that directly bind to the targeted mRNA by penetrating different tissues and cells when modified and attached to a cell-penetrating protein. When an RNA(s) sequence is known to be causative of a specific disease, it is possible to prevent the function of this RNA(s) by introducing different types of antisense nucleic acids in the cell. Many different types of nucleic acids, such as PS-DNA, LNA, PNA, and other modified DNA oligomers, can be employed in various antisense therapeutic strategies. These methods are generally based on Watson-Crick's complementary base-pairing between the ASOs and the targeted mRNA. We can promptly design and synthesize such antisense oligonucleotides. Furthermore, well-established methods exist for antisense oligonucleotide delivery in various cell types.

Moreover, we use various bioinformatics databases to find the most suitable (specific) part of the targeted mRNA. Such databases include KEGG for biochemical pathways, GeneBank for DNA and RNA sequences, Rfam, and Rswitch [99]. This will allow us to achieve a high selective antisense oligonucleotide-based inhibition, which can avoid non-specifically targeting other RNAs and, therefore, may reduce many adverse effects of our particular ASOs. Thus, we apply rational approaches to select our RNA targets [10].

In addition, we have established computational algorithms [11] and software [100] for the design of allosteric ribozymes and postulated rational rules for the design of ASOs that have all been proven to be over 90% successful [64]. They are all based on computing secondary RNA structures and DNA/RNA hybridization using the partition function for RNA folding in conjunction with thermodynamic parameters.

Since synthesizing the first ASOs in the 1960s, a few drugs based on antisense technology have been approved for patient treatment. The first approved drug is Fomivirsen (Vitravene), a 21 nt-long PS-modified oligonucleotide. Its role was local cytomegalovirus (CMV) retinitis treatment in patients with acquired immunodeficiency syndrome (AIDS) by targeting CMV mRNA and inhibiting essential viral proteins [101]. However, in 2002, it was withdrawn from the European Union market for commercial reasons [102].

The second drug is mipomersen (Kynamro), a second-generation 20 nt-long chimeric ASO approved in 2013 and accu{ulated in the liver (Table 1) [103,104]. It inhibits apolipoprotein B-100 and increases the survival of patients with a rare genetic disease called homozygous familial hypercholesterolemia (HoFH). HoFH is an autosomal dominant disease that leads to increased low-density lipoprotein (LDL) and higher risks for atherosclerosis and cardiovascular disease in approximately 1/1,000,000 people in Western Europe [105]. While it has been approved only for the homozygous form of the disease, it is also being tested for its therapeutic role in the heterozygous form of HoFH.

A new antisense drug already applied to a rolling submission to the FDA is alicaforsen to treat pouchitis. It is a 20-base oligonucleotide that targets the intracellular adhesion molecule-1 (ICAM-1) mRNA. It shows promising results in patients with pouchitis and other inflammatory diseases, such as left-sided ulcerative colitis or proctitis.

Many antisense oligonucleotides are being designed and tested for their therapeutic effects in cancer, neurodegenerative diseases, and cardiovascular or metabolic diseases. As of this moment, one of the biggest pharmaceutical companies, Ionis (previously known as ISIS), has over a thousand patents on RNAi and antisense oligonucleotides and 47 ASO drugs (according to the Ionis Pharmaceutical pipeline website) under different phases of clinical trials, including Volanesorsen, Inotersen (applied for NDA in November 2017) and IONIS-HTTRx. The ASOs are in the cardio-renal, metabolic, neurological, infectious diseases, rare cancer, ophthalmology, pulmonary and allergy, hematology, and other therapeutic areas. Currently, there are 16 FDA-approved drugs based on oligonucleotides. Ten are based on ASOs, with two withdrawn (Table 1), 5 are based on siRNAs, and 1 is based on an aptamer and is withdrawn. ASO-based drugs have the highest number among all oligonucleotide-based FDA-approved drugs. The main reason for that is the single-stranded nature of ASO in contrast to siRNA and the lack of secondary and tertiary structures in contrast to the aptamers.

Regarding antibacterial resistance and overgrowing global problems, antisense oligonucleotides inhibit the expression of crucial genes in pathogenic bacteria, leading to their death [106]. Examples of such ASOs are third-generation PNA and PMO, which, combined with CPP, have a much increased cellular effect in vitro and in vivo [8,107]. Therefore, there are reasonable expectations that some ongoing preclinical experiments and clinical trials will successfully produce approved medicines.

In recent years, artificial intelligence (AI) has had an increasing number of applications in drug discovery. Various techniques, such as reasoning, solution search, and machine learning (ML), are parts of AI, and ML applies algorithms that recognize patterns in a database. An essential area of ML is deep learning (DL) based on artificial neural networks (ANNs) [108]. AI algorithms such as solution search and ML can establish promising RNA targets in different diseases using ASOs or ribozymes. ML is applied for drug design and target discovery [109].

Table 1. ASO-based drugs approved by the FDA. There are 10 ASO-based drugs approved, of which the first 2 are withdrawn.

No.	Names	Target	Year of Approval	Administration	Chemical Modification	Company
1	Fomivirsen (Vitravene®)	Cytomegalovirus—the gene for CMV immediate-early 2 protein	1998 Withdrawn	Intravitreal	PS	Ionis (Carlsbad, CA, USA)
2	Mipomersen (Kynamro®)	Hypercholesterolemia (FH)—the gene APOB encoding apolipoprotein B	2016 Withdrawn	Subcutaneous	2'-O-MOE, PS	Genzyme (Cambridge, MA, USA)
3	Eteplirsen (Exondys 51®)	Duchenne muscular dystrophy (DMD)—Rescue the expression of dystrophin through exon-51	2016	Intravenous	PMO	Sarepta (Cambridge, MA, USA)
4	Nusinersen	exon-7 inclusion of the mRNA of SMN2 gene	2016	Intrathecal	2'-O-MOE, PS, 5-methyl cytosine	Biogen (Cambridge, MA, USA)
5	Inotersen (Tegsedi®)	Hereditary transthyretin (TTR) amyloidosis	2018	Subcutaneous	2'-O-MOE, PS	Ionis (Carlsbad, CA, USA)
6	Milasen	DMD—dystrophin through exon-45	2018	Intrathecal	2'-O-MOE, PS, 5-methyl cytosine	Boston Children's Hospital (Cambridge, MA, USA)
7	Golodirsen (Vyondys 53®)	DMD—rescue the expression of dystrophin through exon-53 of DMD gene	2019	Intravenous	PMO	Sarepta (Cambridge, MA, USA)
8	Waylira (Volanesorsen)	Apolipoprotein C3	2019	Intravenous	2'-O-MOE	Akcea Therapeutics (Cambridge, MA, USA)
9	Viltolarsen (Viltepso)	Exon 53 of DMD	2020	Intravenous	PMO	NS Pharma (Kyoto, Japan)
10	Casimersen (Amondys 45)	Exon 53 of DMD	2021	Intravenous	PMO	Sarepta (Cambridge, MA, USA)

Moreover, such AI algorithms can be employed for side effects and toxicity prediction of ASOs, which are significant problems in light of the broad applications of ASOs as therapeutic agents. In addition, HTS and HCS arrays can be used to test side effects and the general and specific toxicity of many ASOs [110]. Such arrays are also applicable for fully automated evaluation of the efficiency of various methods for ASO delivery, general toxicity, and specific RNA inhibition in various cells.

Several issues are using ASOs to develop new drugs, including the half-life of ASOs in vivo, toxicity, accuracy, and delivery methods that can be tackled rationally. For instance, the half-life of ASOs in vivo can be increased by increasing their molecular weight by reducing the renal filtration rate of ASOs. The main advantage of ASO technology is that all these issues can be tackled rationally and systemically because the primary mechanism of action of ASOs is based on DNA/RNA hybridization with Watson–Krick hydrogen bonding that is easy to predict and engineer. The ASOs can quickly be delivered in the cell if coupled with CPP [3,97].

The AI and genome-wide analyses can be used to find and avoid the mis-hybridization of ASOs to unintended RNAs. To address this problem, thermodynamic and kinetic parameters can be computed [11] for the gap between the perfectly matching ASO and its RNA target and the unintended RNA(s). In addition, the non-specific binding of some thiol-modified ASOs from the first generation to proteins can be limited by reducing the number of thiol-modified nucleotides or applying second or third generations of ASOs.

Kidney filtration removes the ASOs from the bloodstream within several hours, which worsens their pharmacokinetic properties to increase the molecular weight of the ASOs and decrease the rate of their kidney filtration; glycoproteins can be attached to them. There are many different glycoprotein types; some aggregate with other proteins, causing problems. Therefore, the glycoproteins used for attachment to ASOs must be chosen wisely, considering the possibility of binding to other proteins in the cell. It is also possible to use proteins that target a specific cell type. Apart from that, there are three other theoretical possibilities for the cell to develop resistance against the ASO that are very difficult to make because more than one mutation in many genes is needed for the cell to degrade the ASO quickly to export it outside the cell, etc.

To achieve significant inhibition, the type of ASO must be carefully chosen following the targeted RNA expression level. For instance, if the targeted RNA has a relatively low expression level, a single-turnover acting ASOs of the second or third generation can be employed. On the contrary, if the targeted RNA has a relatively high expression level, multi-turnover acting ASOs via RNase H of first or chimeric of first and second-generation can be applied. Moreover, such ASOs can also work via RNAse P if three nucleotides CCA at the 3'-terminus of ASOs do not hybridize with the targeted RNA. In addition, the ASOs must not self-hybridize and form stable secondary structures to achieve high inhibition efficiency because that will prevent them from hybridizing with the targeted RNA.

The targeted site of the RNA has to be single-stranded to be fully accessible for hybridization with the ASO. This can be assessed with programs for the computation of RNA secondary structures to reduce the possibility of mutations in the targeted RNA site that are non-complementary to the ASO, thus the targeted RNA sequence must be highly conserved. However, mutations in the targeted RNA can arise, rendering the ASO cab inefficient. When this happens, the targeted RNA can be sequenced, and the ASO sequence can be altered to complement its targeted RNA site.

Administration and delivery methods are essential in applying ASOs in vivo [111]. ASOs can be used locally via topical administration or intramuscular or intravenous injections. ASOs can enter the cell via attached cell-penetrating oligopeptides (CPPs) and various nanoparticles. Some of the carriers can have specificity to particular cells. For instance, CPPs enter only bacterial cells, reducing the side effects of antibacterial ASOs on human cells. There are 5 siRNA-based drugs and only 1 aptamer-based drug, which is withdrawn (Table 2).

Table 2. siRNA and aptamer-based drugs approved by the FDA. There are 5 siRNA-based approved drugs and only 1 aptamer-based drug, which is withdrawn.

Type	Drug	FDA Approval	Company	Disease
siRNA	Patisiran	2018	Ionis (Carlsbad, CA, USA)	Hereditary transthyretin-mediated amyloidosis
	Givosiran	2019	Alnylam (Carlsbad, CA, USA)	Acute hepatic porphyria
	Lumasiran	2020	Alnylam (Carlsbad, CA, USA)	Primary hyperoxaluria type 1
	Inclisiran	2021	Novartis (Basel. Switzerland)	Primary hypercholesterolemia
	Vutrisiran	2022	Alnylam (Carlsbad, CA, USA)	Hereditary transthyretin-mediated amyloidosis
Aptamer	Pegaptanib	2004 (withdrawn)	Pfizer/Eyetech (New York City, NY, USA)	Neovascular (wet) age-related macular degeneration

8. Conclusions

Functional and antisense nucleic acids are essential molecules for drug discovery and development. They can be used as drug targets and discovery and development tools. The results from the Human Genome Project showed that only ~2% of the human genome encodes for proteins; the rest are noncoding RNAs. Many efficient methods exist for delivering nucleic acid oligomers in vitro and in vivo. Modern nucleic acid chemistry lets us synthesize various oligomers, inducing modified DNAs and RNAs, LNAs, and PNAs [112]. These four oligonucleotides possess different thermodynamic stabilities when hybridizing to target RNA. They have other methods for administration, half-life time in the cell, and pharmacokinetic properties. Therefore, antisense nucleic acid technologies offer flexible tools that can successfully adapt to a broad range of clinical trials. These nucleic acids can be used as ASOs based on Watson-Crick's complementary base pairing to target any mRNAs in the cell.

Since mRNAs are present in all life forms, antisense technologies can be regarded as versatile tools for drug development. The full potential of these technologies will be reached in the next several years since there are over 20 antisense drug candidates in various phases of clinical trials. These clinical trials tackle various disorders and include antiviral and anti-cancer treatments. Several ASO drugs, such as Mipomersen, Eteplirsen, Vyondys, Viltepso, and Amondys, are in use, and their number is expected to grow. Functional nucleic acids such as riboswitches and ribozymes serve as molecular targets and tools for drug development. At least 28 riboswitches regulate the gene expression of many critical biochemical pathways in 59 human bacterial pathogens [1,113]. Rational designer methods can be employed for all functional and antisense nucleic acids for drug development with a 100% success rate [64] that can benefit the pharmaceutical industry.

Author Contributions: Conceptualization, R.P.; methodology, M.T.; validation, N.P.; writing—original draft preparation, N.P.; writing—review and editing, R.P.; visualization, V.D. and A.V.G.; supervision, R.P.; project administration, R.P.; funding acquisition, R.P. and M.T. All authors have read and agreed to the published version of the manuscript.

Funding: This work was financially supported by the Bulgarian National Science Fund under Grants No. KP-06-H63/1/13.12.2022 and KP-06-M63/6/15.12.2022.

Conflicts of Interest: The authors declare no conflicts of interest.

References

1. Pavlova, N.; Kaloudas, D.; Penchovsky, R. Riboswitch distribution, structure, and function in bacteria. *Gene* **2019**, *708*, 38–48. [CrossRef]
2. Penchovsky, R.; Miloshev, G.Y.; Pavlova, N.; Popova, K.B.; Valsamatzi-Panagiotou, A.; Otcheva, L.A.; Traykovska, M. Chapter 8—Small RNA-based systems for sensing and therapeutic applications. In *New Frontiers and Applications of Synthetic Biology*; Singh, V., Ed.; Academic Press: Cambridge, MA, USA, 2022; pp. 103–121.
3. Traykovska, M.; Popova, K.B.; Penchovsky, R. Targeting glmS Ribozyme with Chimeric Antisense Oligonucleotides for Antibacterial Drug Development. *ACS Synth. Biol.* **2021**, *10*, 3167–3176. [CrossRef] [PubMed]
4. Penchovsky, R.; Kostova, G.T. Computational selection and experimental validation of allosteric ribozymes that sense a specific sequence of human telomerase reverse transcriptase mRNAs as universal anticancer therapy agents. *Nucleic Acid. Ther.* **2013**, *23*, 408–417. [CrossRef] [PubMed]
5. Penchovsky, R. Engineering integrated digital circuits with allosteric ribozymes for scaling up molecular computation and diagnostics. *ACS Synth. Biol.* **2012**, *1*, 471–482. [CrossRef] [PubMed]
6. Penchovsky, R.; Traykovska, M. Synthetic Approaches to Biology: Engineering Gene Control Circuits, Synthesizing, and Editing Genomes. In *Emerging Research on Bioinspired Materials Engineering*; Bououdina, M., Ed.; IGI Global: Hershey, PA, USA, 2016; pp. 323–351.
7. Blount, K.; Puskarz, I.; Penchovsky, R.; Breaker, R. Development and application of a high-throughput assay for glmS riboswitch activators. *RNA Biol.* **2006**, *3*, 77–81. [CrossRef] [PubMed]
8. Penchovsky, R.; Traykovska, M. Designing drugs that overcome antibacterial resistance: Where do we stand and what should we do? *Expert Opin. Drug Discov.* **2015**, *10*, 631–650. [CrossRef] [PubMed]
9. Penchovsky, R.; Stoilova, C.C. Riboswitch-based antibacterial drug discovery using high-throughput screening methods. *Expert Opin. Drug Discov.* **2013**, *8*, 65–82. [CrossRef] [PubMed]
10. Pavlova, N.; Penchovsky, R. Genome-wide bioinformatics analysis of FMN, SAM-I, glmS, TPP, lysine, purine, cobalamin, and SAH riboswitches for their applications as allosteric antibacterial drug targets in human pathogenic bacteria. *Expert Opin. Ther. Targets* **2019**, *23*, 631–643. [CrossRef]
11. Penchovsky, R.; Breaker, R.R. Computational design and experimental validation of oligonucleotide-sensing allosteric ribozymes. *Nat. Biotechnol.* **2005**, *23*, 1424–1433. [CrossRef]

12. Gong, J.; Ju, Y.; Shao, D.; Zhang, Q.C. Advances and challenges towards the study of RNA-RNA interactions in a transcriptome-wide scale. *Quant. Biol.* **2018**, *6*, 239–252. [CrossRef]
13. Childs, L.; Nikoloski, Z.; May, P.; Walther, D. Identification and classification of ncRNA molecules using graph properties. *Nucleic Acids Res.* **2009**, *37*, e66. [CrossRef] [PubMed]
14. Qadir, M.I.; Bukhat, S.; Rasul, S.; Manzoor, H.; Manzoor, M. RNA therapeutics: Identification of novel targets leading to drug discovery. *J. Cell Biochem.* **2020**, *121*, 898–929. [CrossRef] [PubMed]
15. Weidolf, L.; Björkbom, A.; Dahlén, A.; Elebring, M.; Gennemark, P.; Hölttä, M.; Janzén, D.; Li, X.; Andersson, S. Distribution and biotransformation of therapeutic antisense oligonucleotides and conjugates. *Drug Discov. Today* **2021**, *26*, 2244–2258. [CrossRef] [PubMed]
16. Setten, R.L.; Rossi, J.J.; Han, S.P. The current state and future directions of RNAi-based therapeutics. *Nat. Rev. Drug Discov.* **2019**, *18*, 421–446, Erratum in *Nat. Rev. Drug Discov.* **2020**, *19*, 290 and *Rev. Drug Discov.* **2020**, *19*, 291. [CrossRef] [PubMed]
17. Gheibi-Hayat, S.M.; Jamialahmadi, K. Antisense Oligonucleotide (AS-ODN) Technology: Principle, Mechanism and Challenges. *Biotechnol. Appl. Biochem.* **2020**, *68*, 1086–1094. [CrossRef] [PubMed]
18. Sahu, N.K.; Shilakari, G.; Nayak, A.; Kohli, D.V. Antisense technology: A selective tool for gene expression regulation and gene targeting. *Curr. Pharm. Biotechnol.* **2007**, *8*, 291–304. [CrossRef] [PubMed]
19. Matsuo, M. Antisense Oligonucleotide-Mediated Exon-skipping Therapies: Precision Medicine Spreading from Duchenne Muscular Dystrophy. *JMA J.* **2021**, *4*, 232–240. [CrossRef]
20. Chi, X.; Gatti, P.; Papoian, T. Safety of antisense oligonucleotide and siRNA-based therapeutics. *Drug Discov. Today* **2017**, *22*, 823–833. [CrossRef]
21. Ostergaard, M.E.; Nichols, J.; Dwight, T.A.; Lima, W.; Jung, M.E.; Swayze, E.E.; Seth, P.P. Fluorinated Nucleotide Modifications Modulate Allele Selectivity of SNP-Targeting Antisense Oligonucleotides. *Mol. Ther. Nucleic Acids* **2017**, *7*, 20–30. [CrossRef]
22. Yamamoto, T.; Fujii, N.; Yasuhara, H.; Wada, S.; Wada, F.; Shigesada, N.; Harada-Shiba, M.; Obika, S. Evaluation of multiple-turnover capability of locked nucleic acid antisense oligonucleotides in cell-free RNase H-mediated antisense reaction and in mice. *Nucleic Acid. Ther.* **2014**, *24*, 283–290. [CrossRef]
23. Dowdy, S.F. Overcoming cellular barriers for RNA therapeutics. *Nat. Biotechnol.* **2017**, *35*, 222–229. [CrossRef]
24. Maiti, S.; Sen, K.K. *Bio-Targets and Drug Delivery Approaches*; CRC Press: Boca Raton, FL, USA, 2016.
25. Reuscher, C.M.; Klug, G. Antisense RNA asPcrL regulates expression of photosynthesis genes in Rhodobacter sphaeroides by promoting RNase III-dependent turn-over of puf mRNA. *RNA Biol.* **2020**, *18*, 1445–1457. [CrossRef]
26. Singh, S.K.; Koshkin, A.A.; Wengel, J.; Nielsen, P. LNA (locked nucleic acids): Synthesis and high-affinity nucleic acid recognition. *Chem. Commun.* **1998**, *4*, 455–456. [CrossRef]
27. Obika, S.; Nanbu, D.; Hari, Y.; Morio, K.-i.; In, Y.; Ishida, T.; Imanishi, T. Synthesis of 2′-O,4′-C-methyleneuridine and -cytidine. Novel bicyclic nucleosides having a fixed C3, -endo sugar puckering. *Tetrahedron Lett.* **1997**, *38*, 8735–8738. [CrossRef]
28. Papargyri, N.; Pontoppidan, M.; Andersen, M.R.; Koch, T.; Hagedorn, P.H. Chemical Diversity of Locked Nucleic Acid-Modified Antisense Oligonucleotides Allows Optimization of Pharmaceutical Properties. *Mol. Ther. Nucleic Acids* **2020**, *19*, 706–717. [CrossRef]
29. Fluiter, K.; Mook, O.R.; Vreijling, J.; Langkjaer, N.; Højland, T.; Wengel, J.; Baas, F. Filling the gap in LNA antisense oligo gapmers: The effects of unlocked nucleic acid (UNA) and 4′-C-hydroxymethyl-DNA modifications on RNase H recruitment and efficacy of an LNA gapmer. *Mol. Biosyst.* **2009**, *5*, 838–843. [CrossRef] [PubMed]
30. Jepsen, J.S.; Sorensen, M.D.; Wengel, J. Locked nucleic acid: A potent nucleic acid analog in therapeutics and biotechnology. *Oligonucleotides* **2004**, *14*, 130–146. [CrossRef] [PubMed]
31. Obika, S.; Hemamayi, R.; Masuda, T.; Sugimoto, T.; Nakagawa, S.; Mayumi, T.; Imanishi, T. Inhibition of ICAM-1 gene expression by antisense 2′,4′-BNA oligonucleotides. *Nucleic Acids Res. Suppl.* **2001**, *1*, 145–146. [CrossRef] [PubMed]
32. Kurreck, J.; Wyszko, E.; Gillen, C.; Erdmann, V.A. Design of antisense oligonucleotides stabilized by locked nucleic acids. *Nucleic Acids Res.* **2002**, *30*, 1911–1918. [CrossRef] [PubMed]
33. Summerton, J.; Weller, D. Morpholino antisense oligomers: Design, preparation, and properties. *Antisense Nucleic Acid. Drug Dev.* **1997**, *7*, 187–195. [CrossRef]
34. Verona, M.D.; Verdolino, V.; Palazzesi, F.; Corradini, R. Focus on PNA Flexibility and RNA Binding using Molecular Dynamics and Metadynamics. *Sci. Rep.* **2017**, *7*, 42799. [CrossRef] [PubMed]
35. Rose, M.; Lapuebla, A.; Landman, D.; Quale, J. In Vitro and In Vivo Activity of a Novel Antisense Peptide Nucleic Acid Compound Against Multidrug-Resistant Acinetobacter baumannii. *Microb. Drug Resist.* **2019**, *25*, 961–965. [CrossRef]
36. Moulton, H.M.; Nelson, M.H.; Hatlevig, S.A.; Reddy, M.T.; Iversen, P.L. Cellular uptake of antisense morpholino oligomers conjugated to arginine-rich peptides. *Bioconjug. Chem.* **2004**, *15*, 290–299. [CrossRef]
37. Zhang, G.; Jin, L.Q.; Hu, J.; Rodemer, W.; Selzer, M.E. Antisense Morpholino Oligonucleotides Reduce Neurofilament Synthesis and Inhibit Axon Regeneration in Lamprey Reticulospinal Neurons. *PLoS ONE* **2015**, *10*, e0137830. [CrossRef] [PubMed]
38. Heald, A.E.; Iversen, P.L.; Saoud, J.B.; Sazani, P.; Charleston, J.S.; Axtelle, T.; Wong, M.; Smith, W.B.; Vutikullird, A.; Kaye, E. Safety and pharmacokinetic profiles of phosphorodiamidate morpholino oligomers with activity against ebola virus and marburg virus: Results of two single-ascending-dose studies. *Antimicrob. Agents Chemother.* **2014**, *58*, 6639–6647. [CrossRef]
39. Havens, M.A.; Hastings, M.L. Splice-switching antisense oligonucleotides as therapeutic drugs. *Nucleic Acids Res.* **2016**, *44*, 6549–6563. [CrossRef]

40. Lim, K.R.; Maruyama, R.; Yokota, T. Eteplirsen in the treatment of Duchenne muscular dystrophy. *Drug Des. Devel Ther.* **2017**, *11*, 533–545. [CrossRef] [PubMed]
41. Aartsma-Rus, A.; Krieg, A.M. FDA Approves Eteplirsen for Duchenne Muscular Dystrophy: The Next Chapter in the Eteplirsen Saga. *Nucleic Acid. Ther.* **2017**, *27*, 1–3. [CrossRef]
42. Stein, C.A. Eteplirsen Approved for Duchenne Muscular Dystrophy: The FDA Faces a Difficult Choice. *Mol. Ther.* **2016**, *24*, 1884–1885. [CrossRef]
43. Hoy, S.M. Nusinersen: First Global Approval. *Drugs* **2017**, *77*, 473–479. [CrossRef]
44. Lunn, M.R.; Wang, C.H. Spinal muscular atrophy. *Lancet* **2008**, *371*, 2120–2133. [CrossRef]
45. Wahlestedt, C. Natural antisense and noncoding RNA transcripts as potential drug targets. *Drug Discov. Today* **2006**, *11*, 503–508. [CrossRef] [PubMed]
46. Kubowicz, P.; Zelaszczyk, D.; Pekala, E. RNAi in clinical studies. *Curr. Med. Chem.* **2013**, *20*, 1801–1816. [CrossRef] [PubMed]
47. Aagaard, L.; Rossi, J.J. RNAi therapeutics: Principles, prospects and challenges. *Adv. Drug Deliv. Rev.* **2007**, *59*, 75–86. [CrossRef] [PubMed]
48. Rizk, M.; Tuzmen, S. Update on the clinical utility of an RNA interference-based treatment: Focus on Patisiran. *Pharmgenom. Pers. Med.* **2017**, *10*, 267–278. [CrossRef] [PubMed]
49. Chakraborty, C.; Sharma, A.R.; Sharma, G.; Doss, C.G.P.; Lee, S.S. Therapeutic miRNA and siRNA: Moving from Bench to Clinic as Next Generation Medicine. *Mol. Ther. Nucleic Acids* **2017**, *8*, 132–143. [CrossRef] [PubMed]
50. Hoy, S.M. Patisiran: First Global Approval. *Drugs* **2018**, *78*, 1625–1631. [CrossRef]
51. Wood, H. FDA approves patisiran to treat hereditary transthyretin amyloidosis. *Nat. Rev. Neurol.* **2018**, *14*, 570. [CrossRef]
52. Weng, Y.; Xiao, H.; Zhang, J.; Liang, X.-J.; Huang, Y. RNAi therapeutic and its innovative biotechnological evolution. *Biotechnol. Adv.* **2019**, *37*, 801–825. [CrossRef]
53. Bora, R.S.; Gupta, D.; Mukkur, T.K.; Saini, K.S. RNA interference therapeutics for cancer: Challenges and opportunities (review). *Mol. Med. Rep.* **2012**, *6*, 9–15. [CrossRef]
54. Ma, C.-C.; Wang, Z.-L.; Xu, T.; He, Z.-Y.; Wei, Y.-Q. The approved gene therapy drugs worldwide: From 1998 to 2019. *Biotechnol. Adv.* **2020**, *40*, 107502. [CrossRef]
55. Saxena, V. RNAi-based Cancer Therapeutics: Are we there yet? *J. Pharmacovigil.* **2014**, *1*, 142–151. [CrossRef]
56. Guo, W.; Chen, W.; Yu, W.; Huang, W.; Deng, W. Small interfering RNA-based molecular therapy of cancers. *Chin. J. Cancer* **2013**, *32*, 488–493. [CrossRef] [PubMed]
57. Barrangou, R. The roles of CRISPR-Cas systems in adaptive immunity and beyond. *Curr. Opin. Immunol.* **2015**, *32*, 36–41. [CrossRef]
58. Schultzhaus, Z.; Wang, Z.; Stenger, D. CRISPR-based enrichment strategies for targeted sequencing. *Biotechnol. Adv.* **2021**, *46*, 107672. [CrossRef]
59. Zhen, S.; Hua, L.; Liu, Y.-H.; Sun, X.-M.; Jiang, M.-M.; Chen, W.; Zhao, L.; Li, X. Inhibition of long non-coding RNA UCA1 by CRISPR/Cas9 attenuated malignant phenotypes of bladder cancer. *Oncotarget* **2017**, *8*, 9634–9646. [CrossRef] [PubMed]
60. Wang, F.; Li, X.; Xie, X.; Zhao, L.; Chen, W. UCA1, a non-protein-coding RNA up-regulated in bladder carcinoma and embryo, influencing cell growth and promoting invasion. *FEBS Lett.* **2008**, *582*, 1919–1927. [CrossRef]
61. Wang, H.; Guan, Z.; He, K.; Qian, J.; Cao, J.; Teng, L. LncRNA UCA1 in anti-cancer drug resistance. *Oncotarget* **2017**, *8*, 64638–64650. [CrossRef]
62. Zhang, M.; Du, Y.; Shang, J.; Zhang, D.; Dong, X.; Chen, H. Knockdown of UCA1 restrains cell proliferation and metastasis of diffuse large B-cell lymphoma by counteracting miR-331-3p expression. *Oncol. Lett.* **2021**, *21*, 39. [CrossRef] [PubMed]
63. Park, S.V.; Yang, J.-S.; Jo, H.; Kang, B.; Oh, S.S.; Jung, G.Y. Catalytic RNA, ribozyme, and its applications in synthetic biology. *Biotechnol. Adv.* **2019**, *37*, 107452. [CrossRef]
64. Pavlova, N.; Traykovska, M.; Penchovsky, R. Targeting FMN, TPP, SAM-I, and glmS Riboswitches with Chimeric Antisense Oligonucleotides for Completely Rational Antibacterial Drug Development. *Antibiotics* **2023**, *12*, 1607. [CrossRef]
65. Pley, H.W.; Flaherty, K.M.; McKay, D.B. Three-dimensional structure of a hammerhead ribozyme. *Nature* **1994**, *372*, 68–74. [CrossRef]
66. Popova, K.B.; Penchovsky, R. General and Specific Cytotoxicity of Chimeric Antisense Oligonucleotides in Bacterial Cells and Human Cell Lines. *Antibiotics* **2024**, *13*, 122. [CrossRef]
67. Rossi, J.J.; Sarver, N. RNA enzymes (ribozymes) as antiviral therapeutic agents. *Trends Biotechnol.* **1990**, *8*, 179–183. [CrossRef] [PubMed]
68. Kowalski, P.; Stein, U.; Scheffer, G.L.; Lage, H. Modulation of the atypical multidrug-resistant phenotype by a hammerhead ribozyme directed against the ABC transporter BCRP/MXR/ABCG2. *Cancer Gene Ther.* **2002**, *9*, 579–586. [CrossRef] [PubMed]
69. Citti, L.; Rainaldi, G. Synthetic hammerhead ribozymes as therapeutic tools to control disease genes. *Curr. Gene Ther.* **2005**, *5*, 11–24. [CrossRef]
70. Yamada, M.; Tanaka, Y. Structure-activity relationship of pseudoknot-type hammerhead ribozyme reveals key structural elements for enhanced catalytic activity. *Nucleosides Nucleotides Nucleic Acids* **2020**, *39*, 245–257. [CrossRef]
71. Mao, X.; Li, X.; Mao, X.; Huang, Z.; Zhang, C.; Zhang, W.; Wu, J.; Li, G. Inhibition of hepatitis C virus by an M1GS ribozyme derived from the catalytic RNA subunit of *Escherichia coli* RNase P. *Virol. J.* **2014**, *11*, 86. [CrossRef]

72. Moreno, P.M.; Pego, A.P. Therapeutic antisense oligonucleotides against cancer: Hurdling to the clinic. *Front. Chem.* **2014**, *2*, 87. [CrossRef]
73. Bitko, V.; Oldenburg, A.; Garmon, N.E.; Barik, S. Profilin is required for viral morphogenesis, syncytium formation, and cell-specific stress fiber induction by respiratory syncytial virus. *BMC Microbiol.* **2003**, *3*, 9. [CrossRef] [PubMed]
74. Juliano, R.L. The delivery of therapeutic oligonucleotides. *Nucleic Acids Res.* **2016**, *44*, 6518–6548. [CrossRef]
75. Akbarzadeh, A.; Rezaei-Sadabady, R.; Davaran, S.; Joo, S.W.; Zarghami, N.; Hanifehpour, Y.; Samiei, M.; Kouhi, M.; Nejati-Koshki, K. Liposome: Classification, preparation, and applications. *Nanoscale Res. Lett.* **2013**, *8*, 102. [CrossRef]
76. Nakase, I.; Akita, H.; Kogure, K.; Graslund, A.; Langel, U.; Harashima, H.; Futaki, S. Efficient intracellular delivery of nucleic acid pharmaceuticals using cell-penetrating peptides. *Acc. Chem. Res.* **2012**, *45*, 1132–1139. [CrossRef]
77. Margus, H.; Padari, K.; Pooga, M. Cell-penetrating peptides as versatile vehicles for oligonucleotide delivery. *Mol. Ther.* **2012**, *20*, 525–533. [CrossRef]
78. Du, L.; Kayali, R.; Bertoni, C.; Fike, F.; Hu, H.; Iversen, P.L.; Gatti, R.A. Arginine-rich cell-penetrating peptide dramatically enhances AMO-mediated ATM aberrant splicing correction and enables delivery to brain and cerebellum. *Hum. Mol. Genet.* **2011**, *20*, 3151–3160. [CrossRef] [PubMed]
79. Ranade, V.V. Drug delivery systems—2. Site-specific drug delivery utilizing monoclonal antibodies. *J. Clin. Pharmacol.* **1989**, *29*, 873–884. [CrossRef] [PubMed]
80. Shi, N.; Boado, R.J.; Pardridge, W.M. Antisense imaging of gene expression in the brain in vivo. *Proc. Natl. Acad. Sci. USA* **2000**, *97*, 14709–14714. [CrossRef] [PubMed]
81. Dowdy, A.D.S.a.S.F. GalNAc-siRNA Conjugates: Leading the Way for Delivery of RNAi Therapeutics. *Nucleic Acid Ther.* **2018**, *28*, 109–118. [CrossRef]
82. Huang, L.; Liu, Y. In vivo delivery of RNAi with lipid-based nanoparticles. *Annu. Rev. Biomed. Eng.* **2011**, *13*, 507–530. [CrossRef] [PubMed]
83. De Paula, D.; Bentley, M.V.; Mahato, R.I. Hydrophobization and bioconjugation for enhanced siRNA delivery and targeting. *RNA* **2007**, *13*, 431–456. [CrossRef] [PubMed]
84. Miller, C.M.; Harris, E.N. Antisense Oligonucleotides: Treatment Strategies and Cellular Internalization. *RNA Dis.* **2016**, *3*, e1393. [CrossRef]
85. Ho, S.P.; Britton, D.H.; Stone, B.A.; Behrens, D.L.; Leffet, L.M.; Hobbs, F.W.; Miller, J.A.; Trainor, G.L. Potent antisense oligonucleotides to the human multidrug resistance-1 mRNA are rationally selected by mapping RNA-accessible sites with oligonucleotide libraries. *Nucleic Acids Res.* **1996**, *24*, 1901–1907. [CrossRef] [PubMed]
86. Frazier, K.S. Antisense oligonucleotide therapies: The promise and the challenges from a toxicologic pathologist's perspective. *Toxicol. Pathol.* **2015**, *43*, 78–89. [CrossRef] [PubMed]
87. Senn, J.J.; Burel, S.; Henry, S.P. Non-CpG-containing antisense 2′-methoxyethyl oligonucleotides activate a proinflammatory response independent of Toll-like receptor 9 or myeloid differentiation factor 88. *J. Pharmacol. Exp. Ther.* **2005**, *314*, 972–979. [CrossRef] [PubMed]
88. Flood, B.A.; Higgs, E.F.; Li, S.; Luke, J.J.; Gajewski, T.F. STING pathway agonism as a cancer therapeutic. *Immunol. Rev.* **2019**, *290*, 24–38. [CrossRef] [PubMed]
89. Asada, K.; Ito, K.; Yui, D.; Tagaya, H.; Yokota, T. Cytosolic Genomic DNA functions as a Natural Antisense. *Sci. Rep.* **2018**, *8*, 8551. [CrossRef] [PubMed]
90. Ahn, J.; Barber, G.N. STING signaling and host defense against microbial infection. *Exp. Mol. Med.* **2019**, *51*, 1–10. [CrossRef] [PubMed]
91. Deigan, K.E.; Ferre-D'Amare, A.R. Riboswitches: Discovery of drugs that target bacterial gene-regulatory RNAs. *Acc. Chem. Res.* **2011**, *44*, 1329–1338. [CrossRef] [PubMed]
92. Mehdizadeh Aghdam, E.; Hejazi, M.S.; Barzegar, A. Riboswitches: From living biosensors to novel targets of antibiotics. *Gene* **2016**, *592*, 244–259. [CrossRef]
93. Liu, X.; Cao, B.; Yang, L.; Gu, J.-D. Biofilm control by interfering with c-di-GMP metabolism and signaling. *Biotechnol. Adv.* **2022**, *56*, 107915. [CrossRef]
94. Pavlova, N.; Penchovsky, R. Bioinformatics and Genomic Analyses of the Suitability of Eight Riboswitches for Antibacterial Drug Targets. *Antibiotics* **2022**, *11*, 1177. [CrossRef]
95. Traykovska, M.; Penchovsky, R. Targeting SAM-I Riboswitch Using Antisense Oligonucleotide Technology for Inhibiting the Growth of *Staphylococcus aureus* and *Listeria monocytogenes*. *Antibiotics* **2022**, *11*, 1662. [CrossRef]
96. Traykovska, M.; Penchovsky, R. Engineering Antisense Oligonucleotides as Antibacterial Agents That Target FMN Riboswitches and Inhibit the Growth of *Staphylococcus aureus*, *Listeria monocytogenes*, and *Escherichia coli*. *ACS Synth. Biol.* **2022**, *11*, 1845–1855. [CrossRef]
97. Traykovska, M.; Otcheva, L.A.; Penchovsky, R. Targeting TPP Riboswitches Using Chimeric Antisense Oligonucleotide Technology for Antibacterial Drug Development. *ACS Appl. Bio Mater.* **2022**, *5*, 4896–4902. [CrossRef] [PubMed]
98. Pedrolli, D.B.; Nakanishi, S.; Barile, M.; Mansurova, M.; Carmona, E.C.; Lux, A.; Gartner, W.; Mack, M. The antibiotics roseoflavin and 8-demethyl-8-amino-riboflavin from *Streptomyces davawensis* are metabolized by human flavokinase and human FAD synthetase. *Biochem. Pharmacol.* **2011**, *82*, 1853–1859. [CrossRef] [PubMed]

99. Penchovsky, R.; Pavlova, N.; Kaloudas, D. RSwitch: A Novel Bioinformatics Database on Riboswitches as Antibacterial Drug Targets. *IEEE/ACM Trans. Comput. Biol. Bioinform.* **2021**, *18*, 804–808. [CrossRef]
100. Kaloudas, D.; Pavlova, N.; Penchovsky, R. GHOST-NOT and GHOST-YES: Two programs for generating high-speed biosensors with randomized oligonucleotide binding sites with NOT or YES Boolean logic functions based on experimentally validated algorithms. *J. Biotechnol.* **2023**, *373*, 82–89. [CrossRef]
101. Kozak, I.; McCutchan, J.A.; Freeman, W.R. *Retina*, 5th ed.; Elsevier: Amsterdam, The Netherlands, 2013; Volume 2, pp. 1441–1472.
102. Spada, S.; Walsh, G. *Directory of Approved Biopharmaceutical Products*; CRC Press: Boca Raton, FL, USA, 2004.
103. Wong, E.; Goldberg, T. Mipomersen (kynamro): A novel antisense oligonucleotide inhibitor for the management of homozygous familial hypercholesterolemia. *Pharm. Ther.* **2014**, *39*, 119–122.
104. Geary, R.S.; Baker, B.F.; Crooke, S.T. Clinical and preclinical pharmacokinetics and pharmacodynamics of mipomersen (Kynamro®): A second-generation antisense oligonucleotide inhibitor of apolipoprotein B. *Clin. Pharmacokinet.* **2015**, *54*, 133–146. [CrossRef]
105. Hair, P.; Cameron, F.; McKeage, K. Mipomersen sodium: First global approval. *Drugs* **2013**, *73*, 487–493. [CrossRef] [PubMed]
106. Kamaruzzaman, N.F.; Kendall, S.; Good, L. Targeting the hard to reach: Challenges and novel strategies in the treatment of intracellular bacterial infections. *Br. J. Pharmacol.* **2017**, *174*, 2225–2236. [CrossRef]
107. Bai, H.; You, Y.; Yan, H.; Meng, J.; Xue, X.; Hou, Z.; Zhou, Y.; Ma, X.; Sang, G.; Luo, X. Antisense inhibition of gene expression and growth in gram-negative bacteria by cell-penetrating peptide conjugates of peptide nucleic acids targeted to rpoD gene. *Biomaterials* **2012**, *33*, 659–667. [CrossRef]
108. Paul, D.; Sanap, G.; Shenoy, S.; Kalyane, D.; Kalia, K.; Tekade, R.K. Artificial intelligence in drug discovery and development. *Drug Discov. Today* **2021**, *26*, 80–93. [CrossRef]
109. You, Y.; Lai, X.; Pan, Y.; Zheng, H.; Vera, J.; Liu, S.; Deng, S.; Zhang, L. Artificial intelligence in cancer target identification and drug discovery. *Signal Transduct. Target. Ther.* **2022**, *7*, 156. [CrossRef]
110. Fan, Y.; Yen, C.W.; Lin, H.C.; Hou, W.; Estevez, A.; Sarode, A.; Goyon, A.; Bian, J.; Lin, J.; Koenig, S.G.; et al. Automated high-throughput preparation and characterization of oligonucleotide-loaded lipid nanoparticles. *Int. J. Pharm.* **2021**, *599*, 120392. [CrossRef] [PubMed]
111. Crooke, S.T.; Baker, B.F.; Crooke, R.M.; Liang, X.-H. Antisense technology: An overview and prospectus. *Nat. Rev. Drug Discov.* **2021**, *20*, 427–453. [CrossRef] [PubMed]
112. Qi, S.; Duan, N.; Khan, I.M.; Dong, X.; Zhang, Y.; Wu, S.; Wang, Z. Strategies to manipulate the performance of aptamers in SELEX, post-SELEX and microenvironment. *Biotechnol. Adv.* **2022**, *55*, 107902. [CrossRef] [PubMed]
113. Lozena, A.; Pavlova, N.; Popova, K.B.; Traykovska, M.; Penchovsky, R. Why Some Riboswitches are Suitable Targets for Antibacterial Drug Discovery? *EC Microbiol.* **2020**, *16*, 48–51.

Disclaimer/Publisher's Note: The statements, opinions and data contained in all publications are solely those of the individual author(s) and contributor(s) and not of MDPI and/or the editor(s). MDPI and/or the editor(s) disclaim responsibility for any injury to people or property resulting from any ideas, methods, instructions or products referred to in the content.

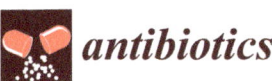

Article

Design, Synthesis, and Structure–Activity Relationship Studies of New Quinone Derivatives as Antibacterial Agents

Juan Andrades-Lagos [1,2,*,†], Javier Campanini-Salinas [2,3,*,†], América Pedreros-Riquelme [2], Jaime Mella [4,5], Duane Choquesillo-Lazarte [6], P. P. Zamora [7], Hernán Pessoa-Mahana [8], Ian Burbulis [9] and David Vásquez-Velásquez [2,*]

1. Facultad de Medicina y Ciencia, Universidad San Sebastián, Santiago 7510157, Chile
2. Drug Development Laboratory, Faculty of Chemical and Pharmaceutical, Sciences, Universidad de Chile, Santiago 8380492, Chile
3. Facultad de Medicina y Ciencia, Universidad San Sebastián, Puerto Montt 5501842, Chile
4. Instituto de Química y Bioquímica, Facultad de Ciencias, Universidad de Valparaíso, Playa Ancha, Valparaíso 2360102, Chile
5. Centro de Investigación Farmacopea Chilena (CIFAR), Facultad de Farmacia, Universidad de Valparaíso, Playa Ancha, Valparaíso 2360102, Chile
6. Laboratorio de Estudios Cristalográficos, IACT (CSIC-UGR), Av. de las Palmeras 4, 18100 Armilla, Spain
7. Departamento de Química y Biología, Facultad de Ciencias Naturales, Universidad de Atacama, Copiapó 1530000, Chile
8. Departamento de Química Orgánica y Fisicoquímica, Facultad de Ciencias Químicas y Farmacéuticas, Universidad de Chile, Santiago 8380492, Chile
9. Centro de Investigación Biomédica, Facultad de Medicina y Ciencias, Universidad San Sebastián, Sede de la Patagonia, Puerto Montt 5501842, Chile
* Correspondence: juan.andrades@uss.cl (J.A.-L.); javier.campanini@uss.cl (J.C.-S.); dvasquez@ciq.uchile.cl (D.V.-V.); Tel.: +56-02-2978-2887 (D.V.-V.)
† These authors contributed equally to this work.

Abstract: Resistance to antibacterial agents is a growing global public health problem that reduces the efficacy of available antibacterial agents, leading to increased patient mortality and morbidity. Unfortunately, only 16 antibacterial drugs have been approved by the FDA in the last 10 years, so it is necessary to develop new agents with novel chemical structures and/or mechanisms of action. In response to this, our group takes up the challenge of designing a new family of pyrimidoisoquinolinquinones displaying antimicrobial activities against multidrug-resistant Gram-positive bacteria. Accordingly, the objective of this study was to establish the necessary structural requirements to obtain compounds with high antibacterial activity, along with the parameters controlling antibacterial activity. To achieve this goal, we designed a family of compounds using different strategies for drug design. Forty structural candidates were synthesized and characterized, and antibacterial assays were carried out against high-priority bacterial pathogens. A variety of structural properties were modified, such as hydrophobicity and chain length of functional groups attached to specific carbon positions of the quinone core. All the synthesized compounds inhibited Gram-positive pathogens in concentrations ranging from 0.5 to 64 µg/mL. Two derivatives exhibited minimum inhibitory concentrations of 64 µg/mL against *Klebsiella pneumoniae*, while compound 28 demonstrated higher potency against MRSA than vancomycin.

Keywords: synthesis; antibacterial agents; quinonic-antibiotics; structure–activity relationships; Craig plot; methicillin-resistant *Staphylococcus aureus*; *Enterococcus faecium*; *Klebsiella pneumoniae*; antibacterial activity; drug discovery; quinone-antibiotics; Free-Wilson

Citation: Andrades-Lagos, J.; Campanini-Salinas, J.; Pedreros-Riquelme, A.; Mella, J.; Choquesillo-Lazarte, D.; Zamora, P.P.; Pessoa-Mahana, H.; Burbulis, I.; Vásquez-Velásquez, D. Design, Synthesis, and Structure–Activity Relationship Studies of New Quinone Derivatives as Antibacterial Agents. *Antibiotics* **2023**, *12*, 1065. https://doi.org/10.3390/antibiotics12061065

Academic Editor: Charlotte A. Huber

Received: 1 June 2023
Revised: 13 June 2023
Accepted: 14 June 2023
Published: 16 June 2023

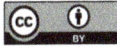

Copyright: © 2023 by the authors. Licensee MDPI, Basel, Switzerland. This article is an open access article distributed under the terms and conditions of the Creative Commons Attribution (CC BY) license (https://creativecommons.org/licenses/by/4.0/).

1. Introduction

Resistance to antibacterial agents is a global problem that often eliminates treatment options in remote locations for several infectious diseases to directly increase mortality [1].

There will be approximately 10 million increased deaths caused by resistant microorganisms by 2050 if no initiatives solve this problem [2]. Investment in creating new antimicrobials has steadily decreased over the last ten years despite the alarming increase in drug resistance [3]. The development of compounds with new mechanisms of action has also decreased in the last decade [3,4]. This problem is worsened by a general lack of interest from the pharmaceutical industry in this market [5,6]. The insufficient investment can be attributed to the perceived low economic return for these types of drugs compared to other pharmacological targets, including treatments for chronic diseases [3,6]. Moreover, this lack of interest is further compounded by various factors. These factors include the focus on short-term curative treatments [3,6], the strict control and restricted use of new antibiotics [7,8], the emergence of generic forms after the expiration of intellectual property patents [6], increased demands by the FDA to demonstrate the efficacy of new antibacterial agents [7], and lastly, the occurrence of drug resistance prior to or shortly after their introduction to the market. Each of these reasons contributes to a decrease in their use and expected economic return [5]. This sentiment is reflected in the fact that only 16 antibacterial compounds have been introduced to the market since 2013 [9–11].

To address this problem, public and non-governmental organizations (NGOs) have started more than 50 initiatives to develop new antibacterial drugs based on known compounds that would likely never be developed in the private pharmaceutical sector. These public-private initiatives include the Joint Programming Initiative on Antimicrobial Resistance (JPIAMR), the Innovative Medicines Initiative's (IMI's) New Drugs for Bad Bugs (ND4BB) Program, the Biomedical Advanced Research and Development Authority's (BARDA) Broad Spectrum Antimicrobials Program, and the Combating Antibiotic Resistant Bacteria Biopharmaceutical Accelerator (CARB-X) [12]. The World Health Organization (WHO) published a list of priority pathogens to guide R&D efforts in the development of new antibacterial drugs called [10].

Within the critical priority group are bacteria such as *Pseudomonas aeruginosa* and enterobacteria (such as *Escherichia coli* and *Klebsiella* sp.) resistant to carbapenems and third-generation cephalosporins. On the other hand, bacteria such as vancomycin-resistant *Enterococcus faecium* and methicillin- and vancomycin-resistant *Staphylococcus aureus* are still under-served and remain classified as high-priority pathogens [10].

In this context, we previously described the synthesis and evaluation of a collection of arylmercaptoquinonic derivatives that exhibit activity against vancomycin-resistant *Enterococcus faecium* (VREF) and methicillin-resistant *Staphylococcus aureus*. These compounds demonstrated 128-fold higher activity against clinical isolates of VREF compared to vancomycin while not affecting the viability of HeLa, HTC-116, SH-SY5Y, or Vero cells in toxicity assays [13,14]. However, there is still a significant gap in our understanding regarding how modifications to the quinone core can impact their biological activity. Based on this, we designed an extensive series of new pyrimidoisoquinolinquinone derivatives and synthesized them to test their antibacterial activities against high-priority pathogens declared by the WHO. The objective of this study was to investigate the structure–activity relationship of this novel family of antibiotic compounds.

To explore this possibility, we designed an extensive series of new pyrimidoisoquinolinquinone derivatives, carrying out their synthesis and testing antibacterial activities using high-priority pathogens declared by the WHO.

The structural requirements necessary to obtain compounds with high antibacterial activity were identified together with the defined parameters that modulated antibacterial profiles. Computational chemistry and crystallographic studies were incorporated to explain the obtained results. The structure–function relationships of these compounds were explored in the context of developing lead drugs for further investigation.

2. Results and Discussion

2.1. Drug Design

Recently, we reported a new kind of quinone-antibiotic exhibiting anti-infective properties against different Gram-positive pathogens [13]. In this study, only a few modifications on the thiophenolic ring substituent were carried out; this reason led us to develop extents on the study of the structure–activity relationship considering a rational design, synthesis, and evaluation of the antibacterial activity of novel compounds of general structure pyrimidoisoquinolinquinone. The **P1** structure (Table 1) was selected as a prototype for further optimization using five optimization strategies. First, the Craig model allowed us to analyze the influence of para-aromatic substituents on biological activity. To contextualize the chemical activities of the derivatives, we grouped theoretical structures in a cartesian graph whose X and Y axes corresponded to the lipophilicity (π) and Hammett substituent constant (σ) parameters of the substituents. For the development of this strategy, we used the compounds previously synthesized in Campanini et al. work [13]. We created a theoretical derivative space in which all possible substituent combinations in the four quadrants of π and σ were displayed in the para position. We calculated molar refractivity (MR) to evaluate the steric influence of substituents on antibacterial activity. Next, we tested classic isosteric replacement by substituting the sulfur atom with nitrogen to determine whether another heteroatom could be used in this position. Third, we performed double substitutions on the thiophenolic ring using a Free-Wilson analysis as a tool to evaluate if the disubstituted compounds had antibacterial activity. Fourth, we performed three homology substitution studies to explore: (1) the effect of the distance between the aromatic ring and the sulfur atom, (2) the effect of the addition of thioalkyl derivatives instead of thioaryl substitutions with the purpose of determining whether the compounds with alkylic chain possess antibacterial activity and the influence of its carbon chain length on the activity, and (3) the effect of modifying position 6 of the tricyclic quinone core on overall activity. We finally added a second chemical group to the tricyclic quinone core to create homodisubstituted derivatives in positions 8 and 9.

A summary of the modifications performed is shown in Figure 1.

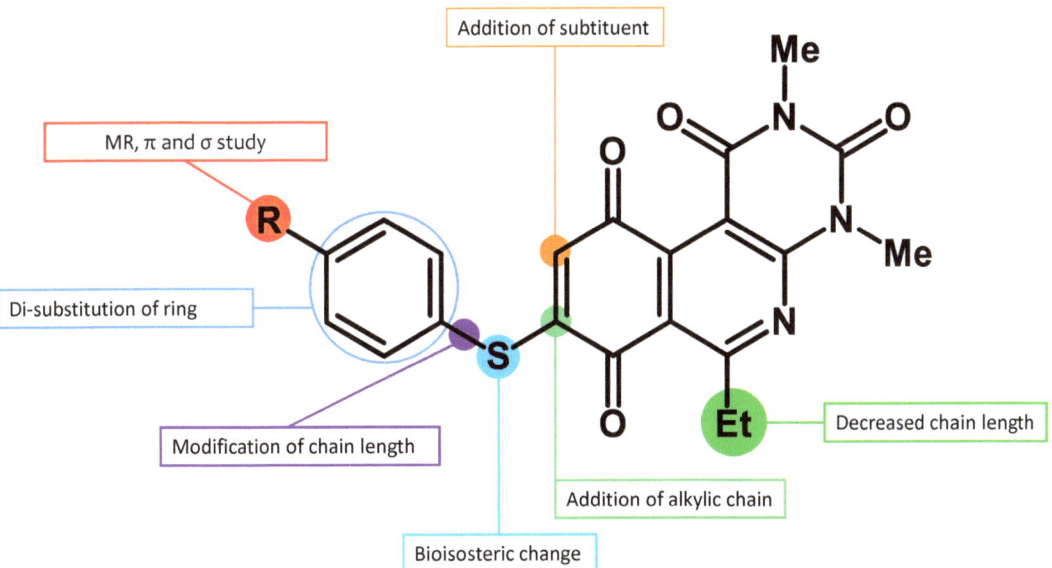

Figure 1. A summary of the structural modifications to the SAR study.

2.2. Synthesis

The compounds were synthesized in two consecutive stages. In the first stage, the tricyclic quinone cores **3**, **4**, and **5** were obtained according to the general procedure A, described by Valderrama et al. [15] and Campanini et al. [13]. This step proceeds via a 'one-pot' reaction, starting with the oxidation of the respective hydroquinone precursor to the quinone ring with silver oxide I at room temperature. The activated quinone reacted with the aminouracil via [3 + 3] cyclization giving rise to the tricyclic hydroquinone intermediate, which was rapidly oxidized aerobically to the respective quinone core. The proposed reaction mechanism is shown in Figure 2.

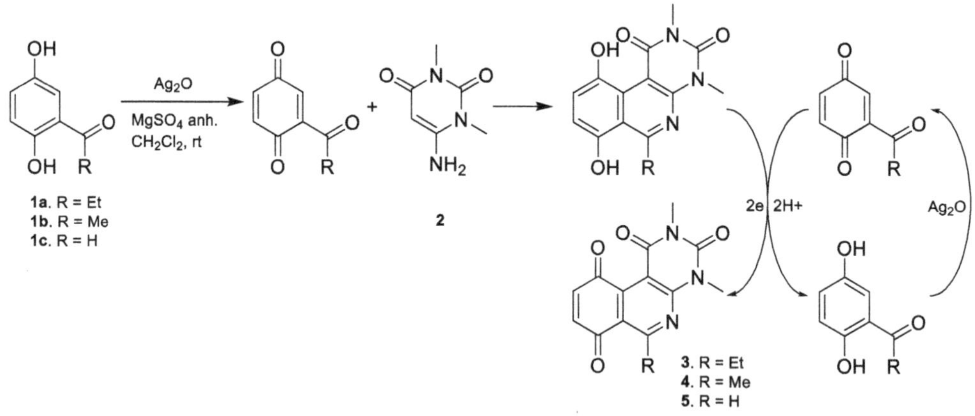

Figure 2. Reaction mechanism proposed for obtaining quinone tricyclic core by one-pot reaction.

In the second stage, regioselective addition to the quinone is performed using four different procedures based on the reactivity of the precursors. For compounds with aniline derivatives, the direct addition of the complete reagent, in equimolar amounts relative to the tricyclic quinone, to the reaction mixture resulted in the predominant formation of only the C-8 regioisomer, corresponding to the derivative with the nitrogen atom attached to the 8-position of the tricyclic quinone core. In this way, the addition of higher proportions of reagent to quinone (2:1) did not generate diaddition products (substituted in 8- and 9-positions). The C-9 regioisomer was not detected in any case. On the other hand, compounds with thiophenol and alkylthio derivatives were slowly added dropwise to the reaction mixture in order to avoid the formation of diaddition compounds. Through this procedure, it was observed that the major products corresponded to the C-8 regioisomers. Similar to the compounds with aniline derivatives, the formation of the C-9 regioisomer was not observed. Finally, considering the possibility of diaddition with thiophenol or alkylthio derivatives, a new procedure ("D") was developed to obtain compounds C-8 and C-9 substitution in order to include this type of structure in the analysis of structure–activity relationship. A summary of the general procedures for obtaining the compounds is shown in Figure 3, and the Supplementary Materials in Figures S1–S4.

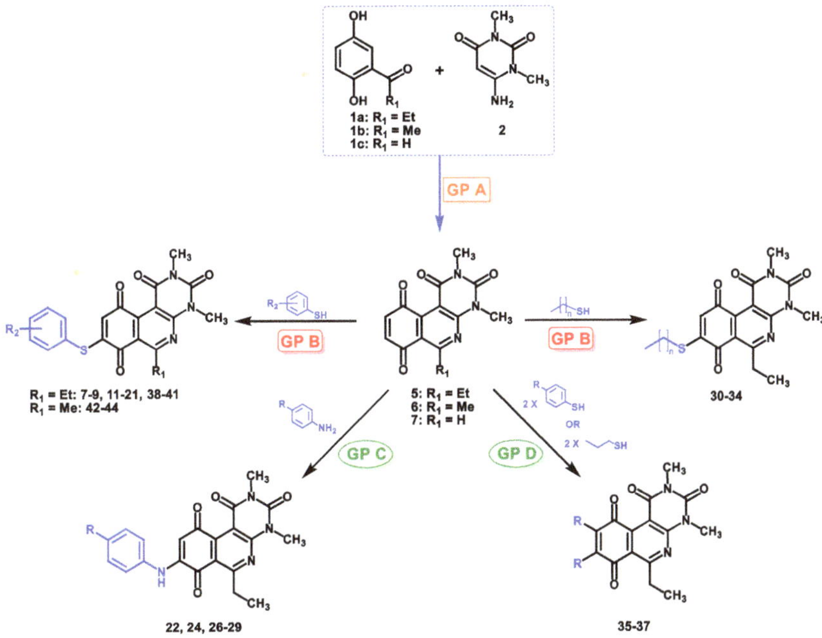

Figure 3. General scheme for obtaining target compounds through the general procedures used.

The regioselectivity observed in these reactions with quinones **3** and **4** can be explained by the effect of the cerium ion, which acts as a catalyst [16] that favors the nucleophilic attack at position C-8 by coordination with the nitrogen heteroatom and/or with the carbonyl group at position C-10, favoring its electron-attractor character and thus allowing the nucleophilic substitution at C-8 [17]. With these results, general procedure B was employed for the thiophenolic compounds **7–9**, **11–21**, **30–34**, and **38–47**, and general procedure C for the arylamines compounds **22**, **24**, and **26–29**. Given the synthetic possibility of obtaining homodisubstituted compounds via aerobic oxidation, the general procedure D was developed, affording compounds **35–37**.

Interestingly, the synthetic route described in general procedure B for the tricyclic quinonic core **5** produced a mixture of C-8 and C-9 isomers in a 73:27 ratio. These results were similar to those reported by Valderrama et al., who studied the addition of cycloalkyl-, n-alkyl-, and arylamines to the phenanthridin-7,10-quinone core [18].

Additionally, compound **11** was subjected to an aryl nitro reduction reaction with iron powder in an acidic medium which allowed obtaining compound **6** [18]. Due to the reactivity of the precursors, some modifications to the corresponding general procedures were necessary to obtain compounds **10**, **23**, and **25**.

2.3. Antibacterial Activity

Compounds target were tested in vitro against *Staphylococcus aureus* methicillin-susceptible strain (ATCC® 29213), *Staphylococcus aureus* methicillin-resistant strain (ATCC® 43300), *Enterococcus faecalis* (ATCC® 29212), *Escherichia coli* (ATCC® 25922), *Pseudomonas aeruginosa* (ATCC® 27853), and *Klebsiella pneumoniae* (ATCC® 700603) by minimum inhibitory concentration (MIC) using microbroth dilutions technique using Müeller–Hinton broth, according to recommendations of the Clinical and Laboratory Standards Institute (CLSI) [13].

The screening results of these new compounds for antibacterial activity in vitro are reported in Table 1. Previously synthesized compounds are designated by the letter P.

Table 1. Antibacterial activities of compounds 3–43, **P1–P7**, and antibiotics controls.

		Compounds			MIC (µg/mL)					
Label	SP [a]	R₁	R₂	R₃	MSSA (ATCC 29213)	MRSA (ATCC 43300)	E. faecalis (ATCC 29212)	E. coli (ATCC 25922)	P. aeruginosa (ATCC 27853)	K. pneumoniae (ATCC 700603)
3	A	H	H	Et	>32	>32	>32	>32	>32	>32
4	A	H	H	Me	>32	>32	>32	>32	>32	>32
5	A	H	H	H	>32	>32	>32	>32	>32	>32
6	_[b]	H₂N-C₆H₄-S-	H	Et	>32	>32	32	>32	>32	>32
7	B	H₃COCHN-C₆H₄-S-	H	Et	16	16	16	>32	>32	>32
8	B	HO-C₆H₄-S-	H	Et	16	16	16	>32	>32	>32
9	B	NC-C₆H₄-S-	H	Et	8	8	8	>32	>32	>32
10	_[b]	HOOC-C₆H₄-S-	H	Et	32	16	32	>32	>32	>32
11	B	O₂N-C₆H₄-S-	H	Et	8	8	8	>32	>32	64
12	B	(H₃C)₂N-C₆H₄-S-	H	Et	16	8	16	>32	>32	>32
13	B	(H₃C)S-C₆H₄-S-	H	Et	>32	>32	>32	>32	>32	>32
14	B	Et-C₆H₄-S-	H	Et	4	4	8	>32	>32	>32
15	B	F₃C-C₆H₄-S-	H	Et	>32	4	>32	>32	>32	>32
16	B	(H₃C)₂HC-C₆H₄-S-	H	Et	>32	>32	>32	>32	>32	>32
17	B	(H₃C)₃C-C₆H₄-S-	H	Et	>32	>32	>32	>32	>32	>32

Table 1. Cont.

Compounds				MIC (µg/mL)					
Label	SP [a]	R_1	R_2	R_3	MSSA (ATCC 29213)	MRSA (ATCC 43300)	E. faecalis (ATCC 29212)	E. coli (ATCC 25922)	P. aeruginosa (ATCC 27853)	K. pneumoniae (ATCC 700603)
18	B	benzyl-S-	H	Et	>64	>64	64	>64	>64	>64
19	B	phenethyl-S-	H	Et	>32	>32	>32	>32	>32	>32
20	B	4-Cl-benzyl-S-	H	Et	>32	>32	>32	>32	>32	>32
21	B	benzothiazol-2-yl-S-	H	Et	>32	>32	>32	>32	>32	>32
22	C	PhNH-	H	Et	>32	>32	>32	>32	>32	>32
23	-[b]	4-H$_2$N-C$_6$H$_4$-NH-	H	Et	>32	>32	>32	>32	>32	>32
24	C	4-H$_3$COOC-C$_6$H$_4$-NH-	H	Et	>16	>16	>16	>16	>16	>16
25	-[b]	4-HOOC-C$_6$H$_4$-NH-	H	Et	>32	>32	>32	>32	>32	>32
26	C	4-F-C$_6$H$_4$-NH-	H	Et	>32	>32	>32	>32	>32	>32
27	C	4-Cl-C$_6$H$_4$-NH-	H	Et	1	1	4	>32	>32	>32
28	C	4-Br-C$_6$H$_4$-NH-	H	Et	0.5	0.5	4	>32	>32	>32
29	C	4-I-C$_6$H$_4$-NH-	H	Et	>32	>32	>32	>32	>32	>32
30	B	Et-S-	H	Et	>8	>8	>8	>8	>8	>8
31	B	n-Pr-S-	H	Et	8	4	8	>32	>32	>32

Table 1. Cont.

		Compounds			MIC (µg/mL)					
Label	SP [a]	R_1	R_2	R_3	MSSA (ATCC 29213)	MRSA (ATCC 43300)	E. faecalis (ATCC 29212)	E. coli (ATCC 25922)	P. aeruginosa (ATCC 27853)	K. pneumoniae (ATCC 700603)
32	B	n-butyl-S-	H	Et	4	4	4	>32	>32	>32
33	B	n-pentyl-S-	H	Et	>16	>16	>16	>16	>16	>16
34	B	n-hexyl-S-	H	Et	>16	>16	>16	>16	>16	>16
35	D	PhS-	PhS-	Et	>16	>16	>16	>16	>16	>16
36	D	4-Cl-C6H4-S-	4-Cl-C6H4-S-	Et	>16	>16	>16	>16	>16	>16
37	D	n-propyl-S-	n-propyl-S-	Et	>32	>32	>32	>32	>32	>32
38	B	4-Cl-2-Br-C6H3-S-	H	Et	>4	4	>4	>4	>4	NT
39	B	2,6-diMeO-C6H3-S-	H	Et	2	2	2	>64	>64	>64
40	B	4-Br-2-MeO-C6H3-S-	H	Et	>32	>32	>32	>32	>32	>32
41	B	3,5-diCl-C6H3-S-	H	Et	>64	4	32	>64	>64	64
42	B	PhS-	H	Me	8	8	8	>32	>32	>32
43	B	4-MeO-C6H4-S-	H	Me	8	8	8	>32	>32	>32
44	B	4-F-C6H4-S-	H	Me	4	8	8	>32	>32	>32
P1		PhS-	H	Et	8	8	8	>32	>32	NT

Table 1. Cont.

Compounds					MIC (µg/mL)					
Label	SP [a]	R_1	R_2	R_3	MSSA (ATCC 29213)	MRSA (ATCC 43300)	E. faecalis (ATCC 29212)	E. coli (ATCC 25922)	P. aeruginosa (ATCC 27853)	K. pneumoniae (ATCC 700603)
P2		4-MeO-C6H4-S-	H	Et	16	16	16	>32	>32	NT
P3		4-Me-C6H4-S-	H	Et	4	4	16	>32	>32	NT
P4		4-F-C6H4-S-	H	Et	8	8	8	>32	>32	NT
P5		4-Cl-C6H4-S-	H	Et	4	4	4	>32	>32	NT
P6		4-Br-C6H4-S-	H	Et	4	8	8	>32	>32	NT
P7		2-Br-C6H4-S-	H	Et	4	1	2	>32	>32	NT
VAN [c]					1	1	2	NT	NT	NT
GEN [d]					NT	NT	NT	0.5	1	2

[a] SP = Structure Procedure. [b] See section of structural procedures. [c] vancomycin, quality control for Gram-positive ATCC® strains is 0.5–2 µg/mL against MRSA and MSSA; 1–4 µg/mL against E. faecalis according to CLSI [19]. [d] gentamicin, quality control for Gram-negative ATCC® strains are 0.25–1 µg/mL against E. coli and 0.25–2 against P. aeruginosa according to CLSI [19]. NT = Not tested; MIC = Minimum inhibitory concentration; VAN = vancomycin; GEN = gentamicin.

The results show that the compounds present antibacterial activity on Gram-positive bacteria within the range of 0.5 to 64 µg/mL. The most active compounds of the series correspond to molecules **28**, **27**, **39**, **32**, and **14**, with activities 0.5, 1, 2, 4, and 4 µg/mL, respectively, for MSSA and MRSA. On the other hand, for *E. faecalis*, the same molecules presented activities of 4, 4, 2, 4, and 8 µg/mL, respectively. On the other hand, no activity was observed against Gram-negative bacteria except for compounds **11** and **41** which were active against *K. pneumoniae* ATCC® 700603 at a concentration of 64 µg/mL.

A detailed study of the structure–activity relationship of the compounds is presented as follows.

3. Structure–Activity Relationship

3.1. Craig Model

For the development of the Craig model [20], p-substituted compounds **6–17** were used, including the previously reported compounds **P1–P6**.

First, p-substituted target compounds were designed using substituents from the four quadrants of a Craig plot to explore the electronic and hydrophobic space around the benzylthio moiety and their effect on activity. We added previously synthesized compounds to this list to expand the landscape to compare these new derivatives. Our results showed that the lipophilic character of the substituent in the para position increases the antibacterial activity of these compounds against Gram-positive bacteria with two outlier compounds (**10** and **13**). These data establish a maximum value of lipophilicity for the substituents in compounds **14** (4-ethyl) and **15** (4-CF$_3$). The compounds with the most lipophilic substituents, **16** (4-iso-propyl) and **17** (4-tert-butyl), did not exhibit antibacterial activity at the concentrations tested (>32 µg/mL).

We observed that the electronic character (Hammett substituent constant) of the substituent had a minimal influence on the antibacterial activity. For example, when comparing compounds **6** (4-NH$_2$) and **12** (4-N(CH$_3$)$_2$), which present similar values of σ and different values of π present MIC values of >32 and 8 µg/mL, respectively, in MRSA. On the other hand, compounds such as **P1** (4-H), **P4** (4-F), and **11** (4-NO$_2$), which have similar π values, have the same MIC value (8 µg/mL) in all the Gram-positive bacteria studied. Additionally, the volume of the substituent, calculated through the molar refractivity parameter, does not show a direct relationship with the antibacterial activity of these compounds. Thus, the lipophilic p-thiophenolic substitution would favor the antibacterial activity of this series of a compound.

3.2. Bioisosteric Replacement

For the bioisosteric replacement analysis, the antibacterial activity of compounds bearing a sulfur atom **P1**, **6**, **10**, and **P4–P6** were compared with the compounds having a nitrogen atom in **22**, **23**, **25–28**, respectively.

The replacement of the sulfur atom by nitrogen (**22–28**) caused the loss of activity for compounds **22–26**. In contrast, derivatives **27** (*p*-Cl aniline) and **28** (*p*-Br aniline) showed activity in Gram-positive bacteria in a range of 0.5–4 µg/mL, establishing themselves as the most active compounds of the entire series. It is observed that the aniline derivatives (**27–28**) are between 2 and 16 times more potent than their thiophenolic analogs, **P5** and **P6**, respectively. In addition, the antibacterial activity of compound **28** is twice that of vancomycin (0.5 µg/mL vs. 1 µg/mL) in MSSA and MRSA.

To study the effect of bioisosteric replacement on the geometry of the compounds, the compounds with nitrogen atoms **23**, **27**, and **28** were crystallized and resolved by X-ray diffraction to compare them with the compounds with sulfur atoms **P5** and **P6**. The data for compound **P5** were extracted from the study by Campanini et al. [13]. (Figure 4).

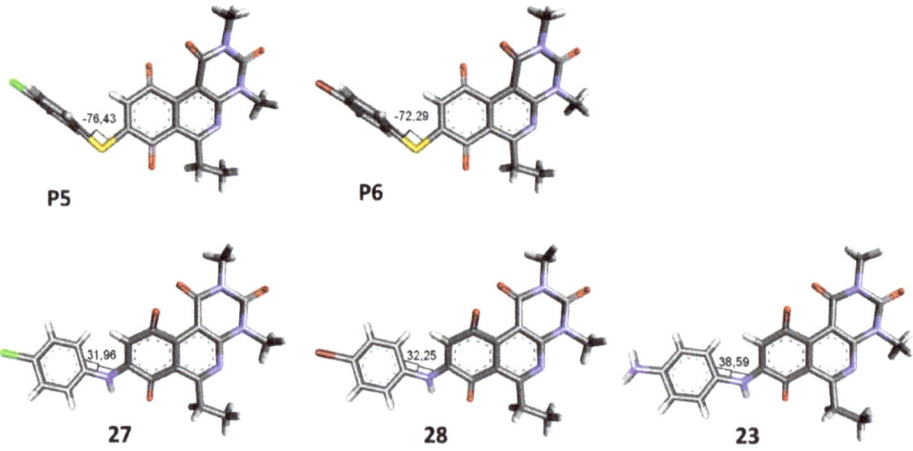

Figure 4. The 3D-dimensional models obtained by X-ray diffraction of individual crystals of compounds **P5**, **P6**, **23**, **27**, and **28**. The dihedral angle of each compound is shown.

The three-dimensional models showed that the dihedral angle of the sulfur derivatives is 76.4° and 72.3° for the compounds **P5** and **P6**, respectively, while for the compounds with nitrogen, they correspond to 31.9° and 32.3°, respectively. Since compounds **27** and **28** are at least four times more active than their bioisosteres **P5** and **P6**, this result suggests that the activity improves when both aromatic systems are more coplanar, probably due to the conjugation between the benzene ring and the aromatic system aromatic of the quinone core. In addition, it is interesting to note that within the series of compounds with a nitrogen atom, the presence of an electron-attracting group, as is the case of the chlorine and bromine atoms in the 4′ position of the benzene ring, since a monovalent bioisosteric replacement by an amino group (compound **23**), maintains the dihedral angle (38.6°) close to compounds **27** and **28** but eliminates the activity completely.

In addition, considering the results of the Craig plot and the bioisosteric change, it was decided to synthesize the derivative 6-ethyl-8-((4-iodophenyl)amino)-2,4-dimethylpyrimido [4,5-c]isoquinolin-1,3,7,10(2H,4H)-tetraone (compound **29**). This compound did not present activity in the evaluated bacteria (MIC > 32 µg/mL), which can be explained by the fact that the hydrophobicity value of iodine is higher than that of the ethyl and CF_3 groups, established as the substituents with the highest hydrophobicity allowed for the series of thiophenolic compounds.

Thus, bioisosteric replacement allowed the generation of the two most active compounds of the series against Gram-positive bacteria, presenting in vitro antibacterial activity similar to vancomycin against MRSA.

3.3. Free-Wilson Study

Considering the clinical relevance of MRSA infections, this antibacterial data was selected for use in the Free-Wilson statistical analysis to understand the contribution of each substituent in the aromatic ring with the aim of generating new active compounds. A Free-Wilson analysis is a numerical method that directly relates structural features with biological properties [21]. In our case, we have correlated the presence or absence of the different substituents in *ortho*, *meta*, and *para* positions on the benzene ring with the biological activity of every compound expressed as pMIC (−logMIC, in Molar units). For this purpose, we constructed a matrix in which the presence of a substituent (Me, MeO, F, Cl, or Br) is represented by 1 and absent a 0. Then, through a multilinear regression, we correlated the biological activity (dependent variable) with the matrix of 1 and 0. The results of the Free-Wilson analysis are shown in Table 2.

Table 2. Summary of the Free-Wilson coefficients analysis.

	Coef. FW				
R	Me	MeO	F	Cl	Br
2′ (*ortho*)	−0.9653	0.255	0	0	0.602
3′ (*meta*)	−0.0622	−0.046	−0.0581	0.2594	0.301
4′ (*para*)	−0.0622	−0.6481	−0.3591	−0.0416	0
Intercept: 5.0849					

The coefficient will be positive for the presence of a substituent that improves the biological activity when it is placed in that position and is the opposite when the coefficient is negative. As can be seen in Table 2, the worst substituents are Me in the *ortho*, and MeO in the *para* position; therefore, such substituents should be avoided to improve anti-MRSA activity. On the other hand, the best substituents are MeO in the ortho position, Cl and Br in the *meta* position, and Br in the para position. This could be explained by both the increase in the lipophilicity of the compounds and by the capacity of these halogens to establish electrostatic interactions with their target.

Based on these results, the following compounds were synthesized to challenge the model Table 3.

Table 3. Compounds designed from the Free-Wilson analysis.

Compound	38	39	40	41
Structure	(structure)	(structure)	(structure)	(structure)
FWc	2'-Br = 0.602 4'-Cl = −0.0416	2'-OMe = 0.255	2'-OMe = 0.255 3'-Br = 0.301	3'-Cl = 0.2594
		FWc = Free-Wilson coefficient.		

The antibacterial activity results showed that compounds **38**, **39**, and **41** exhibited antibacterial activities of 4, 2, and 4 µg/mL against MRSA. In addition, compound **39** exhibited activity against MSSA and *E. faecalis* at 2 µg/mL, and compound **41** was active against *E. faecalis* at 32 µg/mL. This compound stands out for presenting activity against *K. pneumoniae* at 64 µg/mL. Compound **40** did not exhibit activity against the bacteria tested (>32 µg/mL). To explore the structural aspects of these derivatives, we crystallized compound **38** and compared it with compounds **P5** and **P7** reported in the study by Campanini et al. [13] (Figure 5A).

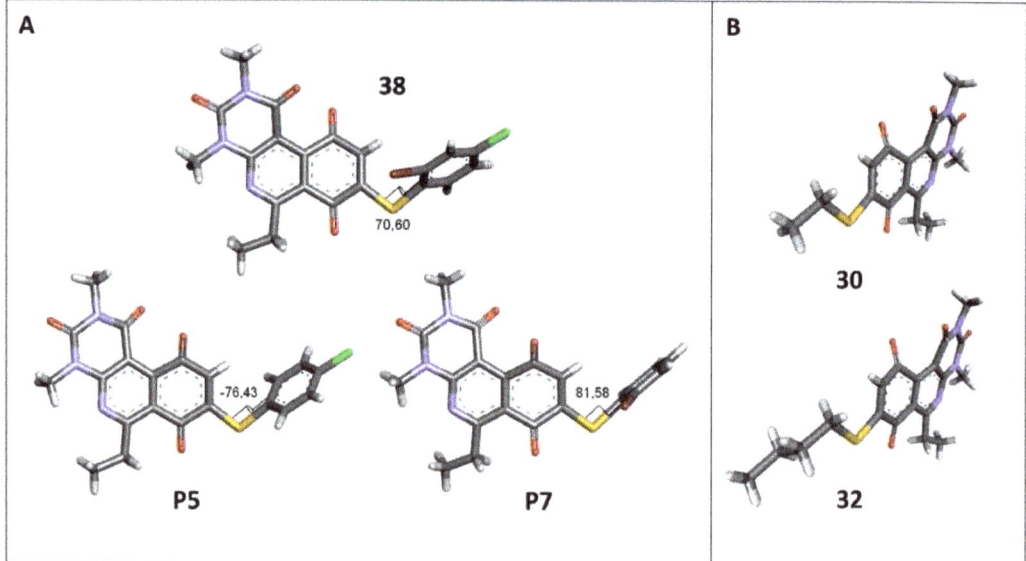

Figure 5. Three-dimensional models obtained by X-ray diffraction of individual crystals of compounds **30**, **32**, **38**, **P5**, and **P7**. (**A**) Comparison of dihedral angles among derived thiophenolic compounds; (**B**) Comparison of geometry of alkylthiol derivatives.

We observed that the dihedral angle of compound **38** is 70.6°, minor than **P5** and **P7**, which correspond to 76.4° and 81.5°. Due to the low solubility of these compounds, it is possible to only observe antimicrobial activity in MRSA with a value of 4 µg/mL, which is similar for **P5** but low for **P7**, which presents 4 and 1 µg/mL, respectively. These results indicated that it is possible to perform a second substitution on the thiophenolic ring to obtain active compounds.

3.4. Homology Study

Three chain extensions were performed in different sections of the structure to understand its relationship with activity. In the first scenario, the compounds **P1** (p-H) and **P5** (p-Cl) [13] were used as references for studying the effect of the distance between the phenyl ring and the sulfur atom on the antibacterial activity. The comparison of **P1** with **18** shows that homologation by one methylene group decreased the antibacterial activity of de 8 µg/mL (**P1**) a 64 µg/mL (**18**) in *E. faecalis* and produced the loss of activity (>64 µg/mL) in MRSA and MSSA. When the distance was extended by inserting a second methylene group, the solubility decreased (**18** vs. **19**) and resulted in the complete loss of antibacterial activity (>64 µg/mL). For the substituted p-Cl pair **P5** and **20**, the loss of antibacterial activity from 4 µg/mL (**P5**) to >32 µg/mL (**20**) is reproducible when a methylene group is added between the thioether and the aromatic ring. These results suggest that extending the distance between the thioether and the aromatic ring and thus increasing the degrees of freedom of the molecule has a deleterious effect on antibacterial activity in the three Gram-positive bacteria evaluated, possibly due to the loss of conjugation between the aromatic system and quinonic nucleus.. The addition of a benzo[d]thiazole-2-thiol derivative was performed to determine the effect on the biological activity if increasing the size and rigidity of the system was associated with a change. In this way, we synthesized compound **21**, which did not exhibit antibacterial activity (>32 µg/mL) in any of the bacteria tested. Thus, the optimal antibacterial activity was obtained when there were no carbon atoms between the thiophenolic ring and the tricyclic quinone core.

The second homology study sought to evaluate the addition of thioalkyl chains from 2 to 6 carbon atoms (**30–34**) to core **3** as an alternative to thiophenolic derivatives. This gave rise to two active compounds, derivatives **31** (3C) and **32** (4C), which presented antibacterial activity in Gram-positive bacteria with MIC values between 4 and 8 µg/mL, establishing the ideal number of carbons as 4. The compounds with fewer carbon atoms (**30**) or more (**33** and **34**) did not present antibacterial activity in any of the bacteria evaluated.

Chemical models obtained by crystallography showed that compounds **30** and **32** do not adopt differences in the structural geometry of the quinone nucleus or in the alkyl chain (Figure 5B). This evidence indicated that the activity exhibited by **32** is due mainly to the increase in lipophilicity of the molecule. It is important to note that alkyl substitutions at position 8 of the tricyclic quinone core can be considered only if their length is 3 or 4 carbons. Other chain lengths generate inactive compounds.

Finally, the impact of the alkyl chain at position 6 of the tricyclic quinone core was evaluated. In such a sense, compounds **42–44** (Series 6-Me) were synthesized from compound **4**. When comparing the 6-Et vs. 6-Me series, no differences in antimicrobial activity were observed, showing that shortening of the alkyl radical a methylene group does not affect activity. To extend the analysis and consider the obtaining of the tricyclic quinone core **5**, procedure B was carried out in an exploratory manner to obtain the 6-H series, with the thiophenol, 4-methoxy-thiophenol, and 4-fluoro-thiophenol substituents. NMR analysis showed the presence of a mixture of isomers of C-8 y C-9 in a 73:27 ratio (data not shown). When evaluating the activity of these isomer mixtures, we observed antibacterial activity (data not shown). These findings open the possibility of characterizing the antimicrobial activity of the different isomers, which until now has not been possible due to the regioselective addition of the substituents.

3.5. Homodisubstitution Study

The addition of a second substitution in the quinone tricyclic core gives rise to the compounds called homodisubstituted, whose positions 8 and 9 are occupied. From derivatives **P1**, **P5**, and **31**, compounds **35**, **36**, and **37**, respectively, were synthesized. These results indicated that homodisubstitution resulted in the loss of antibacterial activity.

4. Conclusions

We used drug optimization tools to establish the structure–activity relationship of this new family of 2,4-dimethylpyrimido[4,5-c]isoquinoline-1,3,7,10(2H,4H)-tetraone derivatives with antimicrobial activity. Nineteen compounds exhibited antibacterial activity against ATCC® Gram-positive bacteria in a range of 0.5 to 64 µg/mL, with compound **28** being the most active of the series. Compound **28** was twice as potent as vancomycin on MRSA. In addition, compounds **11** and **41** showed activity against K. pneumoniae ATCC® 700603 at a concentration of 64 µg/mL. This work supports the conclusion that rational drug design can provide useful insights to guide derivative synthesis that accelerates new drug discovery with potentially novel targets of bioactivity.

For compounds with the bridging sulfur atom bearing a para-substituted benzene ring, the antimicrobial activity is favored when the lipophilicity of the molecule increases. A second substitution on the benzene ring generates active compounds; however, these compounds do not show greater activity than the monosubstituted derivatives. Both the introduction of carbons between the sulfur atom and the benzene ring, as well as the replacement of the aromatic ring by an alkyl chain, annuls the activity of the compounds. The replacement of an ethyl group by a methyl group at the C-6 position of the quinone tricyclic core generates active compounds with similar activity. On the other hand, the elimination of the group in position 6 modifies the reactivity of the quinone tricyclic core, generating a mixture of isomers exhibiting less antimicrobial activity. Homo disubstitution of thiophenolic or thioalkyl groups on the quinone core generated inactive compounds.

In addition, the bioisosteric replacement of the sulfur atom by one of nitrogen produced a change in the geometry by reducing the dihedral angle between the substituted benzene ring and the quinone nucleus. This change increased the activity when the benzene ring presented an electro-attracting atom such as chlorine or bromine; on the other hand, the presence of electron donor groups such as amines lowered the activity.

These results showed that this new family of compounds displayed a high potential for improvement in their performance as potent antimicrobial drugs against Gram-positive bacteria. Finally, it is important to highlight the bioactivity of compounds 11 and 41, which open the way for studying new active structures on K. pneumoniae, a pathogen considered a priority by the WHO.

5. Materials and Methods

5.1. Materials

All reagents were purchased from AK-scientific, Union City, United States; Enamine, Kyiv, Ukraine; Merck, Darmstadt, Germany; or Sigma–Aldrich, Burlington, United States and were used without purification. Melting points (mp) were determined on a Stuart Scientific SMP3 apparatus and were uncorrected. ^{1}H-NMR spectra were recorded on Bruker AM-400 instruments in deuterochloroform (CDCl$_3$) or dimethylsulfoxide (DMSO-d$_6$). ^{13}C-NMR spectra were obtained in CDCl$_3$ or DMSO-d$_6$ at 100 MHz. The assignments of chemical shifts are expressed in ppm downfield relative to tetramethylsilane (TMS, δ scale), and the coupling constants (J) are reported in Hertz. Silica gel (70–230 and 230–400 mesh) and TLC aluminum foil 60 F254 (Merck, Darmstadt, Germany) were used for preparative column chromatography and analytical TLC, respectively. High-resolution mass spectra were obtained on a mass spectrometer with flight time analyzer (TOF) and Triwave® system model SYNAPT™ G2 (WATERS, Milford, MA, USA), using atmospheric pressure ionization with electro spray (ESI+/−), Capillarity 3.0, source temperature 100 °C, desolvation temperature 500 °C.

5.2. Chemical Synthesis

5.2.1. General Procedure A for the Synthesis of 3–5

A suspension of hydroquinone precursor corresponding (**1a–1c**) (1.90 mmol), 6-amino-1,3-dimethyl-2,4(1H,3H)-pyrimidinedione (**2**) (1.90 mmol), Ag$_2$O (5.7 mmol) and anhydrous MgSO$_4$ (5.7 mmol), in 40 mL of dichloromethane was stirred vigorously at room temperature for 3 h. The mixture was filtered with celite and washed with dichloromethane. The solvent was removed under reduced pressure, and the crude reaction was purified using 65 g of silica gel (230–400 mesh) using a mix of dichloromethane and ethyl acetate = 9:1 as eluent. The resulting solution was concentrated to dryness under reduced pressure. The obtained products were yellow solids for all tricyclic quinone cores.

5.2.2. General Procedure B for Synthesis of 8-Thioaryl (thioalquil)-pyrimidoisoquinolinequinones Derivatives (7–9, 11–21, 30–34, 38–47)

A solution of 3 (150 mg, 0.4909 mmol 1.0 equiv.) and $CeCl_3 \cdot 7H_2O$ (5% mmol respect to 3) in a mix of ethanol: dichloromethane = 1:1 (10 mL) was added dropwise slowly a solution of benzenethiol or alquilthiol derivate (0.5 equiv.) in ethanol: dichloromethane = 1:1 (30 mL). The reaction mixture was stirred at room temperature for 16 h. The progress of the reaction was followed by thin-layer chromatography (TLC). The reaction mixture was concentrated under reduced pressure, and the crude of the reaction was purified using 65 g of silica gel (70–230 mesh) and a mix of dichloromethane, light petroleum, and ethyl acetate as an eluent in determinate proportions. The resulting solution was concentrated to dryness under reduced pressure.

5.2.3. General Procedure C for Synthesis of 8-Arylamino-pyrimidoisoquinolinequinones Derivatives (22, 24, 26–29)

A solution of 3 (150 mg, 0.4909 mmol 1.0 equiv.), the required amine (2 equiv.), $CeCl_3 \cdot 7H_2O$ (5% mmol respect to 3), in a mix of ethanol: dichloromethane = 1:1 (10 mL), was left with stirring at room temperature until completion of the reaction indicated by thin-layer chromatography (TLC). The reaction mixture was concentrated under reduced pressure. The crude reaction was purified by column chromatography using 65 g of silica gel (70–230 mesh) and a mix of dichloromethane, chloroform, light petroleum and/or ethyl acetate as eluent in different proportions. The resulting solution was concentrated to dryness under reduced pressure.

5.2.4. General Procedure D for Synthesis of 8,9-Bisthioaryl (Thioalquil)-pyrimidoisoquinolinequinones Derivatives (35–37)

The bis-substituted derivatives were achieved by preparing a solution of 3 (150 mg, 0.4909 mmol 1.0 equiv.), the corresponding thiophenol derivative (2.5 equiv.), and $CeCl_3 \cdot 7H_2O$ (5% mol of 3) in ethanol (40 mL) under reflux conditions for 1–4 h, the progress of the reaction was followed by thin-layer chromatography (TLC). Once the reaction was over, the mixture was cooled to room temperature and stirred under aerobic conditions for 18 h. The reaction mixture was concentrated under reduced pressure, and the crude was purified by column chromatography using 65 g of silica gel (70–230 mesh) using a mix of dichloromethane, light petroleum, and ethyl acetate as eluent in determined proportions. The resulting solution was concentrated to dryness under reduced pressure.

5.2.5. Structural Characterization for Compounds (3–47)

The 6-Ethyl-2,4-dimethylpyrimido[4,5-c]isoquinoline-1,3,7,10(2H,4H)-tetraone(3): Prepared from 1-(2,5-dihydroxyphenyl)propan-1-one **1a** and **2**; yellow solid; mp 167.6–167.9 °C; ^{1}H-NMR (CDCl$_3$, 400 MHz) δ 7.11 (d, J = 10.3 Hz, 1H, H-9), 6.81 (d, J = 10.3 Hz, 1H, H-8), 3.76 (s, 3H, 2-NCH$_3$), 3.47 (s, 3H, 4-NCH$_3$), 3.40 (q, J = 7.3 Hz, 2H, 6-C$\underline{H}_2$CH$_3$), 1.34 (t, J = 7.3 Hz, 3H, 6-CH$_2$C$\underline{H}_3$); ^{13}C-NMR (CDCl$_3$,100 MHz) δ 185.0 (1C, C-10), 183.9 (1C, C-7), 171.2 (1C, C-6), 159.0 (1C, C-4a), 152.9 (1C, C-1), 151.5 (1C, C-3), 146.6 (1C, C-10a), 138.7 (1C, C-8), 138.7 (1C, C-9), 121.2 (1C, C-6a), 105.4 (1C, C-10b), 32.0 (1C, 6-$\underline{C}$H$_2$CH$_3$), 30.6 (1C, 2-NCH$_3$), 29.5 (1C, 4-NCH$_3$), 12.5 (1C, 6-CH$_2$$\underline{C}H_3$); HRMS m/z 299.09070 (Calculated for C$_{15}$H$_{13}$N$_3$O$_4$ [M]$^+$, 299.09061); purified in column chromatography with dichloromethane: ethyl acetate = 9:1; yield: 84%.

The 2,4,6-Trimethylpyrimido[4,5-c]isoquinoline-1,3,7,10(2H,4H)-tetraone (4): Prepared from 1-(2,5-dihydroxyphenyl)ethan-1-one **1b** and **2**; yellow solid; mp 197.5–198.5 °C (d); ^{1}H-NMR (CDCl$_3$,400 MHz) δ 7.13 (d, J = 10.5 Hz, 1H, 8-H), 6.83 (d, J = 10.5 Hz, 1H, 9-H),

3.75 (s, 3H, 2-NCH$_3$), 3.47 (s, 3H, 4-NCH$_3$), 2.99 (s, 3H, 6-CH$_3$); ^{13}C-NMR (CDCl$_3$,100 MHz) δ 184.2, 183.4, 166.2, 158.3, 152.3, 150.9, 145.8, 138.4, 138.1, 121.1, 105.2, 30.1, 28.9, 26.6; HRMS m/z 285.0828 (Calculated for C$_{14}$H$_{11}$N$_3$O$_4$ [M + H]$^+$: 286.0832); purified by column chromatography, dichloromethane: ethyl acetate = 9:1; yield: 86%.

The 2,4-Dimethylpyrimido[4,5-c]isoquinoline-1,3,7,10(2H,4H)-tetraone (**5**): Prepared from 2,5-dihydroxybenzaldehyde **1c** and **2**; yellow solid; mp 203.5–205.5 °C (d); ^{1}H-NMR (400 MHz, CDCl$_3$) δ 9.30 (s, 1H, 6-H), 7.15 (d, J = 10.5 Hz, 1H, 9-H), 6.88 (d, J = 10.5 Hz, 1H, 8-H), 3.79 (s, 3H, 2-NCH$_3$), 3.51 (s, 3H, 4-NCH$_3$); ^{13}C-NMR (100 MHz, CDCl$_3$) δ 182.8, 182.1, 158.2, 154.8, 153.1, 150.8, 142.9, 140.6, 136.3, 122.6, 106.3, 30.5, 29.1; HRMS m/z 272.0671 (Calculated for C$_{13}$H$_9$N$_3$O$_4$ [M + H]$^+$: 272.06); purified by column chromatography with a mixture of dichloromethane: ethyl acetate = 9:1; yield: 86%.

The 8-(4-Aminobenzenethio)-6-ethyl-2,4-dimethylpyrimido[4,5-c]isoquinoline-1,3,7,10 (2H,4H)-tetraone (**6**). A suspension of **11** (150.0 mg, 0.33 mmol), iron powder (370 mg, 6.63 mmol) in a 1:1:1 mixture of water/methanol/acetic acid (30 mL) was stirred for 1 h at 50–60 °C. The mixture was neutralized with NaHCO$_3$ and then extracted with ethyl acetate (2 × 15 mL). The organic extract was dried over anhydrous Na$_2$SO$_4$, filtered, and evaporated under reduced pressure. The organic crude was purified using 45g of silica gel 60 (230–400 mesh). The resulting solution was concentrated to dryness under reduced pressure; brown solid; mp > 250 °C; ^{1}H-NMR (400 MHz, CDCl$_3$) δ 7.24 (d, J = 8.5 Hz, 2H, 3'-H y 5'-H), 6.73 (d, J = 8.5 Hz, 2H, 2'-H y 6'-H), 6.22 (s, 1H, 9-H), 4.01 (s, 2H, 4'-NH$_2$), 3.74 (s, 3H, 2-NCH$_3$), 3.42 (s, 3H, 4-NCH$_3$), 3.40 (q, J = 7.3 Hz, 2H, 6-CH$_2$CH$_3$), 1.35 (t, J = 7.3 Hz, 3H, 6-CH$_2$CH$_3$); ^{13}C-NMR (100 MHz, CDCl$_3$): δ 181.5, 181.2, 170.7, 158.5, 158.1, 152.7, 151.1, 148.9, 147.5, 137.0 (2C), 127.7, 120.8, 116.3 (2C), 113.4, 105.4, 31.7, 30.2, 29.0, 12.2. HRMS m/z 423.1125 (Calculated for C$_{21}$H$_{19}$N$_4$O$_4$S [M + H]$^+$: 423.1127); purified by column chromatography with a mixture of dichloromethane: ethyl acetate: petroleum ether = 9:1:1; yield: 31%.

The 8-(4-Acetamidobenzenethio)-6-ethyl-2,4-dimethylpyrimido[4,5-c]isoquinoline-1,3,7,10 (2H,4H)-tetraone (**7**): Prepared from **3** and 4-acetamidothiophenol using general procedure B; orange solid; mp 170.2–173.0 °C; ^{1}H-NMR (400 MHz, CDCl$_3$) δ 7.99 (s, 1H, NHCO), 7.69 (d, J = 8.3 Hz, 2H, 3'-H and 5'-H), 7.43 (d, J = 8.4 Hz, 2H, 2'-H and 6'-H), 6.15 (s, 1H, 9-H), 3.75 (s, 3H, 2-NCH$_3$), 3.42 (s, 3H, 4-NCH$_3$), 3.40 (q, J = 7.5 Hz, 2H, 6-CH$_2$CH$_3$), 2.21 (s, 3H, COCH$_3$), 1.36 (t, J = 7.3 Hz, 3H, 6-CH$_2$CH$_3$); ^{13}C-NMR (100 MHz, CDCl$_3$): δ 181.3, 180.8 (2C), 170.8, 168.9, 158.5, 157.2, 152.7, 151.0, 147.2, 140.6, 136.5 (2C), 127.7, 121.1 (2C), 120.6, 105.4, 31.7, 30.2, 29.1, 24.7, 12.1; HRMS m/z 465.1246 (Calculated for C$_{23}$H$_{21}$N$_4$O$_5$S [M + H]$^+$: 465.1233); purified in column chromatography with dichloromethane: ethyl acetate = 3:1; yield: 69%.

The 8-(4-hydroxybenzenethio)-6-ethyl-2,4-dimethylpyrimido[4,5-c]isoquinoline-1,3,7,10 (2H,4H)-tetraone(**8**): Prepared from **3** and 4-mercaptophenol using general procedure B; orange solid; mp 208–210 °C (d); ^{1}H-NMR (400 MHz, CDCl$_3$) δ 7.38 (d, J = 8.7 Hz, 2H, 3'-H and 5'-H), 6.96 (d, J = 8.7 Hz, 2H, 2'-H and 6'-H), 6.21 (s, 1H, 4'-OH), 6.15 (s, 1H, 9-H), 3.77 (s, 3H, 2-NCH$_3$), 3.46 (s, 3H, 4-NCH$_3$), 3.43 (q, J = 7.3 Hz, 2H, 6-CH$_2$CH$_3$), 1.38 (t, J = 7.3 Hz, 3H, 6-CH$_2$CH$_3$); ^{13}C-NMR (100 MHz, CDCl$_3$) δ 181.5, 181.0, 171.0, 159.1, 158.2, 157.6, 155.8, 152.7, 151.0, 147.4, 137.4 (2C), 127.7, 120.8, 117.6 (2C), 117.0, 31.8, 30.3, 29.2, 12.2. HRMS m/z 424.0963 (Calculated for C$_{21}$H$_{18}$N$_3$O$_5$S [M + H]$^+$: 424.0967); purified in column chromatography with ethyl acetate: petroleum ether = 9:0.8; yield: 72%.

The 4-((6-ethyl-2,4-dimethyl-1,3,7,10-tetraoxo-1,2,3,4,7,10-hexahydropyrimido[4,5-c] isoquinolin-8-yl)thio)benzonitrile (**9**): Prepared from **3** and 4-mercaptobenzonitrile using general procedure B; orange solid; mp 203–205 °C; ^{1}H-NMR (400 MHz, CDCl$_3$) δ 7.80 (d, J = 8.0 Hz, 2H, 3'-H and 5'-H), 7.69 (d, J = 8.0 Hz, 2H, 2'-H and 6'-H), 6.21 (s, 1H, 9-H), 3.76 (s, 3H, 2-NCH$_3$), 3.44 (s, 3H, 4-NCH$_3$), 3.41 (q, J = 7.3 Hz, 2H, 6-CH$_2$CH$_3$), 1.37 (t, J = 7.3 Hz, 3H, 6-CH$_2$CH$_3$); ^{13}C-NMR (100 MHz, CDCl$_3$) δ 181.1, 180.2, 171.0, 158.3, 158.2, 154.6, 152.9, 151.0, 146.9, 136.2 (2C), 134.0, 133.7 (2C) 128.4, 120.3, 117.6, 114.6, 105.5, 31.8, 30.2, 29.1, 12.1; HRMS m/z 433.0892 (Calculated for C$_{22}$H$_{17}$N$_4$O$_4$S [M + H]$^+$: 433.0971); purified in column chromatography with dichloromethane: ethyl acetate = 9:1; yield: 72%.

Synthesis of 8-(4-carboxibenzenethio)-6-ethyl-2,4-dimethylpyrimido[4,5-c]isoquinoline-1,3,7,10(2H,4H)-tetraone (**10**). Prepared from **3** and 4-mercaptobenzoic acid; A solution of **3** (150 mg, 0.4909 mmol) and $CeCl_3 \cdot 7H_2O$ (5% mmol respect to **3**) in a mix of ethanol: dichloromethane = 1:1 (10 mL), was added dropwise slowly a solution of 4-mercaptobenzoic acid (0.5 equiv.) in ethanol: dichloromethane = 1:1 (30 mL). The reaction mixture was stirred at room temperature for 16 h. The progress of the reaction was followed by thin-layer chromatography (TLC). Then, 10 mL of distilled water and NaOH (0.1 M) are added to the solution until pH 10 is reached. The extractions were carried out with ethyl acetate (10 mL × 2), the precipitate solid, filtered under vacuum, and washed with ethanol (15 mL × 3). Finally, the obtained product was recrystallized from ethanol. Orange solid, mp > 250 °C; ^{1}H-NMR (400 MHz DMSO$_6$) δ 13.29 (s, 1H, 4′-COOH), 8.10 (d, 2H, 3′-H and 5′-H), 7.76 (d, 2H, 2′-H and 6′-H), 6.07 (s, 1H, 9-H), 3.59 (s, 3H, 2-NCH$_3$), 3.30 (q, J = 7.3 Hz, 2H, 6-C$\underline{H}_2$CH$_3$) 3.23 (s, 3H, 4-NCH$_3$), 1.29 (t, J = 7.3 Hz, 3H, 6-CH$_2$C$\underline{H}_3$); ^{13}C-NMR (100 MHz DMSO$_6$) δ 181.1, 180.4, 169.3, 167.0, 158.3, 155.1, 152.9, 151.2, 146.4, 135.8, 133.1, 133.0, 131.5 (2C), 127.8 (2C), 120.6, 105.4, 31.4, 30.3, 29.0, 12.3; HRMS m/z 452.0912 (Calculated for $C_{22}H_{18}N_3O_6S$ [M + H]$^+$: 452.0916); yield: 38%.

The 8-(4-nitrobenzenethio)-6-ethyl-2,4-dimethyl-pyrimido[4,5-c]isoquinoline-1,3,7,10(2H,4H)-tetraone (**11**): Prepared from **3** and 4-nitrobenzenethiol using general procedure B; yellow solid; mp 188.8–190.1 °C (d); ^{1}H-NMR (400 MHz, CDCl$_3$) δ 8.34 (d, 2H, 3′-H and 5′-H), 7.75 (d, 2H, 2′-H and 6′-H), 6.24 (s, 1H, 9-H), 3.75 (s, 3H, 2-NCH$_3$), 3.42 (s, 3H, 4-NCH$_3$), 3.40 (q, J = 7.3 Hz, 2H, 6-C$\underline{H}_2$CH$_3$), 1.36 (t, J = 7.3 Hz, 3H, 6-CH$_2$C$\underline{H}_3$); ^{13}C-NMR (100 MHz, CDCl$_3$) δ 181.0, 181.0, 170.9, 158.3, 154.3, 152.9, 151.0, 149.1, 146.9, 136.4 (2C), 136.1, 128.6, 125.1 (2C), 120.2, 105.4, 31.8, 30.3, 29.1, 12.1; HRMS m/z 453.0871 (Calculated for $C_{21}H_{17}N_4O_6S$ [M + H]$^+$: 453.0869); purified in column chromatography with dichloromethane: ethyl acetate: petroleum ether = 10:1:4; yield: 96%.

The 8-(4-dimethylaminobenzenethio)-6-ethyl-2,4-dimethylpyrimido[4,5-c]isoquinoline-1,3,7,10(2H,4H)-tetraone (**12**): Prepared from **3** and 4-(dimethylamino)benzenethiol using general procedure B; burgundy red; mp 134.6–137.0 °C; ^{1}H-NMR (400 MHz, CDCl$_3$) δ 7.31 (d, J = 8.6 Hz, 2H, 2′-H and 6′-H), 6.75 (d, J = 8.6 Hz, 2H, 3′-H and 5′-H), 6.21 (s, 1H, 9-H), 3.74 (s, 3H, 2-NCH$_3$), 3.43 (s, 3H, 4-NCH$_3$), 3.40 (q, J = 7.3 Hz, 2H, 6-C$\underline{H}_2$CH$_3$), 3.03 (s, 6H, 4′-N(CH$_3$)$_2$), 1.36 (t, J = 7.3 Hz, 3H, 6-CH$_2$C$\underline{H}_3$);^{13}C-NMR (100 MHz, CDCl$_3$) δ 181.7, 181.5, 170.7, 158.7, 158.6, 152.8, 151.9, 151.3, 147.7, 136.7 (2C), 127.8, 121.0, 113.6 (2C), 110.6, 105.5, 77.2, 40.3, 31.8, 30.3, 29.2, 12.3; HRMS m/z 451.1447 (Calculated for $C_{23}H_{23}N_4O_4S$ [M + H]$^+$: 451.1440); purified in column chromatography with dichloromethane: ethyl acetate: petroleum ether = 9:0.5:1; yield: 43%.

The 8-(4-(methylthio)benzenethio)-6-ethyl-2,4-dimethylpyrimido[4,5-c]isoquinoline-1,3,7,10(2H,4H)-tetraone (**13**): Prepared from **3** and 4-(methylthio)benzenethiol using general procedure B; red solid; mp 181.6–184.0 °C; ^{1}H-NMR (400 MHz, CDCl$_3$) δ 7.41 (d, J = 8.1 Hz, 2H, 2′-H and 6′-H), 7.33 (d, J = 8.2 Hz, 2H, 2′-H and 6′-H), 6.19 (s, 1H, 9-H), 3.75 (s, 3H, 2-NCH$_3$), 3.43 (s, 3H, 4-NCH$_3$), 3.41 (q, J = 7.4 Hz, 2H, 6-C$\underline{H}_2$CH$_3$), 2.53 (s, 3H, SC$\underline{H}_3$), 1.36 (t, J = 7.3 Hz, 3H, 6-CH$_2$C$\underline{H}_3$); ^{13}C-NMR (100 MHz, CDCl$_3$) δ 181.33, 180.8, 170.7, 158.4, 156.8, 152.7, 151.1, 147.3, 143.1, 135.8 (2C), 127.9, 127.4 (2C), 122.4, 120.6, 105.4, 31.7, 30.2, 29.1, 15.2, 12.1; HRMS m/z 454.0894 (Calculated for $C_{22}H_{20}N_3O_4S_2$ [M + H]$^+$: 454.0895); purified in column chromatography with dichloromethane: ethyl acetate: petroleum ether = 3:2:0.5; yield: 46%.

The 6-ethyl-8-(4-ethylbenzenethio)-2,4-dimethylpyrimido[4,5-c]isoquinoline-1,3,7,10(2H,4H)-tetraone (**14**): Prepared from **3** and 4-ethylbenzenethiol using general procedure B; yellow solid; mp 172–174 °C; ^{1}H-NMR (400 MHz, CDCl$_3$) δ 7.43 (d, J = 7.9 Hz, 2H, 3′-H and 5′-H), 7.33 (d, J = 7.9 Hz, 2H, 2′-H and 6′-H), 6.18 (s, 1H, 9-H), 3.75 (s, 3H, 2-NCH$_3$), 3.43 (s, 3H, 4-NCH$_3$), 3.41 (q, J = 7.3 Hz, 2H, 6-C$\underline{H}_2$CH$_3$), 2.72 (q, J = 7.6 Hz, 2H, 4′-C$\underline{H}_2$CH$_3$), 1.37 (t, J = 7.3 Hz, 3H, 4′-CH$_2$C$\underline{H}_3$), 1.28 (t, J = 7.6 Hz, 3H, 6-CH$_2$C$\underline{H}_3$); ^{13}C-NMR (100 MHz, CDCl$_3$) δ 181.4, 180.9, 170.7, 158.4, 157.2, 152.7, 151.1, 147.4, 135.7 (2C), 130.1 (2C), 127.8, 123.7, 120.6, 105.4, 31.7, 30.2, 29.0, 28.7, 15.3, 12.2; HRMS m/z 436.1253 (Calculated for $C_{23}H_{22}N_3O_4S$

[M + H]$^+$: 436.1331); purified in column chromatography with dichloromethane: ethyl acetate: petroleum ether = 12:0.5:5; yield: 83%.

The 6-ethyl-2,4-dimethyl-8-((4-trifluoromethyl)phenyl)thio)pyrimido[4,5-c]isoquinoline-1,3,7,10(2H,4H)-tetraone(**15**): Prepared from **3** and 4-(trifluoromethyl)benzenethiol using general procedure B; yellow solid; mp 204–206 °C; ^{1}H-NMR (400 MHz, CDCl$_3$) δ 7.77 (d, J = 8.1 Hz, 2H, 3'-H and 5'-H), 6.96 (d, J = 8.1 Hz, 2H, 2'-H and 6'-H), 6.18 (s, 1H, 9-H), 3.76 (s, 3H, 2-NCH$_3$), 3.43 (s, 3H, 4-NCH$_3$), 3.42 (q, J = 7.3 Hz, 2H, 6-C$\underline{H}_2$CH$_3$), 1.37 (t, J = 7.3 Hz, 3H, 6-CH$_2$C$\underline{H}_3$); ^{13}C-NMR (100 MHz, CDCl$_3$) δ 181.2, 181.4, 170.9, 158.3, 155.3, 152.8, 151.0, 147.1, 136.1 (2C), 132.8 (q, J = 33.1 Hz, 1C), 132.2, 128.2, 127.2 (q, J = 3.6 Hz, 2C), 123.5 (q, J = 272.8 Hz, 1C), 120.4, 105.5, 31.8, 30.2, 29.1, 12.1; HRMS m/z 476.0814 (Calculated for C$_{22}$H$_{17}$F$_3$N$_3$O$_4$S [M + H]$^+$: 476.0812); purified in column chromatography with dichloromethane: ethyl acetate: petroleum ether = 12:0.5:5; yield: 89%.

The 8-(4-(isopropyl)benzenethio)-6-ethyl-2,4-dimethylpyrimido[4,5-c]isoquinoline-1,3,7,10(2H,4H)-tetraone (**16**): Prepared from **3** and 4-isopropylbenzenethiol using general procedure B; orange solid; mp 134.6–137.0 °C; ^{1}H-NMR (400 MHz, CDCl$_3$) δ 7.43 (d, J = 8.0 Hz, 2H, 3'-H and 5'-H), 7.35 (d, J = 8.0 Hz, 2H, 2'-H and 6'-H), 6.17 (s, 1H, 9-H), 3.74 (s, 3H, 2-NCH$_3$), 3.42 (s, 3H, 4-NCH$_3$), 3.40 (q, J = 7.3 Hz, 2H, 6-C$\underline{H}_2$CH$_3$), 3.03–2.90 (m, 1H, 4'-C$\underline{H}$(CH$_3$)$_2$), 1.36 (t, J = 7.3 Hz, 3H, 6-CH$_2$C$\underline{H}_3$), 1.28 (d, J = 6.9 Hz, 6H, 4'-CH(C$\underline{H}_3$)$_2$); ^{13}C-NMR (100 MHz, CDCl$_3$) δ 181.6, 181.0, 170.8, 158.5, 157.3, 152.8, 152.1, 151.2, 147.5, 135.8(2C), 128.7 (2C), 127.9, 123.9, 120.7, 105.5, 34.2, 31.8, 30.2, 29.1, 23.9 (2C), 12.2; HRMS m/z 450.1499 (Calculated for C$_{24}$H$_{24}$N$_3$O$_4$S [M + H]$^+$: 450.1488); purified in column chromatography with dichloromethane: ethyl acetate: petroleum ether = 12:0.5:1; yield: 43%.

The 8-(4-(tertbutyl)benzenethio)-6-ethyl-2,4-dimethylpyrimido[4,5-c]isoquinoline-1,3,7,10(2H,4H)-tetraone (**17**): Prepared from **3** and 4-(*tert*-butyl)benzenethiol using general procedure B; orange solid, mp 157.6–160.7 °C; ^{1}H-NMR (400 MHz, CDCl$_3$) δ 7.52 (d, J = 8.2 Hz, 2H, 3'-H and 5'-H), 7.45 (d, J = 8.1 Hz, 2H, 2'-H and 6'-H), 6.19 (s, 1H, 9-H), 3.75 (s, 3H, 2-NCH$_3$), 3.43 (s, 3H, 4-NCH$_3$), 3.42 (q, J = 7.3 Hz, 2H, 6-C$\underline{H}_2$CH$_3$), 1.37 (t, J = 7.4 Hz, 3H, 6-CH$_2$C$\underline{H}_3$), 1.36 (s, 9H, 4'-C(C$\underline{H}_3$)$_3$); ^{13}C-NMR (100 MHz, CDCl$_3$) δ 181.7, 181.0, 170.9, 158.6, 157.3, 154.4, 152.8, 151.2, 147.5, 135.5(2C), 128.0, 127.9, 127.7, 126.2, 123.7, 120.7, 105.5, 35.1, 31.8, 31.4, 31.3, 30.3, 29.2, 12.3; HRMS m/z 464.1653 (Calculated for C$_{25}$H$_{26}$N$_3$O$_4$S [M + H]$^+$: 464.1644); purified in column chromatography with dichloromethane: ethyl acetate: petroleum ether = 12:0.5:5; yield: 61%.

The 8-(benzylthio)-6-ethyl-2,4-dimethylpyrimido[4,5-c]isoquinoline-1,3,7,10(2H,4H)-tetraone (**18**): Prepared from **3** and phenylmethanethiol using general procedure B; orange solid; mp 181.0–182.0 °C; ^{1}H-NMR (400 MHz, CDCl$_3$) δ 7.40–7.28 (m, 5H, C$_6$H$_5$), 6.76 (s, 1H, 9-H), 4.06 (s, 2H, Ph-C$\underline{H}_2$-S), 3.74 (s, 3H, 2-NCH$_3$), 3.44 (s, 3H, 4-NCH$_3$), 3.36 (q, J = 7.3 Hz, 2H, 6-C$\underline{H}_2$CH$_3$), 1.33 (t, J = 7.3 Hz, 3H, 6-CH$_2$C$\underline{H}_3$); ^{13}C-NMR (100 MHz, CDCl$_3$) δ 180.8 (2C), 170.8, 158.5, 154.6, 152.8, 151.2, 147.1, 134.0, 129.1 (2C), 129.0 (2C), 128.2, 127.1, 120.7, 105.4, 35.8, 31.8, 30.2, 29.1, 12.2. HRMS m/z 422.1171 (Calculated for C$_{22}$H$_{20}$N$_3$O$_4$S [M + H]$^+$: 422.1175); purified in column chromatography with dichloromethane: ethyl acetate: petroleum ether = 9:1:3; yield: 66%.

The 8-(phenethylthio)-6-ethyl-2,4-dimethyl-pyrimido[4,5-c]isoquinoline-1,3,7,10(2H,4H)-tetraone (**19**): Prepared from **3** and 2-phenylethanethiol using general procedure B; yellow solid; mp 170.0–171.0 °C; ^{1}H-NMR (400 MHz, CDCl$_3$) δ 7.33 (t, J = 7.3 Hz, 2H, 3'-H and 5'-H), 7.26–7.24 (m, 3H, 2'-H, 4'-H and 6'-H), 6.70 (s, 1H, 9-H), 3.75 (s, 3H, 2-NCH$_3$), 3.46 (s, 3H, 4-NCH$_3$), 3.37 (q, J = 7.3 Hz, 2H, 6-C$\underline{H}_2$CH$_3$), 3.13–3.00 (m, 4H, Ph-C$_2$H$_4$S), 1.34 (t, J = 7.3 Hz, 3H, 6-CH$_2$C$\underline{H}_3$); ^{13}C-NMR (100 MHz, CDCl$_3$) δ 180.7 (2C), 170.7, 158.5, 154.9, 152.7, 151.1, 147.0, 138.9, 128.8 (2C), 128.5 (2C), 127.0, 126.5, 120.7, 105.4, 33.7, 32.3, 31.7, 30.2, 29.1, 12.1; HRMS m/z 436.1332 (Calculated for C$_{23}$H$_{22}$N$_3$O$_4$S [M + H]$^+$: 436.1331); purified in column chromatography with dichloromethane: ethyl acetate: petroleum ether = 10:1:6; yield: 79%.

The (4-(chlorobenzyl)thio)-6-ethyl-2,4-dimethylpyrimido[4,5-c]isoquinoline-1,3,7,10(2H,4H)-tetraone (**20**): Prepared from **3** and (4-chlorophenyl)methanethiol using general procedure B; orange solid; mp 191.0–191.8 °C; ^{1}H-NMR (400 MHz, CDCl$_3$) δ 7.33 (m, 4H,

2'-H, 3'-H, 5'-H, and 6'-H), 6.72 (s, 1H, 9-H), 4.02 (s, 2H, Ph-CH$_2$-S), 3.74 (s, 3H, 2-NCH$_3$), 3.45 (s, 3H, 4-NCH$_3$), 3.36 (q, J = 7.3 Hz, 2H, 6-C$\underline{H}_2$CH$_3$), 1.33 (t, J = 7.3 Hz, 3H, 6-CH$_2$C$\underline{H}_3$); ^{13}C-NMR (100 MHz, CDCl$_3$) δ 180.7, 180.6, 170.7, 158.4, 154.1, 152.7, 151.0, 146.9, 134.0, 132.4, 130.2 (2C), 129.2 (2C), 127.1, 120.6, 105.4, 35.0, 31.7, 30.2, 29.1, 12.1; HRMS m/z 456.0775 (Calculated for C$_{22}$H$_{19}$ClN$_3$O$_4$S [M + H]$^+$: 456.0785); purified in column chromatography with dichloromethane: ethyl acetate: petroleum ether = 10:1:5; yield: 32%.

The 8-(benzo[d]thiazol-2-ylthio)-6-ethyl-2,4-dimethylpyrimido[4,5-c]isoquinoline-1,3,7,10 (2H,4H)-tetraone(**21**): Prepared from **3** and benzo[d]thiazole-2-thiol using general procedure B; yellow solid; mp > 250 °C; ^{1}H-NMR (400 MHz, CDCl$_3$) δ 8.07 (d, J = 8.1 Hz, 1H, 7'-H), 7.89 (d, J = 8.1 Hz, 1H, 4'-H), 7.54 (d, J = 7.6 Hz, 1H, 5'-H), 7.47 (d, J = 7.6 Hz, 1H, 6'-H), 6.25 (s, 1H, 9-H), 3.74 (s, 3H, 2-NCH$_3$), 3.42 (s, 3H, 4-NCH$_3$), 3.38 (q, J = 7.3 Hz, 2H, 6-C$\underline{H}_2$CH$_3$), 1.34 (t, J = 7.3 Hz, 3H, 6-CH$_2$C$\underline{H}_3$); ^{13}C-NMR (100 MHz, CDCl$_3$) δ 181.5, 179.9, 170.9, 158.2, 156.7, 153.6, 152.9, 151.0, 150.5, 146.8, 136.9, 131.4, 126.7, 123.6, 121.5, 105.4 31.7, 30.2, 29.1, 12.1; HRMS m/z 465.0690 (Calculated for C$_{22}$H$_{17}$N$_4$O$_4$S$_2$ [M + H]$^+$: 465.0691); purified in column chromatography with dichloromethane: ethyl acetate: petroleum ether = 9:1:3; yield: 72%.

The 8-(phenylamino)-6-ethyl-2,4-dimethyl-pyrimido[4,5-c]isoquinoline-1,3,7,10(2H,4H)-tetraone (**22**): Prepared from **3** and aniline using general procedure C; purple solid; mp 189.0–190.0 °C; ^{1}H-NMR (400 MHz, CDCl$_3$) δ 7.60 (s, 1H, NH), 7.42 (t, J = 7.8 Hz, 2H, 3'-H and 5'-H), 7.23 (m, 3H, 2'-H, 4'-H and 6'-H), 6.46 (s, 1H, 9-H), 3.76 (s, 3H, 2-NCH$_3$), 3.47 (s, 3H, 4-NCH$_3$), 3.41 (q, J = 7.3 Hz, 2H, 6-C$\underline{H}_2$CH$_3$), 1.37 (t, J = 7.3 Hz, 3H, 6-CH$_2$C$\underline{H}_3$); ^{13}C-NMR (100 MHz, CDCl$_3$) δ 182.2, 180.0, 170.2, 158.7, 153.1, 151.2, 149.3, 144.6, 137.2, 129.8(2C), 125.8, 122.3(2C), 119.5, 105.9, 103.7, 31.8, 30.2, 29.1, 12.1; HRMS m/z 391.1412 (Calculated for C$_{21}$H$_{19}$N$_4$O$_4$ [M + H]$^+$: 391.1406); purified in column chromatography with dichloromethane: ethyl acetate: petroleum ether = 1:2:4; yield: 76%.

Synthesis of 8-(4-amino-phenylamino)-6-ethyl-2,4-dimethylpyrimido[4,5-c]isoquinoline -1,3,7,10(2H,4H)-tetraone (**23**): A solution of **3** (150 mg, 0.4909 mmol) and CeCl$_3$·7H$_2$O (5% mmol respect to **1**) in a mix of ethanol: dichloromethane = 1:1 (10 mL), was added dropwise slowly a solution of benzene-1,4-phenylendiamine (26.60 mg, 0.2454 mmol) in ethanol: dichloromethane = 1:1 (30mL). The reaction mixture was stirred at room temperature for 16 h. The progress of the reaction was followed by thin-layer chromatography (TLC). The reaction mixture was concentrated under reduced pressure, and the crude reaction was purified using 30 g of silica gel (70–230 mesh) and a mix of chloroform and ethyl acetate as eluent; green solid; mp > 250 °C; ^{1}H-NMR (400 MHz, CDCl$_3$) δ 7.26 (d, J = 8.3 Hz, 2H, 2'-H and 6'-H), 7.26 (s, 1H, NH), 6.75 (d, J = 8.4 Hz, 2H, 3'-H and 5'-H), 6.23 (s, 1H, 9-H), 3.99 (s, 2H, 4'-NH$_2$), 3.75 (s, 3H, 2-NCH$_3$), 3.44 (s, 3H, 4-NCH$_3$), 3.41 (q, J = 7.3 Hz, 2H, 6-C$\underline{H}_2$CH$_3$), 1.36 (t, J = 7.3 Hz, 3H, 6-CH$_2$C$\underline{H}_3$); ^{13}C-NMR (100 MHz, CDCl$_3$) δ 181.5, 181.2, 170.7, 158.5, 158.1, 152.7, 151.1, 148.9, 147.5, 137.0 (2C), 127.7, 120.8, 116.4 (2C), 113.5, 105.4, 31.7, 30.2, 29.0, 12.2; HRMS m/z 406.1528 (Calculated for C$_{21}$H$_{20}$N$_5$O$_4$ [M + H]$^+$: 406.1515); purified in column chromatography with chloroform: ethyl acetate = 8:1; yield: 51%.

The 8-(4-(methoxycarbonyl)phenylamino)-6-ethyl-2,4-dimethylpyrimido[4,5-c]isoquinoline-1,3,7,10(2H,4H)-tetraone (**24**): Prepared from **3** and methyl 4-aminobenzoate using general procedure C; red solid; mp > 250 °C; ^{1}H-NMR (400 MHz, CDCl$_3$) δ 8.10 (d, J = 8.1 Hz, 2H, 3'-H and 5'-H), 7.76 (s, 1H, NH), 7.31 (d, J = 8.1 Hz, 2H, 2'-H and 6'-H), 6.63 (s, 1H, 9-H), 3.93 (s, 3H, 4'-COOCH$_3$), 3.77 (s, 3H, 2-NCH$_3$), 3.47 (s, 3H, 4-NCH$_3$), 3.41 (q, J = 7.3 Hz, 2H, 6-C$\underline{H}_2$CH$_3$), 1.38 (t, J = 7.3 Hz, 3H, 6-CH$_2$C$\underline{H}_3$); ^{13}C-NMR (100 MHz, CDCl$_3$) δ 182.4, 179.6, 170.4, 155.4, 151.9, 143.3, 141.6, 134.5, 132.6 (2C), 131.4, 123.9 (2C), 120.6, 118.9, 110.4, 108.9, 105.5, 57.6, 31.9, 30.2, 29.1, 12.0; HRMS m/z 449.1469 (Calculated for C$_{23}$H$_{21}$N$_4$O$_6$ [M + H]$^+$: 449.1461); purified in column chromatography with chloroform: ethyl acetate = 20:1; yield: 42%.

Synthesis of methyl 4-(6-ethyl-2,4-dimethyl-1,3,7,10-tetraoxo-1,2,3,4,7,10-hexahydropyrimido [4,5-c]isoquinolin-8-yl)amino)benzoic acid (**25**). Prepared from **3** and 4-aminobenzoic acid; A solution of **3** (150 mg, 0.4909 mmol) and CeCl$_3$·7H$_2$O (5% mmol respect to **3**) in a mix of ethanol: dichloromethane = 1:1 (10 mL), was added dropwise slowly a solution of

4-aminobenzoic acid (34.40 mg, 0.2506 mmol) in ethanol: dichloromethane = 1:1 (30 mL). The reaction mixture was stirred at room temperature for 16 h. The progress of the reaction was followed by thin-layer chromatography (TLC). The reaction mixture was concentrated under reduced pressure, and the obtained solid was washed three times with 30 mL of dichloromethane. Finally, the solid was purified using 10 g of silica gel (70–230 mesh) and ethyl acetate as eluent; red solid; mp > 250 °C; ^{1}H-NMR (400 MHz DMSO-d$_6$) δ 9.47 (s, 1H, NH), 7.97 (d, J = 8.6 Hz, 2H, 3′-H and 5′-H), 7.54 (d, J = 8.7 Hz, 2H, 2′-H and 6′-H), 6.40 (s, 1H, 9-H), 3.61 (s, 3H, 2-NCH$_3$), 3.27 (q, J = 7.5 Hz, 2H, 6-C$\underline{H_2}$CH$_3$) 3.23 (s, 3H, 4-NCH$_3$), 1.32 (t, J = 7.3 Hz, 3H, 6-CH$_2$C$\underline{H_3}$); ^{13}C-NMR (400 MHz DMSO$_6$): Not obtained due to low solubility of the compound; HRMS m/z 435.1299 (Calculated for C$_{22}$H$_{19}$N$_4$O$_6$ [M + H]$^+$: 435.1305); purified in column chromatography with ethyl acetate; yield: 12%.

The 6-ethyl-8-((4-fluorophenyl)amino)-2,4-dimethylpyrimido[4,5-c]isoquinoline -1,3,7,10 (2H,4H)-tetraone (**26**): Prepared from **3** and 4-fluoroaniline using general procedure C; burgundy red solid; mp 216.1–216.9 °C (d); ^{1}H-NMR (400 MHz, CDCl$_3$) δ7.49 (s, 1H, NH), 7.22 (dt, $J_{H,H}$ = 7.9, $J_{F,H}$ = 2.6 Hz, 2H, 2′-H and 6′-H), 7.13 (t, $J_{H,H}$ = 8.5, $J_{F,H}$ = 8.5 Hz, 2H, 3′-H and 5′-H), 6.30 (s, 1H, 9-H), 3.76 (s, 3H, 2-NCH$_3$), 3.47 (s, 3H, 4-NCH$_3$), 3.41 (q, J = 7.3 Hz, 2H, 6-C$\underline{H_2}$CH$_3$), 1.37 (t, J = 7.3 Hz, 3H, 6-CH$_2$C$\underline{H_3}$); ^{13}C-NMR (100 MHz, CDCl$_3$) δ 182.1, 179.9, 170.2, 160.4 (d, 1C, $J_{F,C}$ = 253.5 Hz, 4′), 158.8, 153.1, 151.2, 149.3, 145.1, 133.1(d, 1C, $J_{F,C}$ = 2.9 Hz, 1′), 124.7 (d, 2C, $J_{F,C}$ = 8.3 Hz, 2′ and 6′), 119.4, 116.8 (d, 2C, $J_{F,C}$ = 22.8 Hz, 3′ and 5′), 106.0, 103.3, 31.8, 30.2, 29.1, 12.1; HRMS m/z 409.1307 (Calculated for C$_{21}$H$_{18}$FN$_4$O$_4$ [M + H]$^+$: 409.1312); purified in column chromatography with chloroform: ethyl acetate = 9:1; yield: 70%.

The 8-((4-chlorophenyl)amino)-6-ethyl-2,4-dimethylpyrimido[4,5-c]isoquinoline-1,3,7,10 (2H,4H)-tetraone (**27**); Prepared from **3** and 4-chloroaniline using general procedure C; purple solid; mp 206.0–207.0 °C (d); ^{1}H-NMR (400 MHz, CDCl$_3$) δ 7.56 (s,1H, NH), 7.39 (d, J = 8.8 Hz, 2H, 3′-H and 5′-H), 7.20 (d, J = 8.8 Hz, 2H, 2′-H and 6′-H), 6.40 (s, 1H, 9-H), 3.76 (s, 3H, 2-NCH$_3$), 3.47 (s, 3H, 4-NCH$_3$), 3.40 (q, J = 7.3 Hz, 2H, 6-C$\underline{H_2}$CH$_3$), 1.36 (t, J = 7.3 Hz, 3H, 6-CH$_2$C$\underline{H_3}$); ^{13}C-NMR (100 MHz, CDCl$_3$) δ 182.2, 179.8, 170.3, 158.6, 153.1, 151.2, 149.1, 144.3, 135.8, 131.0, 129.3 (2C), 123.5 (2C), 119.3, 105.9, 104.0, 31.8, 30.2, 29.1, 12.1; HRMS m/z 425.1021 (Calculated for C$_{21}$H$_{18}$ClN$_4$O$_4$ [M + H]$^+$: 425.1017); purified in column chromatography with chloroform: ethyl acetate: petroleum ether = 2:1:2; yield: 53%.

The 8-((4-bromophenyl)amino)-6-ethyl-2,4-dimethylpyrimido[4,5-c]isoquinoline-1,3,7,10 (2H,4H)-tetraone (**28**): Prepared from **3** and 4-bromoaniline using general procedure C; red solid; mp > 250.0 °C; ^{1}H-NMR (400 MHz, CDCl$_3$) δ7.55 (s, 1H, NH), 7.54 (d, J = 8.7 Hz, 2H, 3′-H and 5′-H), 7.15 (d, J = 8.7 Hz, 2H, 2′-H and 6′-H), 6.42 (s, 1H, 9-H), 3.76 (s, 3H, 2-NCH$_3$), 3.47 (s, 3H, 4-NCH$_3$), 3.40 (q, J = 7.3 Hz, 2H, 6-C$\underline{H_2}$CH$_3$), 1.36 (t, J = 7.3 Hz, 3H, 6-CH$_2$C$\underline{H_3}$);^{13}C-NMR (100 MHz, CDCl$_3$) δ 182.2, 179.8, 170.3, 158.6, 153.1, 151.2, 149.1, 144.2, 136.4, 132.9 (2C), 123.7 (2C), 119.3, 118.7, 105.9, 104.1, 31.8, 30.2, 29.1, 12.1; HRMS m/z 469.0515 (Calculated for C$_{21}$H$_{18}$BrN$_4$O$_4$ [M + H]$^+$: 469.0511); purified in column chromatography with dichloromethane: ethyl acetate: petroleum ether = 4:1:4; yield: 67%.

The 6-ethyl-8-((4-iodophenyl)amino)-2,4-dimethylpyrimido[4,5-c]isoquinoline-1,3,7,10 (2H,4H)-tetraone (**29**): Prepared from **3** and 4-iodoaniline using general procedure C; purple solid; mp > 250 °C; ^{1}H-NMR (400 MHz, CDCl$_3$) δ 7.73 (d, J = 8.1 Hz, 3H, 3′-H and 5′-H), 7,55 (s, 1H, NH), 7.02 (d, J = 8.2 Hz, 2H, 2′-H and 6′-H), 6.43 (s, 1H, 9-H), 3.76 (s, 3H, 2-NCH$_3$), 3.47 (s, 3H, 4-NCH$_3$), 3.40 (q, J = 7.3 Hz, 2H, 6-C$\underline{H_2}$CH$_3$), 1.36 (t, J = 7.3 Hz, 3H, 6-CH$_2$C$\underline{H_3}$);^{13}C-NMR (100 MHz, CDCl$_3$) δ 182.2, 179.8, 170.3, 158.6, 153.1, 151.2, 149.4, 144.0, 138.8 (2C), 137.1, 123.8 (2C), 119.3, 105.9, 104.3, 89.3, 31.8, 30.2, 29.1, 12.0; HRMS m/z 517.0372 (Calculated for C$_{21}$H$_{18}$IN$_4$O$_4$ [M + H]$^+$: 517.0373); purified in column chromatography with chloroform; yield: 94%.

The 6-ethyl-8-(ethylthio)-2,4-dimethylpyrimido[4,5-c]isoquinoline-1,3,7,10(2H,4H)-tetraone (**30**); Prepared from **3** and ethanethiol; orange solid; mp 171.3–172.8 °C; ^{1}H-NMR (400 MHz, CDCl$_3$) δ 6.67 (s, 1H, 9-H), 3.75 (s, 3H, 2-NCH$_3$), 3.46 (s, 3H, 4-NCH$_3$), 3.37 (q, J = 7.3 Hz, 2H, 6-C$\underline{H_2}$CH$_3$), 2.85 (q, J = 7.4 Hz, 2H, 8-S-C$\underline{H_2}$CH$_3$), 1.43 (t, J = 7.4 Hz, 3H,

8-S-CH$_2$CH$_3$), 1.33 (t, J = 7.3 Hz, 3H, 6-CH$_2$CH$_3$); ^{13}C-NMR (100 MHz, CDCl$_3$) δ 180.8, 180.7, 170.7, 158.5, 155.1, 152.7, 151.1, 147.1, 126.5, 120.8, 105.4, 31.7, 30.2, 29.1, 24.9, 12.5 12.1; HRMS m/z 360.1010 (Calculated for C$_{17}$H$_{18}$N$_3$O$_4$S [M + H]$^+$: 360.1018); purified in column chromatography with dichloromethane: ethyl acetate: petroleum ether = 15:3:4; yield: 48%.

The 6-ethyl-2,4-dimethyl-8-(propylthio)pyrimido[4,5-c]isoquinoline-1,3,7,10(2H,4H)-tetraone (**31**): Prepared from **3** and propane-1-thiol using general procedure B; orange solid; mp 163.8–164.9 °C; ^{1}H-NMR (400 MHz, CDCl$_3$) δ 6.68 (s, 1H, 9-H), 3.76 (s, 3H, 2-NCH$_3$), 3.48 (s, 3H, 4-NCH$_3$), 3.39 (q, J = 7.3 Hz, 2H, 6-CH$_2$CH$_3$), 2.81 (t, J =7.3 Hz, 2H, 8-S-CH$_2$CH$_2$CH$_3$), 1.82 (m, 2H, 8-S-CH$_2$CH$_2$CH$_3$), 1.35 (t, J =7.3 Hz, 3H, 6-CH$_2$CH$_3$), 1.11 (t, J =7.4 Hz, 3H, 8-S-CH$_2$CH$_2$CH$_3$); ^{13}C-NMR (100 MHz, CDCl$_3$) δ 180.84, 180.78, 170.7, 158.6, 155.4, 152.7, 151.1, 147.2, 126.5, 120,8, 105.4, 32.8, 31.7, 30.2, 29.1, 20.9, 13.7, 12.1; HRMS m/z 374.1172 (Calculated for C$_{18}$H$_{20}$N$_3$O$_4$S [M + H]$^+$: 374.1175); purified in column chromatography with dichloromethane: ethyl acetate: petroleum ether = 2:1:4; yield: 40%.

The 8-(butylthio)-6-ethyl-2,4-dimethylpyrimido[4,5-c]isoquinoline-1,3,7,10(2H,4H)-tetraone (**32**): Prepared from **3** and butane-1-thiol using general procedure B; orange solid; mp 158.8–160.5 °C; ^{1}H-NMR (400 MHz, CDCl$_3$) δ 6.67 (s, 1H, 9-H), 3.75 (s, 3H, 2-NCH$_3$), 3.46 (s, 3H, 4-NCH$_3$), 3.37 (q, J = 7.3 Hz, 2H, 6-CH$_2$CH$_3$), 2.82 (t, J = 7.4 Hz, 2H, 8-S-CH$_2$CH$_2$CH$_2$CH$_3$), 1.75 (dt, J = 15.0, J = 7.4 Hz, 2H, 8-S-CH$_2$CH$_2$CH$_2$CH$_3$),1.51 (dq, J = 14.6, J = 7.3 Hz, 2H, 8-CH$_2$CH$_2$CH$_2$CH$_3$), 1.34 (t, J = 7.3 Hz, 3H, 6-CH$_2$CH$_3$), 0.97 (t, J = 7.4 Hz, 3H, 8-CH$_2$CH$_2$CH$_2$CH$_3$); ^{13}C-NMR (100 MHz, CDCl$_3$) δ 180.82, 180.75, 170.7, 158.5, 155.4, 152.7, 151.1, 147.1, 126.4, 120.8, 105.4, 31.7, 30.6, 30.2, 29.3, 29.1, 22.2, 13.5, 12.1; HRMS m/z 388.1326 (Calculated for C$_{19}$H$_{22}$N$_3$O$_4$S [M + H]$^+$: 388.1331); purified in column chromatography with dichloromethane: ethyl acetate: petroleum ether = 4:0.5:3; yield: 58%.

The 8-pentylthio-6-ethyl-2,4-dimethyl-pyrimido[4,5-c]isoquinoline-1,3,7,10(2H,4H)-tetraone (**33**): Prepared from **3** and pentane-1-thiol using general procedure B; orange solid; mp 158.6–160.4 °C; ^{1}H-NMR (400 MHz, CDCl$_3$) δ 6.67 (s, 1H, 9-H), 3.75 (s, 3H, 2-NCH$_3$), 3.46 (s, 3H, 4-NCH$_3$), 3.37 (q, J = 7.3 Hz, 2H, 6-CH$_2$CH$_3$), 2.81 (t, J = 7.3 Hz, 2H, 8-S-CH$_2$CH$_2$CH$_2$CH$_3$), 1.77 (dt, J = 7.5, J = 7.4 Hz, 2H, 8-S-CH$_2$CH$_2$CH$_2$CH$_3$), 1.46 (dt, J = 14.2, J = 6.9 Hz, 2H, 8-S-CH$_2$CH$_2$CH$_2$CH$_2$CH$_3$), 1.37–1.28 (m, 5H, 6-CH$_2$CH$_3$ and 8-S-CH$_2$CH$_2$CH$_2$CH$_2$CH$_3$), 0.97 (t, J = 7.4 Hz, 3H, 8-S-CH$_2$CH$_2$CH$_2$CH$_2$CH$_3$); ^{13}C-NMR (100 MHz, CDCl$_3$) δ 180.95, 180.86, 170.81, 158.64, 155.54, 152.78, 151.23, 147.24, 126.54, 120.93, 105.51, 31.81, 31.26, 30.93, 30.27, 29.17, 27.14, 22.28, 13.99, 12.22; HRMS m/z 402.1483 (Calculated for C$_{20}$H$_{24}$N$_3$O$_4$S [M + H]$^+$: 402.1488); purified in column chromatography with dichloromethane: ethyl acetate: petroleum ether = 12:1:9; yield: 43%.

The 8-hexylthio-6-ethyl-2,4-dimethylpyrimido[4,5-c]isoquinoline-1,3,7,10(2H,4H)-tetraone (**34**): Prepared from **3** and hexane-1-thiol using general procedure B; orange solid; mp 134.6–137.0 °C; ^{1}H-NMR (400 MHz, CDCl$_3$) δ 6.65 (s, 1H, 9-H), 3.73 (s, 3H, 2-NCH$_3$), 3.44 (s, 3H, 4-NCH$_3$), 3.35 (q, J = 7,3 Hz, 2H, 6-CH$_2$CH$_3$), 2.80 (t, J = 7.3 Hz, 2H, 8-S-CH$_2$CH$_2$CH$_2$CH$_2$CH$_2$CH$_3$), 1.74 (q, J = 7.3 Hz, 2H, 8-S-CH$_2$CH$_2$CH$_2$CH$_2$CH$_2$CH$_3$), 1.47 (q, 2H, 8-CH$_2$CH$_2$CH$_2$CH$_2$CH$_2$CH$_3$), 1.47 (m, 4H, 8-CH$_2$CH$_2$CH$_2$CH$_2$CH$_2$CH$_3$ and 8-CH$_2$CH$_2$CH$_2$CH$_2$CH$_2$CH$_3$), 1.32 (t, J = 7.3 Hz, 3H, 6-CH$_2$CH$_3$), 0.88 (t, J = 7.3 Hz, 3H, 8-CH$_2$CH$_2$CH$_2$CH$_2$CH$_2$CH$_3$); ^{13}C-NMR (100 MHz, CDCl$_3$) δ 180.8, 180.7, 170.7, 158.4, 155.4, 152.5, 151.1, 147.1, 126.4, 120.8, 105.4, 31.7 31.2, 30.8, 30.1, 29.0, 28.7, 27.3, 22.5, 14.0, 12.1; HRMS m/z 402.1483 (Calculated for C$_{20}$H$_{24}$N$_3$O$_4$S [M + H]$^+$: 402.1488); purified in column chromatography with dichloromethane: ethyl acetate: petroleum ether = 2:1:4; yield: 52%.

The 6-ethyl-2,4-dimethyl-8,9-bis(phenylthio)pyrimido[4,5-c]isoquinoline-1,3,7,10(2H,4H)-tetraone (**35**): Prepared from **3** and benzenethiol using general procedure D; red solid; mp 188.9–191.5 °C; ^{1}H-NMR (400 MHz, CDCl$_3$) δ 7.58–7.54 (m, 2H, 8-C$_6$H$_5$ or 9-C$_6$H$_5$), 7.43–7.37 (m, 5H, 8-C$_6$H$_5$ or 9-C$_6$H$_5$), 7.34–7.27 (m, 3H, 8-C$_6$H$_5$ or 9-C$_6$H$_5$), 3.71 (s, 3H, 2-NCH$_3$), 3.31 (s, 3H, 4-NCH$_3$), 3.06 (q, J = 7.4 Hz, 2H, 6-CH$_2$CH$_3$), 1.13 (q, J = 7.4 Hz, 3H, 6-CH$_2$CH$_3$); ^{13}C-NMR (100 MHz, CDCl$_3$) δ 179.3, 176.8, 169.9, 157.6, 152.1, 151.1, 150.5, 147.7, 143.7, 133.3, 133.2 (2C), 131.2 (2C), 130.2, 129.4 (2C), 129.3 (2C), 128.9, 127.9, 122.1, 104.8, 31.0, 30.1, 28.8, 12.3; HRMS m/z 516.1058 (Calculated for C$_{27}$H$_{22}$N$_3$O$_4$S$_2$

[M + H]⁺: 516.1052); purified in column chromatography with dichloromethane: ethyl acetate: petroleum ether = 4:1:5; yield: 39%.

The 8,9-bis(4-chlorophenylthio)-6-ethyl-2,4-dimethylpyrimido[4,5-c]isoquinoline-1,3,7,10 (2H,4H)-tetraone (**36**): Prepared from **3** and 4-chlorobenzenethiol using general procedure D; brown solid; mp 207.8–209.8 °C; ^{1}H-NMR (400 MHz, CDCl$_3$) δ 7.49 (d, J = 8.5 Hz, 2H, 2″-H and 6″-H), 7.36 (d, J = 8.6 Hz, 2H, 3″-H and 5″-H), 7.35 (d, J = 8.7 Hz, 2H, 2′-H and 6′-H), 7.29 (d, J = 8.5 Hz, 2H, 3′-H and 5′-H), 3.71 (s, 3H, 2-NCH$_3$), 3.33 (s, 3H, 4-NCH$_3$), 3.10 (q, J = 7.3 Hz, 2H, 6-CH$_2$CH$_3$), 1.17 (t, J = 7.3 Hz, 3H, 6-CH$_2$CH$_3$); ^{13}C-NMR (100 MHz, CDCl$_3$) δ 179.4, 176.40, 170.1, 157.6, 152.1, 151.2, 151.0, 147.8, 142.3, 135.7, 134.8 (2C), 134.3, 132.6 (2C), 131.4, 129.7 (2C), 129.5 (2C), 128.2, 121.7, 104.8, 31.2, 30.1, 28.8, 12.3; HRMS m/z 584.0263 (Calculated for C$_{27}$H$_{20}$Cl$_2$N$_3$O$_4$S$_2$ [M + H]⁺: 548.0272); purified in column chromatography with dichloromethane: ethyl acetate: petroleum ether = 1:1:3; yield: 49%.

The 8,9-bis(propylthio)-6-ethyl-2,4-dimethyl-pyrimido[4,5-c]isoquinoline-1,3,7,10(2H,4H)-tetraone (**37**): Prepared from **3** and propane-1-thiol using general procedure D; red solid; mp 138.9–140.2 °C; ^{1}H-NMR (400 MHz, CDCl$_3$) δ 3.75 (s, 3H, 2-NCH3), 3.46 (s, 3H, 4-NCH3), 3.34 (q, J = 7.3 Hz, 2H, 6-CH$_2$CH$_3$), 3.27 (t, J = 7.2 Hz, 2H, 9-CH$_2$CH$_2$CH$_3$), 3.08 (t, J = 7.3 Hz, 2H, 8-CH$_2$CH$_2$CH$_3$), 1.76 (h, 2H, 9-CH$_2$CH$_2$CH$_3$), 1.60 (h, 2H, 8-CH$_2$CH$_2$CH$_3$), 1.33 (t, J = 7.3 Hz, 3H, 6-CH$_2$CH$_3$), 1.07 (t, J = 7.3 Hz, 3H, 9-CH$_2$CH$_2$CH$_3$), 1.00 (t, J = 7.3 Hz, 3H, 8-CH$_2$CH$_2$CH$_3$); ^{13}C-NMR (100 MHz, CDCl$_3$) δ 180.4, 176.6, 169.8, 158.6, 152.4, 151.8, 151.1, 148.7, 142.2, 122.0, 104.6, 36.0, 35.1, 31.2, 30.1, 28.9, 24.2, 23.9, 13.3, 13.1, 12.5; HRMS m/z 448.1365 (Calculated for C$_{21}$H$_{26}$N$_3$O$_4$S$_2$ [M + H]⁺: 448.1365); purified in column chromatography with dichloromethane: ethyl acetate: petroleum ether = 5:1:14; yield: 86%.

The 8-((2-bromo-4-chlorophenyl)thio)-6-ethyl-2,4-dimethylpyrimido[4,5-c]isoquinoline-1,3,7,10(2H,4H)-tetraone (**38**); Prepared from **3** and 2-bromo-4-chlorobenzenethiol using general procedure B; orange solid; mp 198.4–200.2 °C; ^{1}H-NMR (400 MHz, CDCl$_3$) δ 7.82 (d, J = 1.9 Hz, 1H, 3′-H), 7.59 (d, J = 8.3 Hz, 1H, 6′-H), 7.44 (dd, J = 8.3, J = 1.9 Hz, 1H, 5′-H), 6.06 (s, 1H, 9-H), 3,76 (s, 3H, 2-NCH$_3$), 3,44 (s, 3H, 4-NCH$_3$), 3.42 (q, J = 7.2 Hz, 2H, 6-CH$_2$CH$_3$), 1.37 (t, J = 7.2 Hz, 3H, 6-CH$_2$CH$_3$); ^{13}C-NMR (100 MHz, CDCl$_3$) δ 181.0, 180.5, 170.8, 158.3, 153.4, 152.8, 151.0, 147.1, 138.5, 138.2, 132.3, 131.2, 129.5, 128.0, 127.3, 120.5, 105.5, 31.7, 30.2, 29.1, 12.1; HRMS m/z 519.9739 (Calculated for C$_{21}$H$_{16}$BrClN$_3$O$_4$S [M + H]⁺: 519.9733); purified in column chromatography with dichloromethane: ethyl acetate: petroleum ether = 1:5:4; yield: 70%.

The 8-((2,6-dimethoxyphenyl)thio)-6-ethyl-2,4-dimethylpyrimido[4,5-c]isoquinoline-1,3,7,10(2H,4H)-tetraone (**39**): Prepared from **3** and 2,6-dimethoxybenzenethiol using general procedure B; red solid; mp 223.0–223.7 °C (d); ^{1}H-NMR (400 MHz, CDCl$_3$) δ 7.45 (t, J = 8.4 Hz, 1H, 4′-H), 6.66 (d, 2H, 3′-H and 5′-H), 6.07 (s, 1H, 9-H), 3.84 (s, 6H, 2′-OCH$_3$ and 6′-OCH$_3$), 3.74 (s, 3H, 2-NCH$_3$), 3.43 (s, 3H, 4-NCH$_3$), 3.41 (q, J = 7.2 Hz, 2H, 6-CH$_2$CH$_3$), 1.36 (t, J = 7.3 Hz, 3H, 6-CH$_2$CH$_3$); ^{13}C-NMR (100 MHz, CDCl$_3$) δ 181.3 (2C), 170.5, 161.3 (2C), 158.6, 154.1, 152.6, 151.1, 147.5, 133.2, 126.8, 121.0, 105.4, 104.5 (2C), 102.0, 56.4 (2C), 31.7, 30.2, 29.0, 12.2; HRMS m/z 468.1226 (Calculated for C$_{23}$H$_{22}$N$_3$O$_6$S [M + H]⁺: 468.1229); purified in column chromatography with dichloromethane: ethyl acetate: petroleum ether = 9:1:3; yield: 63%.

The 8-((5-bromo-2-methoxyphenyl)thio)-6-ethyl-2,4-dimethylpyrimido[4,5-c]isoquinoline-1,3,7,10(2H,4H)-tetraone (**40**): Prepared from **3** and 5-bromo-2-methoxybenzenethiol using general procedure B; orange solid; mp 221.0–222.0 °C (d); ^{1}H-NMR (400 MHz, CDCl$_3$) δ 7.63 (q, J = 2.4 Hz, 1H, 6′-H), 7.61 (d, J = 8.7, J = 2.6 Hz, 1H, 4′-H), 6.93 (d, J = 8.6 Hz, 1H, 3′-H), 6.11 (s, 1H, 9-H), 3.85 (s, 3H, 2′-OCH$_3$), 3.75 (s, 3H, 2-NCH$_3$), 3.44 (s, 3H, 4-NCH$_3$), 3.41 (q, J = 7.2 Hz, 2H, 6-CH$_2$CH$_3$), 1.36 (t, J = 7.3 Hz, 3H, 6-CH$_2$CH$_3$); ^{13}C-NMR (100 MHz, CDCl$_3$) δ 181.2, 180.8, 170.7, 159.2, 158.4, 153.8, 152.7, 151.1, 147.2, 139.5, 135.7, 127.7, 120.7, 116.7, 113.5, 113.3, 105.4, 56.4, 31.7, 30.2, 29.1, 12.1; HRMS m/z 516.0237 (Calculated for C$_{22}$H$_{19}$BrN$_3$O$_5$S [M + H]⁺: 516.0229); purified in column chromatography with dichloromethane: ethyl acetate: petroleum ether = 20:1:4; yield: 76%.

The 8-((3,5-dichlorophenyl)thio)-6-ethyl-2,4-dimethylpyrimido[4,5-c]isoquinoline-1,3,7,10 (2H,4H)-tetraone (**41**): Prepared from **3** and 3,5-dichlorobenzenethiol using general procedure B; yellow solid; mp 179.8–182.0 °C; ^{1}H-NMR (400 MHz, CDCl$_3$) δ 7.44 (s, 2H, 2'-H and 6'-H), 7.52 (s, 1H, 4'-H); 6.24 (s, 1H, 9-H), 3.75 (s, 3H, 2-NCH$_3$), 3.43 (s, 3H, 4-NCH$_3$), 3.40 (q, J = 7.3 Hz, 2H, 6-C$\underline{H_2}$CH$_3$), 1.36 (t, J = 7.3 Hz, 3H, 6-CH$_2$C$\underline{H_3}$); ^{13}C-NMR (100 MHz, CDCl$_3$) δ 181.1, 180.3, 170.9, 158.6, 145.9, 152.8, 151.0, 147.0, 136.6, 133.6 (2C), 131.1, 130.5, 128.4 (2C), 120.3, 105.5, 31.7, 30.2, 29.1, 12.1; HRMS m/z 476.0235 (Calculated for C$_{21}$H$_{16}$Cl$_2$N$_3$O$_4$S [M + H]$^+$: 476.0239); purified in column chromatography with dichloromethane: ethyl acetate: petroleum ether = 20:1:7; yield: 69%.

The 8-phenylthio-2,4,6-trimethyl-pyrimido[4,5-c]isoquinoline-1,3,7,10 (2H,4H)-tetraone (**42**): Prepared from **4** and benzenethiol using general procedure B; yellow solid; mp 206.0–208.0 °C (d); ^{1}H-NMR (400 MHz, CDCl$_3$) δ 7.53 (m. 5H, 2'-H, 3'-H, 4'-H, 5'-H and 6'-H), 6.18 (s, 1H, 9-H), 3.74 (s, 3H, 2-NCH$_3$), 3.43 (s, 3H, 4-NCH$_3$), 3.01 (s, 3H, 6-CH$_3$); ^{13}C-NMR (100 MHz, CDCl$_3$) δ 181.1, 180.9, 166.3, 158.3, 156.5, 152.7, 151.0, 146.9, 135.7 (2C), 130.7, 130.5 (2C), 128.1, 127.1, 120.9, 105.7, 30.2, 29.1, 26.9; HRMS m/z 394.0862 (Calculated for C$_{20}$H$_{16}$N$_3$O$_4$S [M + H]$^+$: 394.0862); purified in column chromatography with dichloromethane: ethyl acetate: petroleum ether = 12:1:8; yield: 65%.

The 8-(4-methoxy-phenylthio)-2,4,6-trimethylpyrimido[4,5-c]isoquinoline-1,3,7,10(2H,4H)-tetraone (**43**): Prepared from **4** and 4-methoxybenzenethiol using general procedure B; orange solid; mp 198.0–199.0 °C (d); ^{1}H-NMR (400 MHz, CDCl$_3$) δ 7.43 (d. 2H, 3'-H and 5'-H), 7.02 (d. 2H, 2'-H and 6'-H), 6.16 (s, 1H, 9-H), 3.86 (s, 3H, 4'-OCH$_3$), 3.73 (s, 3H, 2-NCH$_3$), 3.43 (s, 3H, 4-NCH$_3$), 3.00 (s, 3H, 6-CH$_3$); ^{13}C-NMR (100 MHz, CDCl$_3$) δ 181.2, 181.0, 166.2, 161.6, 158.3, 157.3, 152.6, 151.0, 147.0, 137.2 (2C), 128.0, 121.0, 117.2, 116.1 (2C), 105.7, 55.5, 30.2, 29.0, 26.9; HRMS m/z 424.0963 (Calculated for C$_{21}$H$_{18}$N$_3$O$_5$S [M + H]$^+$: 424.0967); purified in column chromatography with dichloromethane: ethyl acetate: petroleum ether = 3:1:4; yield: 69%.

The 8-((4-fluorophenyl)thio)-2,4,6-trimethylpyrimido[4,5-c]isoquinoline-1,3,7,10(2H,4H)-tetraone (**44**): Prepared from **4** and 4-fluorobenzenethiol using general procedure B; yellow solid; mp 211.0–212.0 °C (d); ^{1}H-NMR (400 MHz, CDCl$_3$) δ 7.52 (dd, $J_{H,H}$ = 8.7, $J_{H,H}$ = 5.2 Hz, 2H, 2'-H and 6'-H), 7.21 (t, $J_{H,H}$ = 8.5, $J_{F,H}$ = 8.5 Hz, 2H, 3'-H and 5'-H), 6.15 (s, 1H, 9-H), 3.73 (s, 3H, 2-NCH$_3$), 3.43 (s, 3H, 4-NCH$_3$), 3.01 (s, 3H, 6-CH$_3$); ^{13}C-NMR (100 MHz, CDCl$_3$) δ 181.2, 180.9, 166.4, 164.4 (d, 1C, $J_{F,C}$ = 252.9 Hz, 4'), 158.4, 156.4, 152.8, 151.1, 146.9, 138.0 (d, 2C, $J_{F,C}$ = 8.8 Hz, 2' and 6'), 128.2, 122.5 (d, 1C, $J_{F,C}$ = 3.6 Hz, 1'), 121.0, 118.0 (d, 2C, $J_{F,C}$ = 22.1 Hz, 3' and 5'), 105.8, 30.4, 29.2, 27.0; HRMS m/z 412.0771 (Calculated for C$_{20}$H$_{15}$FN$_3$O$_4$S [M + H]$^+$: 412.0767); purified in column chromatography with dichloromethane: ethyl acetate: petroleum ether = 1:1:2; yield: 69%.

5.3. Crystallography

5.3.1. Preparation of Single Crystals

Single crystals were grown by solvent evaporation at room temperature from the synthesis products. Crystals suitable for X-ray diffraction studies were obtained from crystallization in saturated solutions: tetrahydropyran for **7** and benzene for **16**.

5.3.2. Single Crystal X-ray Diffraction

Crystals were prepared under inert conditions and immersed in perfluoropolyether as a protective oil for manipulation. Suitable crystals were mounted on MiTeGen Micromounts^{TM}, and these samples were used for data collection. Data were collected with a D8 Venture diffractometer CuKα, 298 K (Bruker, Karlsruhe, Germany). The data were processed with the APEX3 program [22] and corrected for absorption using SADABS [23]. The structures were resolved using direct methods [24], which revealed the position of all nonhydrogen atoms. These atoms were refined on F2 by a full-matrix least-squares procedure using anisotropic displacement parameters. All hydrogen atoms were located in different Fourier maps and were included as fixed contributions riding on attached atoms with isotropic thermal displacement parameters 1.2 (C–H) or 1.5 (methyl) times those of the respective atom. CCDC 2023040 (Compound **38**), CCDC 2023047 (Compound **30**), CCDC 2023048 (Compound **27**), CCDC 2023049 (Compound **28**), CCDC 2023045 (Compound **P7**), CCDC

2023064 (Compound **32**), and CCDC 2023061 (Compound **23**) contain the crystallographic data listed in Table S1 and Figures S5–S11. These data can be obtained free of charge from the Cambridge Crystallographic Data Centre.

5.4. Images of 3D-Models

We processed with the BIOVIA Discovery Studio Visualizer software [25] from the .cif files. The 3D models were superimposed considering the quinone tricyclic core as temperate. The dihedral angle was measured by the same software. The images were created with the script/Visualization/Publication Quality.

5.5. Evaluation of Antibacterial Activity

Antimicrobial activity in vitro against *Staphylococcus aureus* methicillin-susceptible strain (ATCC® 29213), *Staphylococcus aureus* methicillin-susceptible strain (ATCC® 43300), *Enterococcus faecalis* (ATCC® 29212), *Escherichia coli* (ATCC® 25922), *Pseudomonas aeruginosa* (ATCC® 25923), and *Klebsiella pneumoniae* (ATCC® 700603) were investigated by minimum inhibitory concentration (MIC) of a broth microdilution method, according to recommendations of the Clinical and Laboratory Standards Institute (CLSI) [26]. All compounds tested were dissolved in dimethyl sulfoxide (DMSO) to levels not exceeding 1% per well. Vancomycin and gentamicin were used as references against the strains, and the results were compared to the MIC ranges reported by the CLSI as a quality control measure [19]. In addition, one well in each plate with medium without antibiotics was used as a positive control for bacterial growth. We also used a well containing only medium without the bacterial inoculum as a sterility control of the procedure. The compounds were tested from the maximum concentration reached and standard drugs since 16 µg/mL. The inoculum was prepared to a turbidity equivalent of an 0.5 McFarland standard, diluted in broth media to give a final concentration of 5×10^5 CFU/mL in the test tray; they were covered and placed in plastic bags to prevent evaporation. The plates were incubated at 35 °C for 18–20 h. The MIC was defined as the lowest concentration of the compound giving complete inhibition of visible growth. All experiments were performed three times in triplicate.

6. Patents

PatentWO2017113031A1, PCT/CL2015003780A1, USAUS11390622B2, EPO EP3404026A4; China CN109121411B. MX/a/2018/008192A titled: "Pyrimidine-Isoquinoline-Quinone Derived Compounds, their Salts, Isomers, Pharmaceutically Acceptable Tautomers; Pharmaceutical Composition; Preparation Procedure; and their Use in the Treatment of Bacterial and Multi-Resistant Bacterial Diseases".

Supplementary Materials: The following supporting information can be downloaded at: https://www.mdpi.com/article/10.3390/antibiotics12061065/s1, Figures S1–S4: General procedures A to D, Table S1: Crystallographic data. Figures S5–S11: Diagrams and crystallographic parameters.

Author Contributions: Conceptualization, J.A.-L. and D.V.-V.; formal analysis, J.A.-L., J.C.-S., A.P.-R., D.C.-L. and H.P.-M.; funding acquisition, D.V.-V.; investigation, J.A.-L., J.C.-S., A.P.-R., J.M. and D.V.-V.; methodology, J.A.-L., J.C.-S., J.M., D.C.-L. and H.P.-M.; resources, J.A.-L., J.C.-S. and D.V.-V.; supervision, J.A.-L.; validation, J.M. and P.P.Z.; visualization, J.C.-S.; writing—original draft, J.A.-L. and D.V.-V.; writing—review and editing, J.A.-L., J.C.-S., J.M., P.P.Z., H.P.-M., I.B. and D.V.-V All authors have read and agreed to the published version of the manuscript.

Funding: This research was funded by FONDECYT No. 11110516, Iniciación en Investigación, Chile; FONDECYT Regular No. 1191737 (IEB) and FONDECYT No. 79100006, Proyecto de Inserción, Chile, and Programa de Estímulo a la Excelencia Institucional PEEI 2017, Universidad de Chile.

Institutional Review Board Statement: Not applicable.

Informed Consent Statement: Not applicable.

Data Availability Statement: Thesis report for the degree of Pharmaceutical Chemist of A.P.-R. https://bibliotecadigital.uchile.cl/permalink/56UDC_INST/llitqr/alma991002956919703936 (accessed on 31 May 2023); Doctoral thesis report of J.A.-L. Link not available due to restricted circulation period.

Acknowledgments: The authors, J.A.L. and J.C.S., thank the CONICYT Beca Doctorado Nacional No. 21130628 and No. 21130643, respectively.

Conflicts of Interest: The authors declare no conflict of interest.

References

1. World Health Organization. *Antimicrobial Resistance: Global Report on Surveillance*; World Health Organization: Geneva, Switzerland, 2014. Available online: https://apps.who.int/iris/handle/10665/112642 (accessed on 15 May 2023).
2. O'Neill, J.I.M. Antimicrobial resistance: Tackling a crisis for the health and wealth of nations. In *Review on Antimicrobial Resistance*; HM Government: London, UK, 2014.
3. Solomon, S.L.; Oliver, K.B. Antibiotic resistance threats in the United States: Stepping back from the brink. *Am. Fam. Physician* **2014**, *89*, 938–941. [PubMed]
4. Renwick, M.; Mossialos, E. What are the economic barriers of antibiotic R&D and how can we overcome them? *Expert Opin. Drug Discov.* **2018**, *13*, 889–892. [PubMed]
5. Spellberg, B.; Guidos, R.; Gilbert, D.; Bradley, J.; Boucher, H.W.; Scheld, W.M.; Bartlett, J.G.; Edwards, J.J. The Epidemic of Antibiotic-Resistant Infections: A Call to Action for the Medical Community from the Infectious Diseases Society of America. *Clin. Infect. Dis.* **2008**, *46*, 155–164. [CrossRef] [PubMed]
6. Norrby, S.R.; Nord, C.E.; Finch, R. Lack of development of new antimicrobial drugs: A potential serious threat to public health. *Lancet Infect. Dis.* **2005**, *5*, 115–119. [CrossRef] [PubMed]
7. White, J.A.C.; Atmar, R.L.; Wilson, J.; Cate, T.R.; Stager, C.E.; Greenberg, S.B. Effects of Requiring prior Authorization for Selected Antimicrobials: Expenditures, Susceptibilities, and Clinical Outcomes. *Clin. Infect. Dis.* **1997**, *25*, 230–239. [CrossRef] [PubMed]
8. McGowan, J.E.; Finland, M. Usage of Antibiotics in a General Hospital: Effect of Requiring Justification. *J. Infect. Dis.* **1974**, *130*, 165–168. [CrossRef] [PubMed]
9. Campanini-Salinas, J.; Andrades-Lagos, J.; Mella-Raipan, J.; Vasquez-Velasquez, D. Novel Classes of Antibacterial Drugs in Clinical Development, a Hope in a Post-antibiotic Era. *Curr. Top. Med. Chem.* **2018**, *18*, 1188–11202. [CrossRef] [PubMed]
10. World Health Organization. *2021 Antibacterial Agents in Clinical and Preclinical Development: An Overview and Análisis*; World Health Organization: Geneva, Switzerland, 2022.
11. Mullard, A. 2022 FDA approvals. *Nat. Rev. Drug Discov.* **2023**, *22*, 83–88. [CrossRef] [PubMed]
12. Simpkin, V.L.; Renwick, M.J.; Kelly, R.; Mossialos, E. Incentivising innovation in antibiotic drug discovery and development: Progress, challenges and next steps. *J. Antibiot.* **2017**, *70*, 1087–1096. [CrossRef] [PubMed]
13. Campanini-Salinas, J.; Andrades-Lagos, J.; Rocha, G.G.; Choquesillo-Lazarte, D.; Dragnic, S.B.; Faúndez, M.; Alarcón, P.; Silva, F.; Vidal, R.; Salas-Huenuleo, E.; et al. A New Kind of Quinonic-Antibiotic Useful Against Multidrug-Resistant *S. aureus* and *E. faecium* Infections. *Molecules* **2018**, *23*, 1776. [CrossRef] [PubMed]
14. Campanini-Salinas, J.; Andrades-Lagos, J.; Hinojosa, N.; Moreno, F.; Alarcón, P.; González-Rocha, G.; Burbulis, I.E.; Vásquez-Velásquez, D. New Quinone Antibiotics against Methicillin-Resistant *S. aureus*. *Antibiotics* **2021**, *10*, 614. [CrossRef] [PubMed]
15. Valderrama, J.A.; Colonelli, P.; Vásquez, D.; González, M.F.; Rodríguez, J.A.; Theoduloz, C. Studies on quinones. Part 44: Novel angucyclinone N-heterocyclic analogues endowed with antitumoral activity. *Bioorg. Med. Chem.* **2008**, *16*, 10172–10181. [CrossRef] [PubMed]
16. Pratt, Y.T. Quinolinequinones. VI. Reactions with Aromatic Amines. *J. Org. Chem.* **1962**, *27*, 3905–3910. [CrossRef]
17. Wang, Z. Béchamp Reduction. In *Comprehensive Organic Name Reactions and Reagents*; Wang, Z., Ed.; Wiley Library: Hoboken, NJ, USA, 2010.
18. Valderrama, J.A.; Ibacache, J.A. Regiochemical control in the amination reaction of phenanthridine-7,10-quinones. *Tetrahedron Lett.* **2009**, *50*, 4361–4363. [CrossRef]
19. Patel, J.B. *Performance Standards for Antimicrobial Susceptibility Testing; Twenty-Fifth Informational Supplement*; Clinical & Laboratory Standards Institute: Wayne, PA, USA, 2015.
20. Craig, P.N. Interdependence between physical parameters and selection of substituent groups for correlation studies. *J. Med. Chem.* **1971**, *14*, 680–684. [CrossRef] [PubMed]
21. Free, S.M.; Wilson, J.W. A Mathematical Contribution to Structure–Activity Studies. *J. Med. Chem.* **1964**, *7*, 395–399. [CrossRef] [PubMed]
22. Francart, T.; van Wieringen, A.; Wouters, J. APEX 3: A multi-purpose test platform for auditory psychophysical experiments. *J. Neurosci. Methods* **2008**, *172*, 283–293. [CrossRef] [PubMed]
23. Sheldrick, G.M.S. *Bruker/Siemens Area Detector Absorption Correction Program*; SADABS: Madison, WI, USA, 2012.
24. Sheldrick, G.M. A short history of *SHELX*. *Acta Crystallogr. A* **2008**, *64*, 112–122. [CrossRef] [PubMed]

25. Biovia, D.S. *Discovery Studio Visualizer*; Dassault Systèmes: San Diego, CA, USA, 2020.
26. Cockerill, F.R. *Methods for Dilution Antimicrobial Susceptibility Tests for Bacteria that Grow Aerobically: Approved Standard*; Clinical and Laboratory Standards Institute: Wayne, PA, USA, 2012.

Disclaimer/Publisher's Note: The statements, opinions and data contained in all publications are solely those of the individual author(s) and contributor(s) and not of MDPI and/or the editor(s). MDPI and/or the editor(s) disclaim responsibility for any injury to people or property resulting from any ideas, methods, instructions or products referred to in the content.

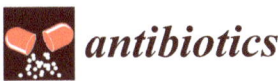

Article

Synthesis, Characterization, Cytotoxicity Analysis and Evaluation of Novel Heterocyclic Derivatives of Benzamidine against Periodontal Disease Triggering Bacteria

Ramasamy Kavitha [1], Mohammad Auwal Sa'ad [1,2], Shivkanya Fuloria [3], Neeraj Kumar Fuloria [3,4,*], Manickam Ravichandran [1,2,5,*] and Pattabhiraman Lalitha [6]

[1] Department of Biotechnology, Faculty of Applied Science, AIMST University, Bedong 08100, Kedah, Malaysia
[2] Centre of Excellence for Vaccine Development (CoEVD), Faculty of Applied Science, AIMST University, Bedong 08100, Kedah, Malaysia
[3] Centre of Excellence for Biomaterials Engineering, Faculty of Pharmacy, AIMST University, Bedong 08100, Kedah, Malaysia
[4] Center for Transdisciplinary Research, Department of Pharmacology, Saveetha Institute of Medical and Technical Sciences, Saveetha Dental College and Hospital, Saveetha University, Chennai 600077, Tamil Nadu, India
[5] Mygenome, ALPS Global Holding, Kuala Lumpur 50400, Malaysia
[6] Department of Biochemistry, Faculty of Medicine, AIMST University, Bedong 08100, Kedah, Malaysia
* Correspondence: neerajkumar@aimst.edu.my (N.K.F.); ravichandran@aimst.edu.my (M.R.)

Abstract: Periodontal disease (PD) is multifactorial oral disease that damages tooth-supporting tissue. PD treatment includes proper oral hygiene, deep cleaning, antibiotics therapy, and surgery. Despite the availability of basic treatments, some of these are rendered undesirable in PD treatment due to side effects and expense. Therefore, the aim of the present study is to develop novel molecules to combat the PD triggering pathogens. The study involved the synthesis of 4-((5-(substituted-phenyl)-1,3,4-oxadiazol-2-yl)methoxy)benzamidine (**5a-e**), by condensation of 2-(4-carbamimidoylphenoxy)acetohydrazide (**3**) with different aromatic acids; and synthesis of 4-((4-(substituted benzylideneamino)-4H-1,2,4-triazol-3-yl)methoxy)benzamidine (**6a-b**) by treatment of **compound 3** with CS_2 followed by hydrazination and a Schiff reaction with different aromatic aldehydes. Synthesized **compounds** were characterized based on the NMR, FTIR, and mass spectrometric data. To assess the effectiveness of the newly synthesized **compound** in PD, new **compounds** were subjected to antimicrobial evaluation against *P. gingivalis* and *E. coli* using the micro-broth dilution method. Synthesized **compounds** were also subjected to cytotoxicity evaluation against HEK-293 cells using an MTT assay. The present study revealed the successful synthesis of heterocyclic derivatives of benzamidine with significant inhibitory potential against *P. gingivalis* and *E. coli*. Synthesized **compounds** exhibited minimal to the absence of cytotoxicity. Significant antimicrobial potential and least/no cytotoxicity of new heterocyclic analogs of benzamidine against PD-triggering bacteria supports their potential application in PD treatment.

Keywords: periodontal disease; periodontitis; heterocyclics; antibacterial; benzamidine

1. Introduction

Periodontal disease (PD) is a noncommunicable oral inflammatory disease that affects the tissue of the teeth, causing severe damage to the periodontal ligament, leading to tooth loss and reducing the quality of life [1]. PD affects around 11% of the global population [2]. Risk factors such as osteoporosis, metabolic disorder, diabetes, and obesity are strongly linked with chronic PD; however, lifestyle (smoking, alcohol consumption, and poor oral hygiene), poor dietary vitamin D, and calcium intake also play a role [3]. Increasing evidence showed that there is a link between PD and other ailments such as

Citation: Kavitha, R.; Sa'ad, M.A.; Fuloria, S.; Fuloria, N.K.; Ravichandran, M.; Lalitha, P. Synthesis, Characterization, Cytotoxicity Analysis and Evaluation of Novel Heterocyclic Derivatives of Benzamidine against Periodontal Disease Triggering Bacteria. *Antibiotics* **2023**, *12*, 306. https://doi.org/10.3390/antibiotics12020306

Academic Editor: Charlotte A. Huber

Received: 13 January 2023
Revised: 30 January 2023
Accepted: 31 January 2023
Published: 2 February 2023

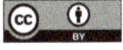

Copyright: © 2023 by the authors. Licensee MDPI, Basel, Switzerland. This article is an open access article distributed under the terms and conditions of the Creative Commons Attribution (CC BY) license (https://creativecommons.org/licenses/by/4.0/).

respiratory infections, adverse pregnancy outcomes, cardiovascular diseases, chronic kidney disease, diabetes, cancer, Alzheimer's, and Parkinson's disease [4–8]. The onset and progression of PD are associated with the synergy among the organisms found in the microbiota, which then interacts with the host immune defense, leading to severe oral inflammation [9]. The oral microbiota is composed of several organisms that are important in the regulation and protection of the oral cavity against the colonization of non-essential organisms. However, dysregulation of these organisms can cause gingivitis which has the potential to progress to PD [10]. PD is known to be associated with diverse species of bacteria, especially *P. gingivalis* and *E. coli* [11,12]; that are strongly linked to and implicated in the initial onset, progression, and severity of PD and its associated systemic diseases [13,14]. The strategies for prevention and treatment of PD are relatively simple, yet difficult to apply. The reduction of risk factors, the use of probiotic agents, and antioxidants, along with mechanical treatment (scaling) and/or a combination of antibiotics such as metronidazole and amoxicillin or metronidazole and ciprofloxacin can greatly contribute to the reduction or elimination of periodontal associated pathogens [15,16]. Furthermore, they aid the treatment of PD associated systemic diseases [17,18]. Although the systematic adjuvant use of mechanical and combination of antibiotics is the best strategy now, other evidence showed that *P. gingivalis* and its related pathogens are developing resistance to commonly available antibiotics and rendering them less effective by degradation using their virulence factors [19–22]. Concerning antibiotic resistance, an alternative treatment strategy for periodontal pathogens is the use of synthetic inhibitors. Recent evidence showed that synthetic molecules have the potential to ease the burden of oral infections caused by *P. gingivalis* with no significant cytotoxicity observed [23,24]. Facts suggest that incorporation of heterocyclic groups into the organic moieties enhances their biological potential [25,26]. A study reported that benzamidine and its derivatives displayed inhibition against gingipains, a major virulence factor produced by *P. gingivalis* [27]. Our previous study showed that benzamidine and its derivatives (ester, hydrazides, and Schiff bases) inhibit *P. gingivalis* and its associated pathogens [12]. Recent studies showed effectiveness of oxadiazoles and triazoles against periodontitis triggering pathogens [28–30]. To combat antibiotic resistance, oxadiazoles have been used due to their sensitive antimicrobial activity [31]. Hence, based on the severity of PD, associated pathogens and their resistance, potential of benzamidine analogs against PD, and the enhancement of inhibitory potential by incorporation of oxadiazoles and triazoles groups in different chemical moieties, researchers are motivated to perform the synthesis, characterization, cytotoxicity analysis, and evaluation of novel heterocyclic derivatives (oxadiazoles and triazoles) of benzamidine against periodontal-disease-triggering bacteria. In the continuation of a previous study, our present study highlights that the synthesis of new oxadiazole and triazole derivatives of benzamidine analogs possess high inhibition potential against triggering bacteria, which makes them the forefront of potential PD treatment.

2. Materials and Methods

2.1. General Information

The reagents, solvents, and chemicals used for the synthesis of compounds in the present study were acquired from Sigma-Aldrich Co. (St. Louis, MO, USA), HmbG® Chemicals, Hamburg, Germany, Friendemann Schmidt Chemical, Washington, DC, USA, Merck KGaA (Darmstadt, Germany), and Qrec Chemicals, Rawang, Malaysia. The Ashless Whattman No. 1 filter paper was used for filtration. To verify compounds' purity, the open capillary tube method was used. The melting points of all synthesized compounds were determined using SMP11 Analogue apparatus. The compounds' characterization was recorded by ^{1}H-NMR and ^{13}C-NMR (NMR 700 MHz ASCEND™ spectrometer) using deuterated DMSO solvent, on a δ value scale as the downfield chemical shift in ppm against tetramethylsilane (TMS). The NMR signals are stated as s, single; d, doublet; t, triplet; m, multiplet. The IR of synthesized compounds was recorded using a Jasco ft/ir-6700 instrument in a wavelength range of 400–4000 cm^{-1}. The analysis of mass spectra was recorded from a Direct Infusion IonTrap MS Full Scan (Thermo Scientific Q Exactive HF-X hybrid quadrupole-Orbitrap mass spectrometer, Waltham, MA, USA). Elemental analysis was performed on a Perkin Elmer 240 B and 240 C. Elemental analysis (C, H, N), indicated by employing element symbols, was within ±0.4% of theoretical values. The purity of compounds and monitoring of reactions were assessed by TLC on aluminum sheets with silica gel 60 F254 (0.2 mm) (Merck Millipore, Darmstadt, Germany) using methanol: chloroform (0.3: 1.7) as a solvent system in a UV chamber using a SPRECTROLINE® CM-26 UV viewing chamber. The 4-hydroxybenzenecarboximidamide analogs were synthesized as per the protocol given by previous authors with slight modifications [32–36].

2.2. Synthesis

2.2.1. General Procedure for the Synthesis of 4-((5-(Substituted-phenyl)-1,3,4-oxadiazol-2-yl)methoxy)benzamidine (5a-e)

To synthesize the oxadiazole derivatives of benzamidine (5a-e), an equal molar concentration of **compound (3)** (0.02 M) and 3-phenoxy benzoic acid was dissolved in 10 mL of phosphoryl chloride and refluxed for 8 h. At the end, the mixture was cooled, washed with ice, filtered, and recrystallized to obtain the pure **compound 5a**. The synthetic scheme for synthesis of **compound 5a-e** is given in Figure 1. During the experiment, anhydrous reaction conditions were maintained, and the recrystallization was done using methanol and activated charcoal. The synthesized **compound 5a** was further characterized based on the spectrometric data (Figures S1–S4). Similarly, other **compounds 5b-e** were synthesized, purified, and characterized.

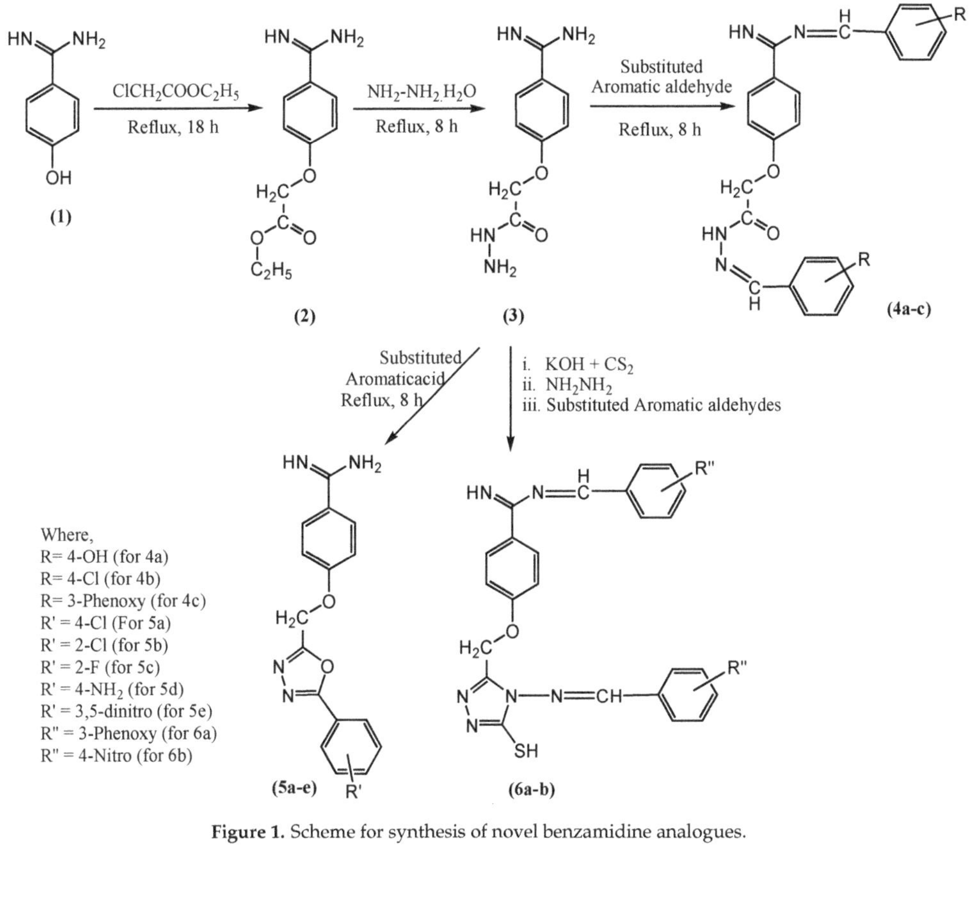

Where,
R= 4-OH (for 4a)
R= 4-Cl (for 4b)
R= 3-Phenoxy (for 4c)
R' = 4-Cl (For 5a)
R' = 2-Cl (for 5b)
R' = 2-F (for 5c)
R' = 4-NH$_2$ (for 5d)
R' = 3,5-dinitro (for 5e)
R'' = 3-Phenoxy (for 6a)
R'' = 4-Nitro (for 6b)

Figure 1. Scheme for synthesis of novel benzamidine analogues.

4-((5-(4-Chlorophenyl)-1,3,4-oxadiazol-2-yl)methoxy)benzamidine (5a)

White crystalline (Yield 73%, m.p. 184 °C); IR (KBr, cm^{-1}): 3051 (Aromatic C–H), 2978 (Aliphatic H–C), 1681 (C=N), 1591, 1425 (Aromatic C=C), 1238, 1066 (C–O–C of oxadiazole ring); ^{1}H-NMR (DMSO-d_6, ppm) δ: 3.21 (s, 2H, O–CH$_2$), 3.71 (brs, 2H, NH$_2$), 7.25–7.79 (m, 8H, Ar–H), 8.41 (s, 1H, C=NH); and ^{13}C–NMR (DMSO, ppm) δ: 68.17 (CH$_2$), 122.93, 128.35, 128.88, 129.29, 130.79, 130.95, 131.432, 133.62, 138.86 (Ar-C), 167.47 (C=N); Mass (m/z): Calcd. 328.75, found 328.4; Anal. Calcd. for C$_{16}$H$_{13}$ClN$_4$O$_2$: C, 58.45; H, 3.99; N, 17.04%, Found: C, 58.53; H, 3.91; N, 17.12%.

4-((5-(2-Chlorophenyl)-1,3,4-oxadiazol-2-yl)methoxy)benzamidine (5b)

Beige crystalline (Yield 70%, m.p. 124 °C); IR (KBr, cm^{-1}): 3065 (Aromatic C–H), 2998, 2888 (Aliphatic C–H), 1682 (C=N), 1569, 1474 (Aromatic C=C), 1265, 1043 (C–O–C of oxadiazole ring); ^{1}H-NMR (DMSO-d_6, ppm) δ: 3.21 (s, 2H, O–CH$_2$), 3.72 (brs, 2H, NH$_2$), 7.46–7.83 (m, 8H, Ar-H), 8.12 (s, 1H, C=NH); ^{13}C-NMR (DMSO, ppm) δ: δ 68.18 (O–CH$_2$), 122.51, 127.64, 131.01, 131.17, 131.50, 131.97, 132.07, 132.93 (Ar-C), 167.24 (C=N); Mass (m/z): Calcd. 328.75, found 328.5; Anal. Calcd. for C$_{16}$H$_{13}$ClN$_4$O$_2$: C, 58.45; H, 3.99; N, 17.04%, Found: C, 58.58; H, 3.93; N, 17.16%.

4-((5-(2-Fluorophenyl)-1,3,4-oxadiazol-2-yl)methoxy)benzamidine (5c)

Light brown crystalline (Yield 75%, m.p. 138 °C); IR (KBr, cm^{-1}): 3051 (Aromatic C–H), 2917 (Aliphatic C–H), 1675 (C=N), 1508, 1426 (Aromatic C=C), 1292, 1067 (C–O–C of oxadiazole ring); ^{1}H-NMR (DMSO-d_6, ppm) δ: 3.20 (s, 2H, CH$_2$), 3.49 (brs, 2H, NH$_2$), 7.30–8.01 (m, 8H, Ar-H), 8.01 (s, 1H, C=NH); ^{13}C-NMR (DMSO, ppm) δ: 68.44 (O-CH$_2$), 115.99, 117.20, 122.63, 123.90, 127.79, 128.77, 129.87, 131.40, 132.35, 134.56 (Ar–C), 164.67 (C=N); Mass (m/z): Calcd. 312.3, found 312.1; Anal. Calcd. for C$_{16}$H$_{13}$FN$_4$O$_2$: C, 61.53; H, 4.20; N, 17.94%, Found: C, 61.61; H, 4.25; N, 17.88%.

4-((5-(4-Aminophenyl)-1,3,4-oxadiazol-2-yl)methoxy)benzamidine (5d)

Brown crystalline (Yield 70%, m.p. 134 °C); IR (KBr, cm^{-1}): 3229 (N–H), 3065 (Aromatic C–H), 2918 (Aliphatic C–H), 1653 (C=N), 1593, 1407 (Aromatic C=C), 1243, 1062 (C–O–C of oxadiazole ring); ^{1}H-NMR (DMSO-d_6, ppm) δ: 3.22 (s, 2H, O-CH$_2$), 3.70–4.20 (brs, 4H, NH$_2$ and Ar–NH$_2$), 7.03–8.11 (m, 8H, Ar-H), 8.12 (s, 1H, C=NH); ^{13}C-NMR (DMSO, ppm) δ: 68.11 (O-CH2), 113.06, 116.17, 119.70, 120.03, 123.24, 130.09, 130.62, 131.82 (Ar–C), 167.19 (C=N); Mass (m/z): Calcd. 384.3, found 384.10; Anal. Calcd. for C$_{16}$H$_{15}$N$_5$O$_2$: C, 62.13; H, 4.89; N, 22.64%, Found: C, 62.22; H, 4.93; N, 22.71%.

4-((5-(3,5-Dinitrophenyl)-1,3,4-oxadiazol-2-yl)methoxy)benzamidine (5e)

Yellowish brown crystalline (Yield 75%, m.p. 130 °C); IR (KBr, cm^{-1}): 3051 (Aromatic C–H), 2919 (Aliphatic C–H), 1680 (C=N), 1589, 1474 (Aromatic C=C), 1310 (N-O), 1242, 1042 (C–O–C of oxadiazole ring); ^{1}H-NMR (DMSO-d_6, ppm) δ: 3.16 (s, 2H, O–CH$_2$), 3.71 (brs, 2H, NH$_2$), 7.41–7.78 (m, 7H, Ar–H), 8.02 (s, 1H, C=NH); ^{13}C-NMR (DMSO, ppm) δ: 67.98 (O–CH$_2$), 122.12, 123.26, 127.7, 128.07, 129.21, 130.56, 131.06, 132.01, 133.28, 134.55 (Ar–C), 167.23 (C=N); Mass (m/z): Calcd. 309.32, Found 309.20; Anal. Calcd. for C$_{16}$H$_{12}$N$_6$O$_6$: C, 50.01; H, 3.15; N, 21.87%, Found: C, 50.12; H, 3.11; N, 21.79%.

2.2.2. General Procedure for the Synthesis of 4-((4-3-Phenoxybenzylideneamino)4-4-nitrobenzylideneamino)-4H-1,2,4-triazole-3-yl methoxy)benzamidine (**6a-b**)

To synthesize the **compound 6a,b**, a mixture of **compound 3** (0.1 M), potassium hydroxide (0.15 M), and CS$_2$ (0.15 M) in absolute ethanol was stirred for 18 h. To the resulting solution, 250 mL of anhydrous ether was added to precipitate potassium dithiocarbazinate. The 0.02 M of dithiocarbazinate was hydrazinated with 0.04 M of hydrazine hydrate. The hydrazinated product was treated with different aromatic aldehydes separately in equimolar concentration. The synthesized **compounds** were recrystallized using absolute ethanol to offer pure **compounds 6a,b**. The synthetic scheme for synthesis of **compound 6a-b** is given in Figure 1. During the experiment, anhydrous reaction conditions were maintained, and the recrystallization was done using methanol and activated charcoal. The synthesized **compound 6a** was further characterized based on spectrometric data (Figures S5, S6, S7a–c and S8). Similarly, **compound 6b** was also synthesized, purified, and characterized.

4-((4-(3-Phenoxybenzylideneamino)-4H-1,2,4-triazole-3-yl)methoxy)benzamidine (**6a**)

Yellow crystalline (Yield 85%, m.p 193 °C); IR (KBr, cm^{-1}): 3034 (Aromatic C–H), 2918 (Aliphatic C–H), 1687 (C=N), 1481, 1447 (Aromatic C=C); ^{1}H-NMR (DMSO-d_6, ppm) δ: 3.35 (s, 2H, O–CH2), 7.06 (s, 1H, S–H), 7.17–7.71 (m, 22H, Ar–H), 9.29 (s, 1H, N=CH), 9.99 (s, 1H, C=NH); ^{13}C-NMR (DMSO, ppm) δ: 67.89 (O–CH2), 117.82, 118.59, 119.75, 119.81, 123.23, 124.52, 124.58, 124.75, 124.89, 125.22, 130.71, 130.77, 130.83, 131.51, 133.30, 138.42, 163.33 (Ar–C), 157.75 (C=N), 167.38 (1H, C=NH), 193.01 (N=C-S); Mass (m/z): Calcd. 624.71, Found 624.20; Anal. Calcd. for $C_{36}H_{28}N_6O_3S$: C, 69.21; H, 4.52; N, 13.45%, Found: C, 69.18; H, 4.59; N, 13.51%.

4-((4-(4-Nitrobenzylideneamino)-4H-1,2,4-triazole-3-yl)methoxy)benzamidine (**6b**)

Yellow crystalline (Yield 88%, m.p 180 °C); IR (KBr, cm^{-1}): 3052 (Aromatic C–H), 2919 (Aliphatic C–H), 1703 (C=N), 1537, 1444 (Aromatic C=C); ^{1}H-NMR (DMSO-d_6, ppm) δ: 3.36 (s, 2H, O–CH2), 7.06 (s, 1H, S–H), 8.16–8.42 (m, 12H, Ar–H), 9.29 (s, 1H, N=CH), 9.98 (s, 1H, C=NH); ^{13}C-NMR (DMSO, ppm) δ: 68.01 (O–CH2), 124.73, 125.32, 127.12, 131.11, 131.57, 135.28, 133.67, 136.59, 138.45, 139.17, 139.82, 140.54 (Ar–C), 151.09 (C=N), 167.82 (C=NH), 192.79 (N=C-S); Mass (m/z): Calcd. 530.52, Found 530.20. Anal. Calcd. for $C_{24}H_{18}N_8O_5S$: C, 54.34; H, 3.42; N, 21.12%, Found: C, 54.29; H, 3.39; N, 21.08%.

2.3. Determination of Antimicrobial Activity

In the present study, the micro-broth dilution method was used to determine the inhibition susceptibility of synthesized **compounds** against *P. gingivalis* (ATCC 33277) and *E. coli* (ATCC 25922). The strain of *P. gingivalis* and *E. coli* were obtained from ATCC. The bacteria were cultured in blood-enriched tryptic soy agar (eTSA) (Merck KGaA, Darmstadt, Germany), supplemented with sterile filtered 5% L-cysteine (Bio-Basic, Markham, ON, Canada), 1% dithiothreitol (Sigma Life Sciences, Burlington, MA, USA), and 0.5 mg/mL vitamin K (Sigma Life Sciences, Burlington, MA, USA) with an adjusted pH of 7.4 [37]. As per CLSI guidelines, the micro broth dilution method was used to determine the minimum inhibition concentration (MIC) of *P. gingivalis*. The synthesized **compounds** were diluted in two-fold serial dilution, starting with the highest concentration at 500 µg/mL, and the lowest concentration at 7.8125 µg/mL. Ampicillin was used as a control (Akum Drugs and Pharmaceuticals, New Delhi, India), with final concentrations of 250 µg/mL to 1.6 µg/mL. All of these dilutions were carried out aseptically. To inoculate bacterial culture for MIC, the 0.5 McFarland standard was used (1.5 × 10^8 CFU/mL) [38,39]. To the microtiter plate, an equal volume of 1.5 × 10^8 CFU/mL of *P. gingivalis* was added, excluding only the negative control. The microtiter plates were incubated in an anaerobic jar (Oxoid, Winchester, UK) supplemented with a gas pack (Merck KGaA, Darmstadt, Germany) that generate 90% N_2, 5% CO_2, and H_2 and a gas indicator (Thermo Fisher Scientific, Waltham, MA, USA) for 46 h at 37 °C.

Cation-adjusted Mueller–Hinton broth (CAMHB) and agar (CAMHA) (HiMedia, Mumbai, India) were used for *E. coli* MIC evaluation. The MIC of *E. coli* was determined using the same method as that of *P. gingivalis*. The final concentration of the ampicillin was 250 µg/mL to 1.6 µg/mL (CSC Pharmaceuticals, Mumbai, India). The microtiter plates were incubated at 37 °C in aerobic conditions for 18 h.

To determine *P. gingivalis* minimum bactericidal concentration, MIC results of the clear wells of samples where there was no visible bacterial growth were aseptically plated on eTSB agar and incubated in an anaerobic jar at 37 °C with a gas indicator and gas pack for 46 h. The MBC of *E. coli* was determined by plating the MIC results of the clear wells on CAMHA and incubating for 18 h at 37 °C according to the guidelines given by CLSI. After incubation, MBC was recorded as the lowest concentration of a **compound** with no visible growth of bacteria with agar clarity, the same as that of the negative control. All experiments were performed in triplicate.

2.3.1. Cell Viability Assay

MTT is the most common cell viability assay used and it depends on the conversion of substrate to a chromogenic product by live cells. This assay involves the conversion of the water-soluble MTT [3-(4,5-dimethylthiazol-2-yl)-2,5-diphenyltetrazolium bromide] to an insoluble formazan by the action of mitochondrial reductase. The solubilized formazan concentration is then determined by an optical density at 570 nm [40]. To determine cell viability, HEK 293 cells obtained from ATCC were revived and cultured using DMEM (Dulbecco's modified Eagle medium) supplemented with 5% fetal bovine serum (FBS) (Sigma life science, Burlington, MA, USA) and 1% antibiotic (GIBCO, Waltham, MA, USA) and incubated at 37 °C, with 5% CO_2, and relative humidity of about 95% (Heal Force/HF90, Hong Kong, China).

2.3.2. Cell Counting

Cells were counted using the hemocytometer (Hirschmann Laborgerate, Darmstadt, Germany) counting technique. Here, cells were washed with PBS (First base, Axil Scientific, Singapore), treated with trypsin (Sigma life science, Burlington, MA, USA), and incubated at 37 °C to detach them from the flask surface. After trypsinization, 0.1 mL of cells were added to 0.9 mL of 0.2% trypan blue (Sigma life science, Burlington, MA, USA) in a sterile microcentrifuge tube. A 10 µL sample of stained cells were loaded into both sides of the chamber of the hemocytometer, covered with microscopic cover glass, and cells were viewed under the inverted microscope (Olympus/CK40-F200, Shinjuku, Japan). The viable cells were not stained with trypan blue, whereas the dead cells were stained [41]. Using Equations (1) and (2), the total viable cells were calculated:

$$\text{Total number of viable cells} = \frac{\text{Total number of cells from 4 grids}}{4} \quad (1)$$

$$\text{Number of live cells} = \text{Total number of viable cells} \times \text{Dilution factor} \times 10^4/\text{mL} \quad (2)$$

2.3.3. Cell Treatment

After 24 h of incubation, the counted cells were treated with different concentrations (50–7.8125 µg/mL) of the synthesized **compounds**. All seeded cells were treated with synthesized **compounds** except the controls, and cells were further incubated until MTT analysis [42].

2.3.4. 3-[4,5-Dimethylthiazol-2-yl]2,5-diphenyl Tetrazolium Bromide (MTT) Assay

A 20 µL sample of MTT reagent (0.5 mg/mL) (Sigma life science, Burlington, MA, USA) in PBS was added to each well, including the controls, and the plates were covered with aluminum foil paper and incubated at 37 °C for 4 h. After incubation, the cells were treated with MTT detergent (DMSO) (Sigma life science, Burlington, MA, USA) and further incubated for 1 h. After 1 h of incubation, the sample OD was measured at 570 nm with the reference of 630 nm using Infinite 200 PRO (Tecan Microplate Reader, Mannedorf, Switzerland). A triplicate experiment was carried out for all synthesized **compounds**. Below is the formula used for calculating the percentage (%) of cell viability:

$$\text{Cytotoxicity (\%)} = \frac{\text{Sample Absorbance (mean)}}{\text{Control Absorbance (mean)}} \quad (3)$$

2.3.5. Statistical Analysis

GraphPad Prism software version 5 (GraphPad Software, Inc., San Diego, CA, USA) was used to analyze cytotoxicity statistical data. One-way analysis of variance (ANOVA) followed by Dunnett's post-hoc test to determine the source of significant difference between the groups using SPSS software (IBM SPSS Statistics, Version 25). Results are presented as mean ± standard error of experiment performed in triplicate.

3. Results and Discussion
3.1. Chemistry

In a previous study, the authors of the present study, described the synthesis of **compounds 2, 3,** and **4a-c**, that involved preparation of ethyl-2-(4-carbamimidoylphenoxy)acetate 2, by esterification of 4-hydroxybenzenecarboximidamide (**1**), followed by hydrazination to form 2-(4-carbamimidoylphenoxy)acetohydrazide (**3**), which was further treated with different aromatic aldehydes to offer N-(substituted benzylidene)-2-(4-(N-(4-ydroxybenzylidene) carbamimidoyl)phenoxy)acetohydrazide (**4a-c**) [12].

In the current study, **compound 3** was subjected to different types of reactions. In one part of the experiment, **compound** (**3**) was treated with different aromatic acids (4-chlorobenzoic acid, 2-chlorobenzoic acid, 4-flurobenzoic acid, 4-aminobenzoic acid, and 3,5-dinitrobenzoic acid) in the presence of $POCl_3$ to offer new oxadiazoles derivatives of benzamidine (**5a-e**). The stated experiment involved cyclo-condensation reaction of aromatic acids with hydrazide (**3**) in the presence of $POCl_3$ to form **compound 5a-e**. The physical and chemical properties of newly synthesized **compounds** in the present study are also supported by other investigations [43,44]. Whereas, in another part of the experiment, **compound** (**3**) was treated with carbon disulfide in the presence of potassium hydroxide to offer potassium dithiocarbazinate, which was further subjected to hydrazination followed by treatment with different aromatic aldehydes to offer **compounds** (**6a,b**) [45–47]. The synthetic scheme for all new **compounds 5a-e** and **6a-b** is given in Figure 1.

Figure 1 shows synthetic route of novel analogs obtained in this study. The purity of synthesized **compounds** was determined based on melting point, single spot TLC (thin-layer chromatography) pattern, and CHN analysis. In the present study, the spectrometric analysis of synthesized **compounds** using mass spectrometry, FTIR, ^1H, and ^{13}C-NMR confirmed the structure of **compounds 5a-e** and **6a-b**. The successful synthesis of **compound 5a-e** was confirmed based on the presence of the characteristic IR bands at 1042–1295 (C–O–C of oxadiazole ring), disappearance of ^1H-NMR signals at 8.27, appearance of extra 13C-NMR signals for aromatic carbons raging between 113 and 166, and the appearance of a mass spectrum ion peak ranging between 309 and 384 confirmed the structure of the synthesized **compounds 5a-e**. The successful synthesis of the **compound** (**6a-b**) was confirmed based on the appearance of the characteristic IR bands at 1687 and 1703 (C=N), ^1H-NMR signals at 7.06 (1H, s, S-H), 9.2 (N=CH), 9.9–10.17 (C=NH), ^{13}C-NMR signals at 193 (N=C–S), and the appearance of mass signals at 624 and 530.

3.2. Biological Activity
3.2.1. In Vitro Antibacterial Activity of Synthesized Compounds

In vitro antibacterial assay consists of numerous biological assays such as agar dilution, well-diffusion, disk-diffusion, and broth dilution methods [48]. The antibacterial screening of all synthesized **compounds 5a-e** and **6a,b** against *P. gingivalis* and *E. coli* resulted in a minimum inhibition concentration (MIC) between 31 µg/mL and 250 µg/mL (Table 1). However, not all the synthesized **compounds** yielded a result for minimum bactericidal concentration (MBC). The synthesized **compounds 5b, 5d, 5e,** and **6b** have all displayed an MBC against *P. gingivalis* with a range of 250 µg/mL to 125 µg/mL. While for *E. coli*, only **compounds 5c, 5e,** and **6b** have yielded MBC results with a range of 125 µg/mL to 250 ug/mL (Table 2). Moreover, both **compounds 5a** and **6a** displayed no MBC activity against *P. gingivalis* and *E. coli*, respectively. On the contrary, **compounds 5e** and **6b** are the only two **compounds** to yield MBC against both *P. gingivalis* and *E. coli*.

Table 1. MIC values of synthesized compounds.

Compound (µg/mL)	Organisms	
	P. gingivalis	E. coli
1	62.5 ± 0.00 [c]	31.25 ± 0.00 [b]
2	62.5 ± 0.00 [c]	55.5 ± 12.03 [c]
3	62.5 ± 0.00 [c]	31.5 ± 0.00 [b]
5a	62.5 ± 0.44 [c]	250 ± 1.76 [d]
5b	31.25 ± 0.11 [b]	250 ± 0.00 [d]
5c	62.5 ± 0.00 [c]	250 ± 1.76 [d]
5d	31.25 ± 0.00 [b]	250 ± 0.00 [d]
5e	31.25 ± 0.88 [b]	250 ± 1.76 [d]
6a	125 ± 0.00 [d]	250 ± 0.00 [d]
6b	31.25 ± 0.00 [b]	62.5 ± 0.00 [c]
Ampicillin	15.63 + 0.00 [a]	1.600 + 0.00 [a]

MIC: Minimum inhibitory concentration. Data presented as mean ± standard error of each experiment performed in triplicate values. Means with different superscripts (a–d) were significantly different ($p < 0.05$).

Table 2. MBC values of synthesized compounds.

Compound (µg/mL)	Organisms	
	P. gingivalis	E. coli
1	125	-
2	125	-
3	125	-
5a	-	-
5b	125	-
5c	-	250
5d	125	-
5e	125	250
6a	-	-
6b	125	125
Ampicillin	62.5	7.8

MBC: Minimum bactericidal concentration.

The synthesis of oxadiazole compounds in recent years has spiked up tremendously, solely due to their biological activities. Their antibacterial activity against pathogenic microorganisms has exceeded some of the known antibiotics, making them an alternative to combat drug resistance organisms [31]. It was previously reported by [49], that evaluation of scaffold oxadiazoles has resulted in MIC against gram-positive and gram-negative organisms. In addition, multiple other studies have shown that oxadiazoles have suppressed bacterial growth at low concentrations [50–53], similar to the observation that was noted in this study. Although oxadiazoles have broad-spectrum antibacterial activities [54], and their activities have been evaluated in both gram-positive and gram-negatives some of which are associated with oral diseases [55,56], there is no data on its evaluation and inhibition activity against *P. gingivalis*. This study may be the first one to report the ability of oxadiazoles to inhibit *P gingivalis* growth, a putative organism that promotes PD.

In the continuous search for alternatives to antibiotics, triazole Schiff bases derivatives possess the biological properties that inhibit the growth of drug-resistant organisms [57]. In the present study, it is worth knowing that compound 6b has yielded MIC and MBC against both *P. gingivalis* and *E. coli* compared to other synthesized compounds (Tables 1 and 2). But this is not a surprise considering its known activity against pathogenic organisms [58], with some studies reporting that it is twice as active as ciprofloxacin [59], whereas other studies reported that it has activity comparable to that of chloramphenicol [60]. Furthermore, it was reported by [61,62], that triazole Schiff bases have an inhibition activity against multi-drug resistance organisms. Despite triazole Schiff base's diverse antibacterial activity, there's less evaluation of its activities against *P. gingivalis*. Nevertheless, a study showed that synthesized triazoles have the activity to inhibit adherence of *P. gingivalis* [30]. Another study showed that triazole has an inhibitory influence against *HmuY* and *fimA* gene expression (hemin binding proteins) which are responsible for *P. gingivalis* growth [63]. In the present study, all synthesized compounds have yielded antibacterial effects against tested pathogens with some having higher potential than others, making them a promising therapeutic alternative. Although all synthesized compounds exhibited significant activity against *P. gingivalis* and *E. coli*; however, among all, **compound 6b** was found to be most active, as it exhibited the best MIC and MBC values against *P. gingivalis* and *E. coli*.

3.2.2. Cytotoxicity Analysis of Synthesized Compounds

In drug development, cytotoxicity is an important aspect of biological evaluation. In the present study, the MTT assay of all synthesized compounds was evaluated against HEK 293 cells. A previous study suggested that oxadiazole compounds yielded no to less toxicity when tested against NIH/3T3 cells due to cell viability greater than 75% [64]. Testing synthesized compounds of oxadiazoles against A549, L929, and HpG2 cells [65], showed that most synthesized compounds yielded no cytotoxicity against tested cell lines with cell viability greater than 75%, with only a few compounds resulting in cell death. Satisfactory results and minimal cytotoxicity of oxadizoles evaluation were previously described [66,67], which is in agreement with this study. In the current study, it was observed that all synthesized oxadiazoles (**5a-e**) yielded more than 70% cell viability when tested against HEK 293 cells at 62.5 µg/mL (Table 3 and Figure 1). At 125 µg/mL, all synthesized oxadiazoles showed no sign of cytotoxicity, except for **5b**, having only 66% cell viability. At the maximum concentration tested (500 µg/mL), only **compound 5d-e** showed no signs of cytotoxicity compared to other synthesized **compounds (5a-c)**. Hence the minimal cytotoxicity at high concentrations and high antibacterial at low concentrations of these synthesized compounds are their major advantages.

Table 3. Cytotoxicity values of synthesized compounds.

Concentration (µg/mL)	Cell Viability (%)									
	1	2	3	5a	5b	5c	5d	5e	6a	6b
7.8125	122.87 ± 17.59	116.06 ± 19.78	116.06 ± 19.78	97.67 ± 0.90	92.67 ± 1.62 *	92.83 ± 1.35 *	96.00 ± 2.52	93.87 ± 1.78 *	90.53 ± 1.00	86.83 ± 10.09
15.625	105.89 ± 19.53	100.67 ± 29.35	100.67 ± 29.35 *	93.33 ± 2.08	87.93 ± 0.87 *	90.10 ± 2.19 *	89.13 ± 1.35 *	92.80 ± 2.12 *	87.47 ± 1.35 *	82.13 ± 7.81
31.25	94.83 ± 17.46 *	107.65 ± 29.99 *	107.65 ± 29.99	93.53 ± 0.84	82.77 ± 1.40 *	87.37 ± 1.85 *	88.00 ± 1.04 *	90.23 ± 1.19 *	84.83 ± 2.15 *	78.20 ± 6.30 *
62.5	93.56 ± 10.72 *	111.10 ± 16.38 *	111.10 ± 16.38 *	91.03 ± 2.66	76.10 ± 3.72 *	80.23 ± 2.83 *	87.00 ± 1.23 *	88.57 ± 2.11 *	72.80 ± 7.50 *	78.77 ± 10.12 *
125	94.41 ± 9.93	100.71 ± 6.74	100.71 ± 6.74	84 ± 8.22 *	66 ± 1.69 *	72 ± 2.15 *	83 ± 2.05 *	87 ± 2.51 *	62 ± 0.86 *	74 ± 9.77 *
250	96.03 ± 17.65 *	114.80 ± 10.81 *	114.80 ± 10.81	71 ± 8.42 *	62 ± 0.70 *	72 ± 2.48 *	71 ± 4.86 *	74 ± 3.71 *	62 ± 3.06 *	72 ± 11.41 *
Control	100 ± 0.00	100 ± 0.00	100 ± 0.00	100 ± 0.00	100 ± 0.00	100 ± 0.00	100 ± 0.00	100 ± 0.00	100 ± 0.00	100 ± 0.00

Data presented as mean ± standard error with each experiment were performed in triplicate. Mean values having superscript '*' statistically indicates by * $p < 0.05$.

Triazole has exemplary biological activity and due to its minimal cytotoxicity, it is ideal for many biological studies. Triazole Schiff bases have shown to be safe and have relatively less cytotoxicity when tested against HEK-293 and WI-38, respectively [68–70]. Triazole Schiff bases analysis against kidney, red blood cells, and lung cells all yielded no cytotoxicity, hence supporting their minimal cytotoxicity, and it is even suggested to be safer than cisplatin [71–73]. Here in this study, it was observed that **6a-b** resulted in more than 70% cell viability when tested against HEK-293 cells at 62.5 µg/mL (Table 3 and Figure 1). However, at 250 µg/mL, only **6b** resulted in more than 70% cell viability. Among

6a and **6b**, the **compound 6b** is found to be much safer with 68% cell viability (Table 3) at the maximum tested concentration (500 µg/mL).

Based on the resultant MIC data of synthesized **compounds 5a-e** and **6a,b** given in Table 1, the structure of benzamidine and its analogues synthesized in the present study, were related to their inhibitory potential (MIC) against PD triggering bacteria. The study revealed that incorporation of heterocyclic ring (oxadiazole and triazole) increases their inhibitory potential by twofold against *P. gingivalis* in comparison to parent benzamidine **compound 1**. It is observed that incorporation of Cl at ortho, NO_2 at ortho and meta, and NH_2 group at para position of benzene ring that is directly attached to oxadiazole ring containing benzamidine analogues **5b**, **5d**, and **5e**, enhances their inhibitory potential against *P. gingivalis* in comparison to **compound 1**. However, incorporation of Cl at para position of benzene ring in **compound 5a** offers activity similar to **compound 1**. Whereas incorporation of NO_2 group at para position on benzene ring attached to triazole containing benzamidine analogue **6b** further enhances their inhibitory potential against *P. gingivalis* in comparison to **compound 1**. The resultant MBC data of **compound 5b**, **5d**, **5e**, and **6b** given in Table 2, revealed their equipotent MBC value when compared with parent **compound 1**. As per the resultant cyto-toxicity study data given in Table 3 and Figure 2, the **compounds 5a**, **5c-e**, and **6b** can be considered as nontoxic and safer alternatives for the treatment of PD. However, **compound 5a** containing para substituted Cl on benzene and **compound 6a** containing phenoxy group at meta position of benzene offers lesser safety when compared with other synthesized compounds. Free hydroxy group is not essential for the activity, conversion into ether linkage further enhances the inhibitory activity. Based on the MIC, MBC, and cytotoxicity data it is recommended that these synthesized compounds should be further subjected to preclinical and clinical evaluation.

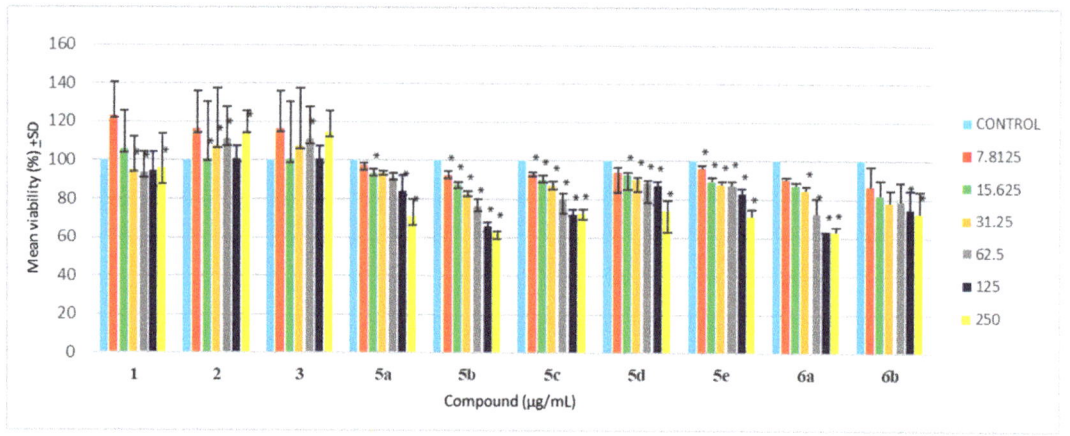

Figure 2. Cytotoxicity analysis of synthesized compounds against HEK-293 cells (Where, * $p < 0.05$).

4. Conclusions

In conclusion, compounds were successfully synthesized by the condensation of hydrazides with different aromatic benzoic acids, and cyclo-condensation of a triazole with imine Schiff bases. The synthesized compounds were further confirmed based on sharp melting point, single spot TLC pattern, and spectral data. All synthesized compounds displayed minimum to high inhibition activity against tested pathogens. Additonally, all the synthesized compounds showed less cytotoxicity when tested against HEK-293 cells. Despite the present study showing the ability of benzamidine derivatives to inhibit the growth of periodontal pathogens with an absence of cytotoxicity of some of these derivatives, additional in-vivo and clinical studies are required to establish their safety and efficacy.

Supplementary Materials: The following supporting information can be downloaded at: https://www.mdpi.com/article/10.3390/antibiotics12020306/s1, Figure S1: FTIR spectrum of **compound 5a**; Figure S2: ^{1}H-NMR spectrum of **compound 5a**; Figure S3: ^{13}C-NMR spectrum of **compound 5a**; Figure S4: MASS spectrum of **compound 5a**; Figure S5: FTIR spectrum of **compound 6a**; Figure S6: ^{1}H-NMR spectrum of **compound 6a**; Figure S7a: ^{13}C-NMR spectrum of **compound 6a**; Figure S7b: ^{13}C-NMR spectrum of **compound 6a**; Figure S7c: ^{13}C-NMR spectrum of **compound 6a**; Figure S4: MASS spectrum of **compound 6a**.

Author Contributions: Conceptualization, N.K.F., S.F., M.R. and P.L.; methodology, M.A.S., R.K., N.K.F., S.F., M.R. and P.L.; investigation, M.A.S., R.K., N.K.F., S.F., M.R. and P.L.; resources, M.A.S., R.K., N.K.F., S.F., M.R. and P.L.; data curation, M.A.S., R.K., N.K.F., S.F., M.R. and P.L.; writing—original draft preparation, M.A.S., R.K., N.K.F., S.F., M.R. and P.L.; writing—review and editing, M.A.S., N.K.F., S.F., M.R. and P.L. All authors have read and agreed to the published version of the manuscript.

Funding: This research was funded by the Ministry of Higher Education (MOHE) Malaysia, grant number FRGS/1/2018/SKK14/AIMST/01/1.

Institutional Review Board Statement: Not applicable.

Informed Consent Statement: Not applicable.

Data Availability Statement: The data presented in this study are available on request from the corresponding author.

Acknowledgments: The authors would like to thank the Ministry of Higher Education (Ref: FRGS/1/2018/SKK14/AIMST/01/1) and AIMST University for financial support and assistance to successfully complete this study.

Conflicts of Interest: The authors declare no conflict of interest.

References

1. Dannewitz, B.; Holtfreter, B.; Eickholz, P. Periodontitis-therapy of a widespread disease. *Bundesgesundheitsblatt* **2021**, *64*, 931–940. [CrossRef] [PubMed]
2. Kwon, T.; Lamster, I.B.; Levin, L. Current Concepts in the Management of Periodontitis. *Int. Dent. J.* **2021**, *71*, 462–476. [CrossRef]
3. Genco, R.J.; Borgnakke, W.S. Risk factors for periodontal disease. *J. Periodontol. 2000.* **2013**, *62*, 59–94. [CrossRef]
4. Bui, F.Q.; Almeida-da-Silva, L.C.; Huynh, B.; Trinh, A.; Liu, J.; Woodward, J.; Asadi, H.; Ojcius, D.M. Association between periodontal pathogens and systemic disease. *Biomed. J.* **2019**, *42*, 27–35. [CrossRef] [PubMed]
5. Lyra, P.; Botelho, J.; Machado, V.; Rota, S.; Walker, R.; Staunton, J.; Proença, L.; Chaudhuri, K.R.; Mendes, J.J. Self-reported periodontitis and C-reactive protein in Parkinson's disease: A cross-sectional study of two American cohorts. *NPJ Park. Dis.* **2022**, *8*, 40. [CrossRef]
6. Preshaw, P.M.; Alba, A.L.; Herrera, D.; Jepsen, S.; Konstantinidis, A.; Makrilakis, K.; Taylor, R. Periodontitis and diabetes: A two-way relationship. *Diabetologia.* **2012**, *55*, 21–31. [CrossRef] [PubMed]
7. Parra-Torres, V.; Melgar-Rodríguez, S.; Muñoz-Manríquez, C.; Sanhueza, B.; Cafferata, E.A.; Paula-Lima, A.C.; Díaz-Zúñiga, J. Periodontal bacteria in the brain-Implication for Alzheimer's disease: A systematic review. *Oral Dis.* **2023**, *29*, 21–28. [CrossRef] [PubMed]
8. Serni, L.; Caroti, L.; Barbato, L.; Nieri, M.; Serni, S.; Cirami, C.L.; Cairo, F. Association between chronic kidney disease and periodontitis. A systematic review and metanalysis. *Oral Dis.* **2023**, *29*, 40–50. [CrossRef]
9. Kinane, D.F.; Stathopoulou, P.G.; Papapanou, P.N. Periodontal diseases. *Nat. Rev. Dis. Prim.* **2017**, *3*, 17038. [CrossRef]
10. Arweiler, N.B.; Netuschil, L. The Oral Microbiota. *Adv. Exp. Med. Biol.* **2016**, *902*, 45–60.
11. Chigasaki, O.; Aoyama, N.; Sasaki, Y.; Takeuchi, Y.; Mizutani, K.; Ikeda, Y.; Gokyu, M.; Umeda, M.; Izumi, Y.; Iwata, T.; et al. *Porphyromonas gingivalis*, the most influential pathogen in red-complex bacteria: A cross-sectional study on the relationship between bacterial count and clinical periodontal status in Japan. *J. Periodontol.* **2021**, *92*, 1719–1729. [CrossRef]
12. Sa'ad, M.A.; Kavitha, R.; Fuloria, S.; Fuloria, N.K.; Ravichandran, M.; Lalitha, P. Synthesis, Characterization and Biological Evaluation of Novel Benzamidine Derivatives: Newer Antibiotics for Periodontitis Treatment. *Antibiotics* **2022**, *11*, 207. [CrossRef]
13. Chopra, A.; Radhakrishnan, R.; Sharma, M. *Porphyromonas gingivalis* and adverse pregnancy outcomes: A review on its intricate pathogenic mechanisms. *Crit. Rev. Microbiol.* **2020**, *46*, 213–236. [CrossRef]
14. Zhao, X.; Liu, J.; Zhang, C.; Yu, N.; Lu, Z.; Zhang, S.; Li, Y.; Li, Q.; Liu, J.; Liu, D.; et al. *Porphyromonas gingivalis* exacerbates ulcerative colitis via *Porphyromonas gingivalis* peptidylarginine deiminase. *Int. J. Oral Sci.* **2021**, *13*, 31. [CrossRef]
15. Scannapieco, F.A.; Gershovich, E. The prevention of periodontal disease-An overview. *Periodontol. 2000.* **2020**, *84*, 9–13. [CrossRef]
16. Slots, J. Primer on etiology and treatment of progressive/severe periodontitis: A systemic health perspective. *Periodontology 2000* **2020**, *83*, 272–276. [CrossRef]

17. Fischer, R.G.; Lira Junior, R.; Retamal-Valdes, B.; Figueiredo, L.C.; de Malheiros, Z.; Stewart, B.; Feres, M. Periodontal disease and its impact on general health in Latin America. Section V: Treatment of periodontitis. *Braz. Oral Res.* **2020**, *34* (Suppl. 1), e026. [CrossRef]
18. Di Domenico, G.L.; Minoli, M.; Discepoli, N.; Ambrosi, A.; de Sanctis, M. Effectiveness of periodontal treatment to improve glycemic control: An umbrella review. *Acta Diabetol.* **2023**, *60*, 101–113. [CrossRef]
19. Pretzl, B.; Sälzer, S.; Ehmke, B.; Schlagenhauf, U.; Dannewitz, B.; Dommisch, H.; Eickholz, P.; Jockel-Schneider, Y. Administration of systemic antibiotics during non-surgical periodontal therapy-a consensus report. *Clin. Oral Investig.* **2019**, *23*, 3073–3085. [CrossRef]
20. Kaufmann, M.; Lenherr, P.; Walter, C.; Thurnheer, T.; Attin, T.; Wiedemeier, D.B.; Schmidlin, P.R. Comparing the Antimicrobial In Vitro Efficacy of Amoxicillin/Metronidazole against Azithromycin—A Systematic Review. *Dent. J.* **2018**, *6*, 59. [CrossRef]
21. Ardila, C.-M.; Bedoya-García, J.A. Antimicrobial resistance of Aggregatibacter actinomycetemcomitans, *Porphyromonas gingivalis* and Tannerella forsythia in periodontitis patients. *J. Glob. Antimicrob. Resist.* **2020**, *22*, 215–218. [CrossRef] [PubMed]
22. Kulik, E.M.; Thurnheer, T.; Karygianni, L.; Walter, C.; Sculean, A.; Eick, S. Antibiotic Susceptibility Patterns of *Aggregatibacter actinomycetemcomitans* and *Porphyromonas gingivalis* Strains from Different Decades. *Antibiotics* **2019**, *8*, 253. [CrossRef] [PubMed]
23. Li, Y.; Miao, Y.S.; Fu, Y.; Li, X.T.; Yu, S.J. Attenuation of *Porphyromonas gingivalis* oral infection by α-amylase and pentamidine. *Mol. Med. Rep.* **2015**, *12*, 2155–2160. [CrossRef] [PubMed]
24. Tan, J.; Patil, P.C.; Luzzio, F.A.; Demuth, D.R. In Vitro and In Vivo Activity of Peptidomimetic **Compounds** That Target the Periodontal Pathogen *Porphyromonas gingivalis*. *Antimicrob. Agents Chemother.* **2018**, *62*, e00400–e00418. [CrossRef]
25. Obradović, D.; Nikolić, S.; Milenković, I.; Milenković, M.; Jovanović, P.; Savić, V.; Roller, A.; Crnogorac, M.Đ.; Stanojković, T.; Grgurić-Šipka, S. Synthesis, characterization, antimicrobial and cytotoxic activity of novel half-sandwich Ru (II) arene complexes with benzoylthiourea derivatives. *J. Inorg. Biochem.* **2020**, *210*, 111164. [CrossRef]
26. Tipparaju, S.K.; Joyasawal, S.; Pieroni, M.; Kaiser, M.; Brun, R.; Kozikowski, A.P. In Pursuit of Natural Product Leads: Synthesis and Biological Evaluation of 2-[3-hydroxy-2-[(3-hydroxypyridine-2-carbonyl) amino] phenyl] benzoxazole-4-carboxylic acid (A-33853) and Its Analogues: Discovery of N-(2-Benzoxazol-2-ylphenyl) benzamides as Novel Antileishmanial Chemotypes. *J. Med. Chem.* **2008**, *51*, 7344–7347.
27. Fröhlich, E.; Kantyka, T.; Plaza, K.; Schmidt, K.H.; Pfister, W.; Potempa, J.; Eick, S. Benzamidine derivatives inhibit the virulence of *Porphyromonas gingivalis*. *Mol. Oral Microbiol.* **2013**, *28*, 192–203. [CrossRef]
28. Desai, N.; Monapara, J.; Jethawa, A.; Khedkar, V.; Shingate, B. Oxadiazole: A highly versatile scaffold in drug discovery. *Arch. Pharm.* **2022**, *355*, 2200123. [CrossRef]
29. Patil, P.C.; Tan, J.; Demuth, D.R.; Luzzio, F.A. 1,2,3-Triazole-based inhibitors of *Porphyromonas gingivalis* adherence to oral streptococci and biofilm formation. *Bioorg. Med. Chem.* **2016**, *24*, 5410–5417. [CrossRef]
30. Patil, P.C.; Tan, J.; Demuth, D.R.; Luzzio, F.A. "Second-generation" 1,2,3-triazole-based inhibitors of *Porphyromonas gingivalis* adherence to oral streptococci and biofilm formation. *MedChemComm* **2019**, *10*, 268–279. [CrossRef]
31. Glomb, T.; Świątek, P. Antimicrobial Activity of 1,3,4-Oxadiazole Derivatives. *Int. J. Mol. Sci.* **2021**, *22*, 6979. [CrossRef] [PubMed]
32. Fuloria, N.K.; Fuloria, S.; Sathasivam, K.; Karupiah, S. Synthesis and discerning of antimicrobial potential of novel oxadiazole derivatives of chloroxylenol moiety. *Acta Pol. Pharm.* **2017**, *74*, 1125-30.
33. Husain, A.; Varshney, M.M.; Parcha, V.; Ahmad, A.; Khan, S.A. Synthesis and biological evaluation of new hydrazide-Schiff bases. *Bangladesh J. Pharmacol.* **2015**, *10*, 23381. [CrossRef]
34. Taha, M.; Imran, S.; Alomari, M.; Rahim, F.; Wadood, A.; Mosaddik, A.; Uddin, N.; Gollapalli, M.; Alqahtani, M.A.; Bamarouf, Y.A. Synthesis of oxadiazole-coupled-thiadiazole derivatives as a potent β-glucuronidase inhibitors and their molecular docking study. *Bioorg. Med. Chem.* **2019**, *27*, 3145–3155. [CrossRef]
35. Fuloria, N.K.; Singh, V.; Shaharyar, M.; Ali, M. Synthesis and Antimicrobial Evaluation of Some New Oxadiazoles Derived from Phenylpropionohydrazides. *Molecules* **2009**, *14*, 1898–1903. [CrossRef]
36. Yang, S.; Ren, C.-L.; Ma, T.-Y.; Zou, W.-Q.; Dai, L.; Tian, X.-Y.; Liu, X.-H.; Tan, C.-X. 1,2,4-Oxadiazole-Based Bio-Isosteres of Benzamides: Synthesis, Biological Activity and Toxicity to Zebrafish Embryo. *Int. J. Mol. Sci.* **2021**, *22*, 2367. [CrossRef] [PubMed]
37. Potempa, J.; Nguyen, K. Purification and Characterization of Gingipains. *Curr. Protoc. Protein Sci.* **2017**, *49*, 21.20.1–21.20.27. [CrossRef]
38. Herrera, H.A.; Franco, O.L.; Fang, L.; Díaz, C.A. Susceptibility of *Porphyromonas gingivalis* and *Streptococcus mutans* to Antibacterial Effect from *Mammea americana*. *Adv. Pharmacol. Sci.* **2014**, 384815.
39. Shetty, S.; Shetty, R.M.; Rahman, B.; Vannala, V.; Desai, V.; Shetty, S.R. Efficacy of Psidium guajava and Allium sativum Extracts as Antimicrobial Agents against Periodontal Pathogens. *J. Pharm. Bioallied Sci.* **2020**, *12* (Suppl. 1), S589–S594. [CrossRef]
40. Kumar, P.; Nagarajan, A.; Uchil, P.D. Analysis of Cell Viability by the MTT Assay. *Cold Spring Harb. Protoc.* **2018**, *6*, 95505. [CrossRef]
41. Green, M.R.; Sambrook, J. Estimation of Cell Number by Hemocytometry Counting. *Cold Spring Harb. Protoc.* **2019**, *2019*, 97980. [CrossRef] [PubMed]
42. Ishteyaque, S.; Mishra, A.; Mohapatra, S.; Singh, A.; Bhatta, R.S.; Tadigoppula, N.; Mugale, M.N. In Vitro: Cytotoxicity, Apoptosis and Ameliorative Potential of *Lawsonia inermis* Extract in Human Lung, Colon and Liver Cancer Cell Line. *Cancer Investig.* **2020**, *38*, 476–485. [CrossRef] [PubMed]

43. Mousa, E.F.; Jassim, I.K. Synthesis and characterization of oxadiazole compounds derived from naproxen. *J. Pharm. Sci. Res.* **2018**, *10*, 3036–3040.
44. Romeo, R.; Giofrè, S.V.; Chiacchio, M.A.; Veltri, L.; Celesti, C.; Iannazzo, D. Synthesis and Biological Evaluation of 2,3,4-Triaryl-1,2,4-oxadiazol-5-ones as p38 MAPK Inhibitors. *Molecules* **2021**, *26*, 1745. [CrossRef] [PubMed]
45. Ayah, A.; Hameed, F.; Hassan, F.X. Synthesis, Characterization and Antioxidant Activity of Some 4-Amino-5-Phenyl-4h-1, 2, 4-Triazole-3-Thiol Derivatives. *KMUTNB Int. J. Appl. Sci. Technol.* **2014**, *4*, 202–211.
46. Beyzaei, H.; Bahabadi, S.E.; Najafi, S.; Sadegh, F.H. Synthesis and Antimicrobial Evaluation of the Potassium Salts of Benzhydrazine Dithiocarbamates. *J. Microbiol. Immunol. Infect.* **2020**, *7*, 15–21. [CrossRef]
47. Jawahar, J.; Sikdar, P.; Antony, S.R.; Byran, G.; Subramanian, G.; Elango, K. Synthesis and biological evaluation of some Schiff bases of [4-(amino)-5-phenyl-4H-1,2,4-triazole-3-thiol]. *Pak. J. Pharm. Sci.* **2011**, *24*, 109–112.
48. Balouiri, M.; Sadiki, M.; Ibnsouda, S.K. Methods for In Vitro evaluating antimicrobial activity: A review. *J. Pharm. Anal.* **2016**, *6*, 71–79. [CrossRef]
49. Bordei, A.T.; Nuță, D.C.; Căproiu, M.T.; Dumitrascu, F.; Zarafu, I.; Ioniță, P.; Bădiceanu, C.D.; Avram, S.; Chifiriuc, M.C.; Bleotu, C.; et al. Design, Synthesis and In Vitro Characterization of Novel Antimicrobial Agents Based on 6-Chloro-9H-carbazol Derivatives and 1,3,4-Oxadiazole Scaffolds. *Molecules* **2020**, *25*, 266.
50. Mansoori, M.H.; Khatik, G.L.; Mishra, V. Synthesis and pharmacological evaluation of pyridinyl-1,3,4-oxadiazolyl-ethanone derivatives as antimicrobial, antifungal and antitubercular agents. *Med. Chem. Res.* **2018**, *27*, 744–755. [CrossRef]
51. Peraman, R.; Varma, R.V.; Reddy, Y.P. Re-engineering nalidixic acid's chemical scaffold: A step towards the development of novel anti-tubercular and anti-bacterial leads for resistant pathogens. *Bioorg. Med. Chem. Lett.* **2015**, *25*, 4314–4319. [CrossRef] [PubMed]
52. Zheng, Z.; Liu, Q.; Kim, W.; Tharmalingam, N.; Fuchs, B.B.; Mylonakis, E. Antimicrobial activity of 1,3,4-oxadiazole derivatives against planktonic cells and biofilm of *Staphylococcus aureus*. *Future Med. Chem.* **2018**, *10*, 283–296. [CrossRef] [PubMed]
53. Zoumpoulakis, P.; Camoutsis, C.; Pairas, G.; Soković, M.; Glamočlija, J.; Potamitis, C.; Pitsas, A. Synthesis of novel sulfonamide-1,2,4-triazoles, 1,3,4-thiadiazoles and 1,3,4-oxadiazoles, as potential antibacterial and antifungal agents. Biological evaluation and conformational analysis studies. *Bioorg. Med. Chem.* **2012**, *20*, 1569–1583. [CrossRef]
54. Tresse, C.; Radigue, R.; Gomes Von Borowski, R.; Thepaut, M.; Hanh Le, H.; Demay, F.; Georgeault, S.; Dhalluin, A.; Trautwetter, A.; Ermel, G.; et al. Synthesis and evaluation of 1,3,4-oxadiazole derivatives for development as broad-spectrum antibiotics. *Bioorg. Med. Chem.* **2019**, *27*, 115097. [CrossRef] [PubMed]
55. Al-Wahaibi, L.H.; Mohamed, A.A.B.; Tawfik, S.S.; Hassan, H.M.; El-Emam, A.A. 1,3,4-Oxadiazole N-Mannich Bases: Synthesis, Antimicrobial, and Anti-Proliferative Activities. *Molecules* **2021**, *26*, 2110. [CrossRef]
56. Aljamali, N.J.; Al-Jammali, Z.S.; Ali, S. Microbial Studying Of (Thiazole, Oxadiazole, Thiadiazole)-Derivatives on Mouth and Teeth Bacteria. *Int. J. Med. Res. Pharm. Sci.* **2016**, *3*, 30–39.
57. Gao, F.; Wang, T.; Xiao, J.; Huang, G. Antibacterial activity study of 1,2,4-triazole derivatives. *Eur. J. Med. Chem.* **2019**, *173*, 274–281. [CrossRef]
58. Deodware, S.A.; Barache, U.B.; Chanshetti, U.B.; Sathe, D.J.; Panchsheela, A.U.; Gaikwad, S.H.; Prasad, K.S. Newly synthesized triazole-based Schiff base ligands and their Co (II) complexes as antimicrobial and anticancer agents: Chemical synthesis, structure and biological investigations. *Results Chem.* **2021**, *3*, 100162. [CrossRef]
59. Login, C.C.; Bâldea, I.; Tiperciuc, B.; Benedec, D.; Vodnar, D.C.; Decea, N.; Suciu, Ş. A Novel Thiazolyl Schiff Base: Antibacterial and Antifungal Effects and In Vitro Oxidative Stress Modulation on Human Endothelial Cells. *Oxidative Med. Cell. Longev.* **2019**, *2019*, 1607903. [CrossRef]
60. Jin, R.Y.; Zeng, C.Y.; Liang, X.H.; Sun, X.H.; Liu, Y.F.; Wang, Y.Y.; Zhou, S. Design, synthesis, biological activities and DFT calculation of novel 1,2,4-triazole Schiff base derivatives. *Bioorg. Chem.* **2018**, *80*, 253–260. [CrossRef]
61. Venugopala, K.N.; Kandeel, M.; Pillay, M.; Deb, P.K.; Abdallah, H.H.; Mahomoodally, M.F.; Chopra, D. Anti-Tubercular Properties of 4-Amino-5-(4-Fluoro-3-Phenoxyphenyl)-4H-1,2,4-Triazole-3-Thiol and Its Schiff Bases: Computational Input and Molecular Dynamics. *Antibiotics* **2020**, *9*, 559. [CrossRef] [PubMed]
62. Gavara, L.; Verdirosa, F.; Legru, A.; Mercuri, P.S.; Nauton, L.; Sevaille, L.; Feller, G.; Berthomieu, D.; Sannio, F.; Marcoccia, F.; et al. 4-(N-Alkyl- and -Acyl-amino)-1,2,4-triazole-3-thione Analogs as Metallo-β-Lactamase Inhibitors: Impact of 4-Linker on Potency and Spectrum of Inhibition. *Biomolecules* **2020**, *10*, 1094. [CrossRef] [PubMed]
63. Mi, L.; Zhang, X.; Hao, W.; Wang, S. Two Transition Metal Coordination Polymers: Luminescent Sensing Properties and Treatment Effect on Chronic Periodontitis by Reducing IL-6 and TNF-α Content. *J. Fluoresc.* **2021**, *31*, 165–173. [CrossRef]
64. Levent, S.; Kaya, Ç.B.; Sağlık, B.N.; Osmaniye, D.; Acar, Ç.U.; Atlı, Ö.; Özkay, Y.; Kaplancıklı, Z.A. Synthesis of Oxadiazole-Thiadiazole Hybrids and Their Anticandidal Activity. *Molecules* **2017**, *22*, 2004. [CrossRef]
65. Paruch, K.; Biernasiuk, A.; Berecka-Rycerz, A.; Hordyjewska, A.; Popiołek, Ł. Biological Activity, Lipophilicity and Cytotoxicity of Novel 3-Acetyl-2,5-disubstituted-1,3,4-oxadiazolines. *Int. J. Mol. Sci.* **2021**, *22*, 13669. [CrossRef]
66. Mamatha, S.V.; Belagali, S.L.; Bhat, M. Synthesis, characterisation and evaluation of oxadiazole as promising anticancer agent. *SN Appl. Sci.* **2020**, *2*, 882. [CrossRef]
67. Tiwari, A.; Gopalan Kutty, N.; Kumar, N.; Chaudhary, A.; Vasanth, R.P.; Shenoy, R.; Mallikarjuna, R.C. Synthesis and evaluation of selected 1,3,4-oxadiazole derivatives for In Vitro cytotoxicity and In Vivo anti-tumor activity. *Cytotechnology* **2016**, *68*, 2553–2565. [CrossRef] [PubMed]

68. Dhawan, S.; Awolade, P.; Kisten, P.; Cele, N.; Pillay, A.S.; Saha, S.; Kaur, M.; Jonnalagadda, S.B.; Singh, P. Synthesis, Cytotoxicity and Antimicrobial Evaluation of New Coumarin-Tagged β-Lactam Triazole Hybrid. *Chem. Biodivers.* **2020**, *17*, 201900462. [CrossRef]
69. Palakhachane, S.; Ketkaew, Y.; Chuaypen, N.; Sirirak, J.; Boonsombat, J.; Ruchirawat, S.; Tangkijvanich, P.; Suksamrarn, A.; Limpachayaporn, P. Synthesis of sorafenib analogues incorporating a 1,2,3-triazole ring and cytotoxicity towards hepatocellular carcinoma cell lines. *Bioorg. Chem.* **2021**, *112*, 104831. [CrossRef]
70. Zampieri, D.; Cateni, F.; Moneghini, M.; Zacchigna, M.; Laurini, E.; Marson, D.; De Logu, A.; Sanna, A.; Mamolo, M.G. Imidazole and 1,2,4-Triazole-based Derivatives Gifted with Antitubercular Activity: Cytotoxicity and Computational Assessment. *Curr. Top. Med. Chem.* **2019**, *19*, 620–632. [CrossRef]
71. Magalhães, T.F.F.; da Silva, C.M.; Dos Santos, L.B.F.; Santos, D.A.; Silva, L.M.; Fuchs, B.B.; Mylonakis, E.; Martins, C.V.B.; de Resende-Stoianoff, M.A.; de Fátima, Â. Cinnamyl Schiff bases: Synthesis, cytotoxic effects and antifungal activity of clinical interest. *Lett. Appl. Microbiol.* **2020**, *71*, 490–497. [CrossRef] [PubMed]
72. Chohan, Z.H.; Sumrra, S.H. Synthesis, characterization and biological properties of thienyl derived triazole Schiff bases and their oxovanadium (IV) complexes. *J. Enzym. Inhib. Med. Chem.* **2012**, *27*, 187–193. [CrossRef] [PubMed]
73. Luo, H.; Lv, Y.F.; Zhang, H.; Hu, J.M.; Li, H.M.; Liu, S.J. Synthesis and Antitumor Activity of 1-Substituted 1,2,3-Triazole-Mollugin Derivatives. *Molecules* **2021**, *26*, 3249. [CrossRef] [PubMed]

Disclaimer/Publisher's Note: The statements, opinions and data contained in all publications are solely those of the individual author(s) and contributor(s) and not of MDPI and/or the editor(s). MDPI and/or the editor(s) disclaim responsibility for any injury to people or property resulting from any ideas, methods, instructions or products referred to in the content.

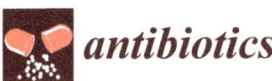

Article

Synthesis and Development of *N*-2,5-Dimethylphenylthioureido Acid Derivatives as Scaffolds for New Antimicrobial Candidates Targeting Multidrug-Resistant Gram-Positive Pathogens

Povilas Kavaliauskas [1,2,3,4], Birutė Grybaitė [1], Rita Vaickelionienė [1], Birutė Sapijanskaitė-Banevič [1], Kazimieras Anusevičius [1,*], Agnė Kriaučiūnaitė [1], Gabrielė Smailienė [1], Vidmantas Petraitis [2,4], Rūta Petraitienė [2,4], Ethan Naing [2], Andrew Garcia [2] and Vytautas Mickevičius [1]

[1] Department of Organic Chemistry, Kaunas University of Technology, Radvilėnų Rd. 19, LT-50254 Kaunas, Lithuania
[2] Transplantation-Oncology Infectious Diseases Program, Division of Infectious Diseases, Department of Medicine, Weill Cornell Medicine of Cornell University, 1300 York Ave., New York, NY 10065, USA
[3] Institute for Genome Sciences, School of Medicine, University of Maryland, 655 W. Baltimore Street, Baltimore, MD 21201, USA
[4] Institute of Infectious Diseases and Pathogenic Microbiology, Birštono Str. 38A, LT-59116 Prienai, Lithuania
* Correspondence: kazimieras.anusevicius@ktu.lt; Tel.: +370-646-21841

Abstract: The growing antimicrobial resistance to last-line antimicrobials among Gram-positive pathogens remains a major healthcare emergency worldwide. Therefore, the search for new small molecules targeting multidrug-resistant pathogens remains of great importance. In this paper, we report the synthesis and in vitro antimicrobial activity characterisation of novel thiazole derivatives using representative Gram-negative and Gram-positive strains, including tedizolid/linezolid-resistant *S. aureus*, as well as emerging fungal pathogens. The 4-substituted thiazoles **3h**, and **3j** with naphthoquinone-fused thiazole derivative **7** with excellent activity against methicillin and tedizolid/linezolid-resistant *S. aureus*. Moreover, compounds **3h**, **3j** and **7** showed favourable activity against vancomycin-resistant *E. faecium*. Compounds **9f** and **14f** showed broad-spectrum antifungal activity against drug-resistant *Candida* strains, while ester **8f** showed good activity against *Candida auris* which was greater than fluconazole. Collectively, these data demonstrate that *N*-2,5-dimethylphenylthioureido acid derivatives could be further explored as novel scaffolds for the development of antimicrobial candidates targeting Gram-positive bacteria and drug-resistant pathogenic fungi.

Keywords: 2-aminothiazoles; antifungal; antibacterial; anticancer activity; hydrazone; benzimidazole; sulphanilamide

1. Introduction

Infections caused by Gram-positive pathogens, such as methicillin-resistant *Staphylococcus aureus* (MRSA) and vancomycin-resistant enterococci (VRE) remain among one of the most common infectious agents worldwide. Infections caused by MRSA and VRE are responsible for increased mortality rates among hospitalised patients with chronic illness [1,2]. Numerous virulence factors are harboured by MRSA and VRE as well as biofilm production often leading to infections in surgically implanted catheters, especially in patients receiving cancer chemotherapy, hematopoietic stem-cell transplantation, and solid-organ transplantation. The profound antimicrobial resistance among MRSA and VRSA shortens the available treatment options, resulting in the systemic manifestation of the pathogen and death. Therefore, it is important to develop and investigate novel compounds with antimicrobial activity directed to MRSA and VRE.

The ability of pathogens to form biofilms on indwelling catheters has previously been associated with greater morbidity [3,4]. Moreover, the formation of interkingdom biofilms, consisting of bacterial pathogens and *Candida* species worsens the clinical prognosis. Despite being the most common fungal pathogen in clinical settings responsible for great morbidity worldwide, *Candida* spp. can form synergistic relationships with *S. aureus* leading to bacterial protection from antimicrobial treatment. Moreover, there is evidence that *S. aureus* provides a niche for *C. albicans* to evade antifungal drugs and thus survive the treatment [5,6]. Moreover, the recent emergence of the highly resistant *C. auris* with an instinctive resistance to azoles remains an increasing hardcore threat. Therefore, it is critical to apply novel concepts and develop multifunctional compounds with the ability to evade pre-existing antimicrobial activity in Gram-positive pathogens and clinically important fungi [7–9].

The development of new antimicrobials is focused on aspects of enhancing antimicrobial properties as well as evading antimicrobial resistance of bacterial and fungal pathogens or restoring the susceptibility of the pathogens to clinically approved antimicrobials [10–15]. In addition, compounds should remain minimally toxic to the host and show good pharmacological properties. However, the main aspect of developing effective drugs is their structural characteristics and the rate of activity. Lipophilicity is a significant physicochemical parameter that influences the membrane's transport and the binding's ability to act [16–19]. The study of lipophilicity-related parameters of thiazole derivatives showed these compounds to be promising drug candidates [20].

Thiazole derivatives are a family of heterocyclic compounds with large-scale biological properties [21] and are well-known in medicinal chemistry as promising drug candidates [22–24]. Synthesis of variously substituted thiazole ring led to novel compounds with numerous interesting pharmacological properties, including antibacterial [25–29], antifungal [15,20,23,30,31], antiviral [32–35], anthelmintic [36], antihypertensive, antihistaminic [37,38] and analgesic [39–41] effect. For instance, a naphthyl-substituted thiazole was established to inhibit the allosteric cysteine in the p10 subunit of caspase-5, thus acting as a cell's protective compound [42]. Furthermore, benzimidazole-thiazole hybrid [43] was shown to be a privileged scaffold with a potent anti-inflammatory effect [40], and benzene sulphonamide thiazoles revealed its potent inhibitory properties against DPP-4 [27].

The 2,5-dimethylphenyl scaffold is a common structural feature in many antimicrobial compounds, particularly in the class of compounds known as phenylpropanoids [44]. These compounds have been found to have antimicrobial activity against a wide range of microorganisms, including bacteria, fungi and viruses [45–47]. They have been the subject of extensive research for the development of new antimicrobial agents, particularly in the fight against antibiotic-resistant infections [48]. Some examples of drugs that have been developed from the 2,5-dimethylphenyl scaffold include antifungal echinocandins and antibacterial agents such as linezolid. Therefore, novel compounds bearing 2,5-dimethylphenyl substituents may pose antimicrobial activity against Gram-positive and Gram-negative pathogens with novel or emerging resistance mechanisms. To explore aminothiazole derivatives as novel candidates targeting clinically important and multidrug-resistant WHO priority pathogens, we generated a series of aminothiazole derivatives bearing N-2,5-dimethylphenyl and β-alanine and characterised their antimicrobial activity using pathogens with defined resistance mechanisms. In addition to that, we characterised anticancer activity using A549 and Caco-2 cell culture models. A SAR investigation of aminothiazole derivatives revealed the influence of modification to a carboxylic acid moiety on the antimicrobial activity of the synthesized compounds [49]. In this paper, we describe the synthesis and in vitro characterisation of antimicrobial and anticancer properties of a series of novel thiazole derivatives bearing 4-quinolone, quinoxaline, naphthoquinone, hydrazone, benzimidazole, and benzenesulphonamide moieties. It is known that thiazoles can be synthesised from α-bromoketone and thiourea via *Hantzsch* thiazole synthesis in high yields.

2. Results and Discussion

2.1. Synthesis

This research work is a continuation of projects on the synthesis and biological evaluation of various thiazole derivatives. 3-(1-(2,5-Dimethylphenyl)thioureido)propanoic acid (**1**) as the starting compound was synthesized by multistep reactions according to the method described in [50]. It is known that thiazoles can be synthesised from α-haloketone and a thioamide via *Hantzsch* thiazole synthesis in high yields [51]. To synthesize thiazolone **2** (Scheme 1), thioureido acid **1** was reacted with monochloroacetic acid in an aqueous 10% potassium carbonate solution at room temperature followed by the acidification with acetic acid to pH 6. In this reaction, the conventional reaction conditions at reflux were not suitable due to the formation of a large number of impurities. A singlet at 3.91 ppm of CH_2 group protons in the ^1H NMR spectrum and resonance lines at 183.3 ppm (C=O) and 187.0 ppm (C=N) in the ^{13}C NMR spectrum of compound **2** confirmed the formation of the thiazolone ring. 2-Amino-1,3-thiazole derivative **3a** was obtained from thioureido acid **1** and a chloroacetaldehyde 50% aqueous solution. The reaction was performed by refluxing acetone for 12 h. Product **3a** was obtained in the form of water-soluble hydrochloride salt [52]. The convenience of the method is the crystallisation of the product from the reaction mixture already during the process. The data of the ^1H and ^{13}C NMR spectra of synthesized compounds **1**, **2 3a** are included in the Supplementary Material (Figures S1–S6).

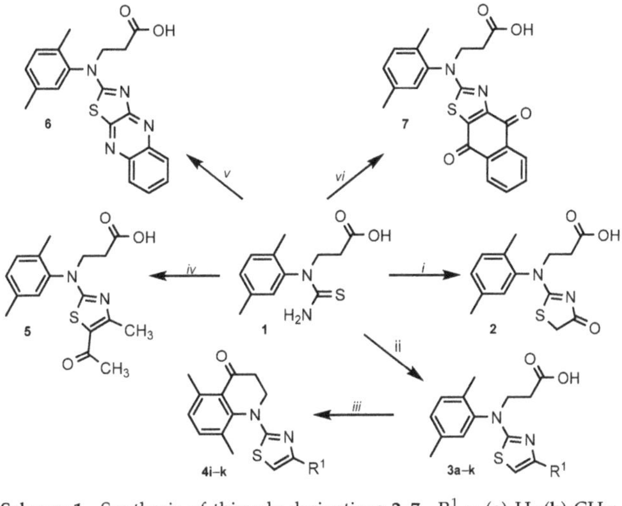

Scheme 1. Synthesis of thiazole derivatives **2–7**. R^1 = (**a**) H; (**b**) CH_3; (**c**) C_6H_5; (**d**) 4-F-C_6H_4; (**e**) 4-CN-C_6H_4; (**f**) 4-Cl-C_6H_4; (**g**) 4-NO_2-C_6H_4; (**h**) 3,4-diCl-C_6H_4; (**i**) 4-Br-C_6H_4; (**j**) naphthalen-2-yl; (**k**) chromenon-3-yl. Reagents and conditions: (i) $ClCH_2COOH$, 10% K_2CO_3, r.t. 24 h, AcOH to pH 6; (ii) **a** 50% $ClCH_2CHO$, acetone, reflux, 12 h; **b** $ClCH_2COCH_3$, water, rt, 24 h, AcONa, heated to boil; **c–k** α-bromoacetophenone, acetone, reflux, 2–5 h, (iii) PPA, 120 °C, 2–3 h, crushed ice; (iv) 3-chloropentane-2,4-dione, acetone, reflux, 2 h; (v) 2,3-dichloroquinoxaline or (vi) 2,3-dichloro-1,4-naphthoquinone, AcOH, AcONa, rt, 24 h, 70–80 °C, 10 h, water.

Next, the 4-methyl substituted thiazole **3b** was synthesized as shown in Scheme 1. Previously, in [53], 4-methyl-2-aminothiazole was prepared in acetone, but for **3b**, the interaction of thioureido acid **1** with chloroacetone proceeded better in water than in acetone. The reaction at room temperature for 24 h and the following addition of sodium acetate to the reaction mixture gave the desired 4-methyl-1,3-thiazole derivative **3b**, the structure of which was easily confirmed by the NMR spectral data (Supplementary Material, Figures S7 and S8).

According to the publication [54], 4-substituted thiazoles and especially those with chromen-3-yl and naphthalen-2-yl moieties demonstrate convincing antibacterial properties. Based on this, we have prepared a library of 4-substituted thiazoles **3c–k**. The well-known *Hantzsch* thiazole synthesis method was applied and the generation of the target products **3c–k** was performed by condensation of thioureido acid **1** with a series of α-bromoacetophenones without the use of a base. The isolated hydrobromide salts were transformed to free-based by dissolving them in 10% aqueous sodium carbonate and acidifying the solutions with acetic acid to pH 6. The structures of the obtained compounds **3c–k** were confirmed by the data of the ^{1}H and ^{13}C NMR spectra (Supplementary Material, Figures S9–S26).

The activity of broad-spectrum quinolone-based antibiotics against both Gram-positive and Gram-negative bacteria, including mycobacteria and anaerobes, promotes the synthesis and development of new quinolone-type compounds which are relevant to the development of knowledge on this topic [55]. Heating of *N*-aryl-β-alanines with strong dehydrating agents such as Eaton's reagent [56], polyphosphoric acid [57,58] or phosphorus pentoxide [59] causes the formation of compounds containing 2,3-dihydroquinolin-4(1*H*)-one moiety. To obtain quinolone-type compounds **4i–k**, thiazoles **3i–k** were treated with polyphosphoric acid at 120 °C. The intramolecular cyclisation occurred over 2–3 h and 2,3-dihydroquinolin-4(1*H*)-ones **4i–k** were obtained in 71–88% yield. The data of the ^{1}H and ^{13}C NMR spectra of synthesized compounds **4i–k** are included in the Supplementary Material (Figures S27–S32).

Compounds bearing a 5-acetyl-4-methylthiazole structure were found to exhibit high cytotoxicity against the MCF-7 cell line [60] as well as demonstrate up-and-coming antimicrobial properties [61,62]. For that purpose, we have included the synthesis of a compound containing this fragment into the goals of our study, and 5-acetyl-4-methylthiazole **5** was prepared by the same technique as for **3c–k**. The product was separated in 75% yield and its structure was confirmed by the methods of IR, NMR spectroscopy and the data of elemental analysis (NMR data are included in the Supplementary Material, Figures S33 and S34).

The previous study [63] on the synthesis and the assessment of biological properties of thiazole derivatives revealed naphthoquinone-fused derivatives to demonstrate good antimicrobial properties against Gram-positive and Gram-negative bacteria strains. The efforts to synthesize quinoxaline- and naphthoquinone-fused thiazoles **6** and **7** by the interaction of thioureido acid **1** with 2,3-dichloroquinoxaline or 2,3-dichloro-1,4-naphthoquinone, respectively, were successful. The stirring of the reaction mixture in glacial acetic acid with the presence of sodium acetate in the mixture at room temperature for 24 h and the additional stirring at the higher temperature of 70–80 °C for 10 h afforded thiazoles **6** and **7** (NMR data are included in the Supplementary Material, Figures S35–S38). An even higher temperature of the reaction mixture strongly reduces the yield of the products due to the formation 1-(2,5-dimethylphenyl)-2-thioxotetrahydropyrimidin-4(1*H*)-one caused by the intramolecular cyclisation of thioureido acid **1** [64]. Noteworthy, Matsuoka et al. state that in some cases the reactions of 2,3-dichloro-1,4-naphthoquinone with thioamides, thiourea and dithiooxamide led to the formation of dibenzo[*b*,*i*]thianthrene-5,7,12,14-tetraone as the main product of the reaction [65–67]. The same by-product was identified in the synthesis route of 3-[(2,5-dimethylphenyl)(4,9-dioxo-4,9-dihydronaphtho [2,3-*d*][1,3]thiazol-2-yl)amino]propanoic acid (**7**).

The carboxyl functional group can be an important constituent of a pharmacophore [68]. Its functionalisation can greatly expand the library of biological properties of compounds [69,70]. To expand the library of thiazole derivatives and to evaluate the influence of substituents on their biological properties, some transformations of the carboxyl group were performed (Scheme 2). Firstly, acid **3f** was esterified with methanol to obtain ester **8f**. No additional catalyst was required for this reaction with hydrobromide analogue. Afterwards, ester **8f** was refluxed in 1,4-dioxane with hydrazine monohydrate and the resulting acid hydrazide **9f** was then condensed with aldehydes and ketones. The structure of **9f** was confirmed by the NMR techniques and microanalysis data. The presence of the CONHNH$_2$ group protons were indicated by the singlets at 9.11 (NH) and 4.07 (NH$_2$) ppm in the ^{1}H NMR spectrum of **9f**, whereas the spectral line of the carbon of the C=O group resonated at the characteristic area of the ^{13}C NMR spectrum, i.e., at 169.4 ppm (Supplementary Material, Figures S39 and S42).

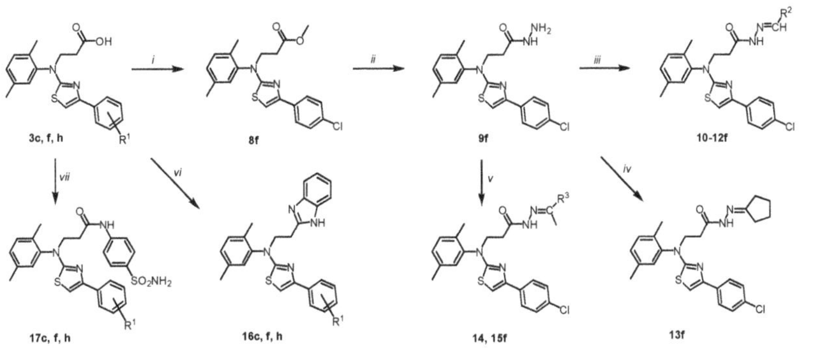

Scheme 2. Chemical transformations of carboxylic acids **3c, f, h** and hydrazide **9f**. (**3, 16, 17c**) R^1 = H; (**3, 16, 17f**) R^1 = 4-Cl; (**3, 16, 17h**) R^1 = 2,4-diCl; (**10f**) R^2 = 5-nitrothiophen-2-yl; (**11f**) R^2 = 5-nitrofuran-2-yl; (**12f**) R^2 = indol-3-yl; (**14f**) R^3 = Et; (**15f**) Hex. Reagents and conditions: (i) MeOH, a few drops of conc. H$_2$SO$_4$, reflux, 4 h; 5% Na$_2$CO$_3$ (ii) N$_2$H$_4$·H$_2$O, 1,4-dioxane, reflux, 5 h; (iii) corresponding aldehyde, 1,4-dioxane, a few drops of glacial acetic acid, reflux, 2–12 h; (iv) cyclopentanone, 1,4-dioxane, a few drops of conc. acetic acid, reflux, 3 h; (v) corresponding ketone, 1,4-dioxane, a few drops of conc. acetic acid, reflux, 4 (**14**) or 8 (**15**) h; (vi) *o*-phenylenediamine, 15% HCl, reflux 72 h, water, 10% K$_2$CO$_3$; (vii) sulphanilamide, TEA, DMF, rt, 0.5 h, HBTU, DMF, argon, r.t. 72 h, 10% K$_2$CO$_3$.

As previously reported in [71], 4-aryl substituted thiazoles bearing hydrazonyl fragments appeared to be an eligible scaffold for the future development of antifungal and antibacterial agents targeting highly resistant pathogenic microorganisms. Further, a series of various hydrazones were synthesized and investigated for their bioactivity. To obtain hydrazones **10–15f**, hydrazide **9f** was condensed with heterocyclic and aliphatic ketones. The products were isolated in a 75–85% yield. The NMR spectra of the synthesized hydrazones **10–15f** showed that in the DMSO-*d*$_6$ solution, they exist as a mixture of E/Z conformers due to the presence of a CO-NH fragment in the molecule and the restricted rotation around it; in the studies [57,72], the Z-form predominate are described NMR data are included in the Supplementary Material, Figures S43–S54).

One of the methods for the synthesis of a benzimidazole heterosystem involves to condensation of carboxylic acids with 1,2-diaminobenzenes. The target compounds **16c, f, h** were synthesized by Phillip's method (heating of both reagents in 4 M hydrochloric acid). The reflux for 72 h gave benzimidazoles **16c, f, h** in good yields (NMR data are in the Supplementary Material, Figures S45–S60).

Finally, amides **17c, f, h** were prepared by direct coupling of acids **3** with the sulphanilamide using HBTU as the coupling reagent and triethylamine as the base (Scheme 2).

The reactions were performed in dimethylformamide at room temperature in an inert argon atmosphere. The products were isolated by the dilution of the reaction mixture with an aqueous 10% potassium carbonate and were characterised using NMR and IR spectroscopy and elemental analysis (NMR data are included in the Supplementary Material, Figures S61–S66).

It is worth noting that the analysis of NMR spectra revealed that the CH$_2$N protons are often observed as two broad singlets. The characteristic splitting of resonances was observed for all compounds except **4i–k**. The literature in [64] suggests that such splitting of the proton resonances of the compounds possessing methyl group in the 2nd position of the benzene ring was caused by the restricted rotation of benzene and other N-substituents around the C(1′)-N(1) bond and the possibility of diastereomers.

2.2. Antibacterial Activity of Compounds 1–17 against Multidrug-Resistant Pathogens

In order to understand the structure-dependent antibacterial activity of novel thiazole derivatives **1–17**, we first used a representative collection of multidrug-resistant Gram-positive and Gram-negative bacterial pathogens with genetically defined antimicrobial resistance profiles [73]. The bacterial strains were selected to represent WHO ESKAPE group pathogens with emerging and challenging antimicrobial resistance mechanisms. To do so, the compounds were screened by using clinically approved minimal inhibitory concentration (MIC) determination by using the Clinical Laboratory Standard Institute (CLSI) recommendations.

Novel thiazole derivatives **1–17** exhibited structure-dependent antibacterial and antifungal activity. Interestingly, compounds **1–17** failed to show antimicrobial activity against multidrug-resistant Gram-negative pathogens, such as K. pneumoniae, P. aeruginosa, A. baumannii and E. coli (MIC > 64 µg/mL), suggesting the possible existence of Gram-positive bacteria-derived targets of compounds **1–17** (Table 1). On the other hand, only 4-substituted thiazoles **3h**, **3j** and ring-fused **7** showed favourable activity against Gram-positive bacteria (S. aureus and E. faecium) harbouring multidrug-resistance profiles (Table 2). Compound **3h** bearing 3,4-diCl-C_6H_3 moiety showed antimicrobial activity against S. aureus TCH 1516 (MIC 8 µg/mL) harbouring *mecA* gene conferring resistance to β-lactam antibiotics [1]. Moreover, **3h** showed one-fold lover antimicrobial activity against E. faecium AR-0783 (MIC 16 µg/mL) strain-harbouring *vanB* gene conferring resistance to vancomycin. The chlorines on the 3,4-diCl-C_6H_4 substituent could pose a synergistic activity by targeting multiple cellular targets on bacterial cells, in comparison to mono chlorine derivatives, thus exerting more potent antimicrobial activity. Moreover, dichloro substitutions could potentially greatly enhance lipophilicity, thus increasing compound penetration to bacterial cells. Finally, chlorine atoms are electron-windrowing groups and diCl substitution can greatly increase the electrophilicity of the compounds, thus greatly increasing reactivity and stronger interaction with microbial targets. Therefore, the chlorines at 3,4-positions of the phenyl ring are important for antimicrobial activity against Gram-positive multidrug-resistant pathogens [53]. The introduction of the 4-Cl-C_6H_4 substitution (**3f**) or the replacement of 3,4-diCl-C_6H_4 with 4-fluoro (**3d**) or 4-bromo (**3i**) phenyl substituents results in a complete loss of antimicrobial activity (MIC >64 µg/mL) against S. aureus and E. faecium suggesting the high importance of 3,4-diCl-C_6H_4 for the antimicrobial activity. Interestingly, the introduction of naphthalen-2-yl substitution (**3j**) greatly enhances the antimicrobial activity against S. aureus and E. faecium (MIC 2 µg/mL).

The replacement of the thiazole ring with the ring-fused structure strongly enhanced the antibacterial activity against S. aureus TCH 1516 strain (MIC 1 µg/mL), while the antibacterial activity against E. faecium AR-0783 increased two-fold (MIC 8 µg/mL) if compared to **3h** (Table 1). The antibacterial activity of compound **7** against S. aureus was similar to daptomycin (MIC 1 µg/mL) and twice stronger than vancomycin (MIC 2 µg/mL) and excellent if compared to ampicillin (MIC > 64 µg/mL).

The emerging resistance to oxazolidinones (linezolid and tedizolid) which are last-line antimicrobial pharmaceuticals used to treat infections caused by Staphylococcus remains one of the major healthcare threats worldwide. Therefore, we further evaluated if the most promising thiazole derivatives **3h, 3j** and **7** will be active against linezolid/tedizolid-resistant S. aureus strains (Table 2). The compounds **3h, 3j** and **7** showed promising activity against linezolid/tedizolid-resistant S. aureus strains with MIC ranging from 1 to 32 µg/mL (Table 2). Compound **3j** showed the highest activity against tested strains (MIC 1–2 µg/mL), and its antimicrobial activity was greater than linezolid (8–32 µg/mL).

Table 1. In vitro antibacterial activity of compounds 1–17 against the representative, multidrug-resistant Gram-positive and Gram-negative bacterial strains harbouring genetically defined resistance mechanisms.

Compounds	Minimal Inhibitory Concentration (µg/mL)					
	S. aureus TCH 1516 [1]	E. faecium AR-0783 [2]	K. pneumoniae AR-0139 [3]	E. coli AR-0149 [4]	A. baumannii AR-0037 [5]	P. aeruginosa AR-0100 [6]
1	>64	>64	>64	>64	>64	>64
2	>64	>64	>64	>64	>64	>64
3a	>64	>64	>64	>64	>64	>64
3b	>64	>64	>64	>64	>64	>64
3c	>64	>64	>64	>64	>64	>64
3d	>64	>64	>64	>64	>64	>64
3e	>64	>64	>64	>64	>64	>64
3f	>64	>64	>64	>64	>64	>64
3g	>64	>64	>64	>64	>64	>64
3h	8	16	>64	>64	>64	>64
3i	>64	>64	>64	>64	>64	>64
3j	2	2	>64	>64	>64	>64
3k	>64	>64	>64	>64	>64	>64
4i	>64	>64	>64	>64	>64	>64
4j	>64	>64	>64	>64	>64	>64
4k	>64	>64	>64	>64	>64	>64
5	>64	>64	>64	>64	>64	>64
6	>64	>64	>64	>64	>64	>64
7	1	8	>64	>64	>64	>64
8f	>64	>64	>64	>64	>64	>64
9f	>64	>64	>64	>64	>64	>64
10f	>64	>64	>64	>64	>64	>64
11f	16	>64	>64	>64	>64	>64
12f	>64	>64	>64	>64	>64	>64
13f	>64	>64	>64	>64	>64	>64
14f	>64	>64	>64	>64	>64	>64
15f	>64	>64	>64	>64	>64	>64
16c	>64	>64	>64	>64	>64	>64
16f	>64	>64	>64	>64	>64	>64
16h	>64	>64	>64	>64	>64	>64
17c	>64	>64	>64	>64	>64	>64
17f	>64	>64	>64	>64	>64	>64
17h	>64	>64	>64	>64	>64	>64
Vancomycin	2	64	N/A	N/A	N/A	N/A
Ampicillin	>64	64	>64	64	>64	>64
Daptomycin	1	4	N/A	N/A	N/A	N/A
Aztreonam	N/A	N/A	4	2	2	16
Meropenem	N/A	N/A	8	16	32	32
Imipenem	N/A	N/A	>64	>64	>64	>64

[1] S. aureus TCH 1516 mecA, USA300 lineage. [2] E. faecium AR-0783 VanB. [3] K. pneumoniae AR-0193 ac(6′)-IIa, armA, ARR-3, cmlA1, CMY-4, CTX-M-15, dfrA1, fosA, mph(E), msr(E), NDM-1, oqxA, oqxB, OXA-10, SHV-11, strA, strB, sul1, sul2. [4] E. coli AR-0149 CMY-42, NDM-7. [5] A. baumannii AR-0037 NDM-1, OXA-94, sul2. [6] P. aeruginosa AR-0100 aac(3)-Id, aadA6, dfrB5, OXA-50, PAO, sul1, VIM-2.

Table 2. In vitro antibacterial activity of the most promising thiazole derivatives 3h, 3j and 7 against tedizolid/linezolid resistant S. aureus strains.

Compounds	S. a AR-0701	S. a AR-0702	S. a AR-0703	S. a AR-0704	S. a AR-0705
3h	4	8	8	32	8
3j	2	2	1	2	2
7	4	16	8	8	8
Vancomycin	1	2	1	1	1
Daptomycin	0.5	1	0.5	0.5	1
Linezolid	16	16	32	8	16

Abbreviations: S. a—Staphylococcus aureus (S. aureus).

Collectively, these results demonstrated that substituted thiazoles exert in vitro antibacterial activity against Gram-positive bacterial pathogens harbouring emerging antibacterial resistance profiles. Moreover, 3,4-diCl-C$_6$H$_3$ and naphthalen-2-yl substitutions, as well as naphthothiazoledione moiety, are important for the potent in vitro antibacterial activity against *S. aureus* with challenging resistance mechanisms.

2.3. Antifungal Activity of Thiazoles 1–17 against Drug-Resistant Candida Species

Antifungal drugs of the azole group are one of the most widely used for the treatment of invasive and systemic fungal infections [74]. Candida species are responsible for the majority of fungal infections, as rapidly rising resistance to azole antifungals among Candida species, in particular C. albicans is responsible for increased morbidity and mortality worldwide [75]. We, therefore, evaluated novel thiazoles 1–17 for their in vitro antifungal activity against multidrug-resistant Candida species by exposing the fungal strains with clinically relevant concentrations of each compound or control antifungal drug (Table 3).

Table 3. In vitro antifungal activity of compounds 1–17 against the representative, multidrug-resistant fungal pathogens.

Compounds	Minimal Inhibitory Concentration (µg/mL)				
	C. auris AR-0383	C. albicans	C. glabrata AR-315	C. parapsilosis AR-0335	C. haemulonii AR-395
1	>64	>64	>64	>64	>64
2	>64	>64	>64	>64	>64
3a	>64	>64	>64	>64	>64
3b	>64	>64	>64	>64	>64
3c	>64	>64	>64	>64	>64
3d	>64	>64	>64	>64	>64
3e	>64	>64	>64	>64	>64
3f	>64	>64	>64	>64	>64
3g	>64	>64	>64	>64	>64
3h	>64	>64	>64	>64	>64
3i	>64	>64	>64	>64	>64
3j	>64	>64	>64	>64	>64
3k	>64	>64	>64	>64	>64
4i	>64	>64	>64	>64	>64
4j	>64	>64	>64	>64	>64
4k	>64	>64	>64	>64	>64
5	>64	>64	>64	>64	>64
6	>64	>64	>64	>64	>64
7	>64	>64	>64	>64	>64
8f	2	1	4	8	2
9f	>64	8	4	4	2
10f	>64	>64	>64	>64	>64
11f	>64	>64	>64	>64	>64
12f	>64	>64	>64	>64	>64
13f	>64	>64	>64	>64	>64
14f	>64	8	16	32	32

Table 3. *Cont.*

Compounds	Minimal inhibitory Concentration (µg/mL)				
	C. auris AR-0383	C. albicans	C. glabrata AR-315	C. parapsilosis AR-0335	C. haemulonii AR-395
15f	>64	>64	>64	>64	>64
16c	>64	>64	>64	>64	>64
16f	>64	>64	>64	>64	>64
16h	>64	>64	>64	>64	>64
17c	>64	>64	>64	>64	>64
17f	>64	>64	>64	>64	>64
17h	>64	>64	>64	>64	>64
Amphotericin B	<0.5	<0.5	<0.5	<0.5	<0.5
Fluconazole	32	16	16	8	4
Posaconazole	0.5	1	0.5	1	1

Interestingly, only thiazoles **8f**, **9f** and **14f** showed in vitro antifungal activity against *Candida* strains, expressing the multidrug-resistance phenotype to azoles (Table 3). The transformation of thiazole **3f** (MIC > 64 µg/mL) to ester **8f** was observed to result in striking changes in antifungal activity. (Table 3). The derivative **8f** showed antifungal activity against all tested strains (1–8 µg/mL) including *Candida auris* AR-0383 strains to harbour instinctive resistance to clinically approved antifungal drugs. The ester **8f** transformation to hydrazide **9f** greatly affected the antifungal activity. The hydrazide **9f** was no longer active against *C. auris* (MIC > 64 µg/mL) and had decreased activity against *C. albicans* (MIC 8 µg/mL) in comparison to ester **8f** (MIC 1 µg/mL). Interestingly, despite the loss of activity against *C. auris*, hydrazide **9f** showed increased activity against *C. parapsilosis* AR-0335 (MIC 4 µg/mL). Numerous hydrazones were previously reported to show antifungal activity [76–78]; therefore, we further transformed hydrazide **9f** to the corresponding hydrazones **10–15f** and evaluated their structure-dependent antifungal activity in vitro. Hydrazone **14f** bearing the butan-2-ylidene substitution exhibited antifungal activity against the majority of tested fungi (MIC 8–32 µg/mL) with the exception of *C. auris* (MIC > 64 µg/mL). The substitution of this moiety with a longer octan-2-ylidene carbon chain (**15f**) results in a complete loss of antifungal activity against all tested strains.

Thus, these results demonstrate novel thiazole derivatives **9f**, **14f** and, especially, **8f** with a moderately functionalised carboxyl group exert the most promising antifungal activity against highly multidrug-resistant fungal pathogens. On the other hand, the functionalization of the carboxyl group is important for the broad-spectrum antifungal activity since bulky substitutions result in decreased antifungal activity spectrum or potency in these novel compounds.

2.4. Anticancer Activity of Compounds 1–17

The thiazole scaffold of often explored by medicinal chemists as an attractive pharmacophore for the development of novel antineoplastic drug candidates [79–81]. Therefore, we used two well-described pulmonary (A549) [82] and corectal adenocarcinoma (Caco-2) [83] models to evaluate the anticancer activity of compounds **1–17**. We exposed the cells to 100 µM of each compound or cisplatin (CP) that was used as a clinically approved drug for the neoplastic disease treatment. The treatment was initiated for 24 h and after that, the cellular viability was measured by using MTT assay.

The novel thiazoles **1–17** demonstrated structure-dependent anticancer activity on A549 and Caco-2 cells. Interestingly, Caco-2 corectal adenocarcinoma cells showed significantly higher susceptibility to the treatment compounds in comparison to A549 cells ($p < 0.05$) suggesting the possible existence of selective novel thiazole-response involved targets in Caco-2. The starting compound **1** showed no significant anticancer activity against A549 human pulmonary adenocarcinoma cells. On the other hand, compound **1** significantly decreased the viability of Caco-2 cells (39.8%) in comparison to untreated control (UC) ($p < 0.001$) (Figure 1B). Thiazolone **2** resulted in slightly enhanced anticancer activity against Caco-2 (31.9%) while 2-amino-1,3-thiazole derivative **3a** showed decreased (56.9%) anticancer activity in comparison to UC ($p = 0.0019$). The addition of a 4-methyl group on the 1,3-thiazole ring (**3b**) enhanced the anticancer activity against Caco-2 cells ($p = 0.004$). Interestingly, compounds **2–3b** showed no anticancer activity against A549 cells (Figure 1A).

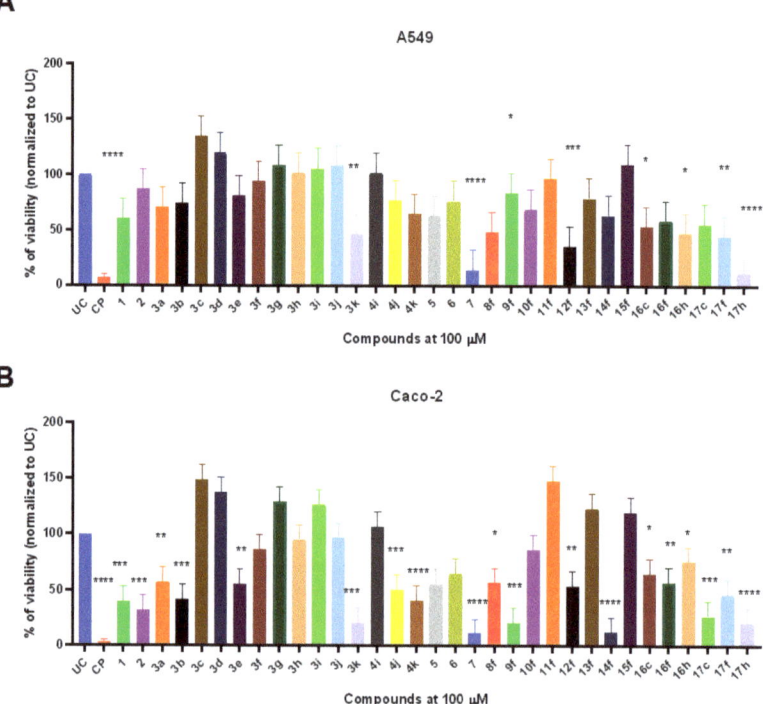

Figure 1. The in vitro anticancer activity of compounds **1–17** on A549 (**A**) and Caco-2 (**B**) adenocarcinoma cell line. Cells were exposed with fixed 100 µM of compounds **1–17** or cisplatin (CP) that served as a cytotoxicity control for 24 h. After the treatment, the remaining viability was determined by using MTT assay. Data represent the mean ± SD of triplicate experiments ($n = 3$). Statistical differences were determined using the Kruskal–Wallis test. * $p < 0.05$; ** $p < 0.01$, *** $p < 0.001$, **** $p < 0.0001$.

Amongst 4-substituted thiazoles, only **3e** bearing 4-CN-C_6H_4 and **3k** with chromenon-3-yl substitutions showed anticancer activity against A549 and Caco-2 cells. Thiazole **3e** (R: 4-CN-C_6H_4) was able to significantly reduce the Caco-2 viability (54.9%) ($p = 0.0011$) while having no significant effect against A549 cells. Interestingly, the incorporation of chromenon-3-yl moiety (**3k**) significantly enhances the anticancer activity against Caco-2 ($p = 0.001$) as well as A549 cells ($p = 0.0084$) (Figure 1A,B).

Quinolone-type compound **4i** bearing 4-Br-C_6H_4 substituent failed to significantly decrease the Caco-2 and A549 viability (106.1 and 101.4%, respectively). The incorporation of naphthalen-2-yl substitution (**4j**) significantly enhanced the anticancer activity against Caco-2 cells ($p = 0.002$) while chromenon-3-yl substitution (**4k**) resulted in significant 40.2% post-treatment viability of Caco-2 cells ($p < 0.001$) (Figure 1B).

5-Acetyl-4-methylthazole **5** did not significantly reduce the viability of A549 or Caco-2, although the compound was able to decrease the viability to 63 and 55%, respectively. Thiazole fusion with quinoxaline (compound **6**) did not result in significant viability reduction, although fusion with naphthoquinone lead to compound **7** with significantly high anticancer activity. Compound **7** exhibited broad-spectrum anticancer activity and was able to reduce A549 and Caco-2 viability to 14.0 and 13.1% compared to UC ($p < 0.001$) (Figure 1A,B).

The carboxyl group transformation to ester **8f** in compound **3f** slightly enhanced the anticancer activity if compared to parent acid **3f** and showed similar anticancer efficacy against A549 and Caco-2 by reducing the viability to 48.1 and 56.4%, respectively. Interestingly subsequent ester **8f** transformation to hydrazide **9f** greatly enhanced the anticancer activity against Caco-2 cells (20.6%) while ameliorating compound-mediated cytotoxic activity against A549 cells (Figure 1A,B).

On the other hand, hydrazones **10–15f** showed highly structure-dependent activity. Hydrazones **10f** and **11f** bearing the 5-nitrothien-2-yl and 5-nitrofuran-2-yl substitutions showed no anticancer activity against both tested cancer cell lines. Compound **12f** containing indol-3-yl substitution demonstrated greater anticancer activity against A549 (35.0%) than Caco-2 (53.1%). The incorporation of cyclopentyl substitution resulted in compound **13f** with a complete loss of anticancer activity against both cell lines, while the incorporation of ethyl radical (**14f**) significantly enhanced the anticancer activity against Caco-2 cells, but not A549. On the other hand, the incorporation of the hexyl chain (**15f**) resulted in a complete loss of anticancer activity against Caco-2, suggesting the importance of ethyl radical in novel thiazole structures (Figure 1A,B).

Benzimidazoles **16c,f,h** demonstrated similar anticancer activity in both A549 and Caco-2 cell lines by decreasing viability to approximately 47–60%. Amide **17c** containing 4-phenyl substituted thiazole showed potent anticancer activity against Caco-2 cells (27.2%) and little activity against A549 cells (55.4%). Compound **17f** bearing 4-Cl-C_6H_4 substituent at 4th position of the thiazole cycle showed similar activity in both cell lines (44.3 and 46.0%, respectively), while the incorporation of 2,4-diCl-C_6H_3 into the same position resulted in strong anticancer activity against both cell lines (Figure 1A,B).

These results demonstrate that novel thiazole derivatives possess strong anticancer activity against different adenocarcinoma cell lines. The structure–activity relation studies showed that naphthoquinone-fusion and 2,4-diCl-C_6H_3 substitution are required for broad-spectrum anticancer activity.

3. Materials and Methods

3.1. Synthesis

All reagents and used solvents were purchased from Sigma-Aldrich (St. Louis, MO, USA) and used as received without any purification. Reaction progress and compound purity were monitored by TLC using aluminium plates precoated with Silica gel with F254 nm (Merck KGaA, Darmstadt, Germany). Melting points were determined in an open capillary with a B-540 melting point apparatus (Büchi Corporation, New Castle, DE, USA) and were uncorrected. A Perkin–Elmer Spectrum BX FT–IR spectrometer (Perkin–Elmer Inc., Waltham, MA, USA) was used to record the IR spectra (v, cm^{-1}) and the pellets were prepared using KBr. The NMR spectra were recorded on Bruker Ascend 400 (^{1}H 400 MHz, ^{13}C 101 MHz) and Bruker Ascend (^{1}H 700 MHz, ^{13}C 176 MHz) spectrometers (Bruker BioSpin AG, Fällanden, Switzerland) using DMSO-d_6 and CDCl$_3$ as solvents and TMS as an internal reference. The spectra data are presented as follows: chemical shift, multiplicity, integration, coupling constant [Hz] and allocation. The Elemental Analyzer CE-440 was used for elemental analyses (C, H, N) in good agreement (± 0.3%) with the calculated values.

3-[Carbamothioyl(2,5-dimethylphenyl)amino]propanoic acid (**1**). The thioureido acid **1** was synthesized according to the method described in the literature [64]. Yield 85%, m.p. 134–135 °C (from water).

IR (KBr): ν 1167 (C=S), 1746 (C=O), 3342 (NH$_2$), 3445 (OH) cm^{-1}.
^{1}H NMR (400 MHz, CDCl$_3$): δ 2.13 (s, 3H, CH$_3$), 2.29 (s, 3H, CH$_3$), 2.49–2.56 (m, 2H, CH$_2$CO), 3.76 (br. s,, 1H, NCH$_2$), 4.44 (br. s, 1H, NCH$_2$), 5.95 (br. s, 1H, NH$_2$), 6.96 (s, 1H, H$_{Ar}$), 7.10 (s, 1H, H$_{Ar}$), 7.21 (s, 1H, H$_{Ar}$), 7.50 (br. s, 1H, NH$_2$), ppm.
^{13}C NMR (101 MHz, CDCl$_3$): δ 16.9 (CH$_3$), 21.6 (CH$_3$), 32.9 (CH$_2$CO), 50.3 (NCH$_2$), 128.4, 130.3, 132.1, 132.3, 138.1, 138.9 (C$_{Ar}$), 176.9 (COOH), 181.6 (C=O) ppm.
Anal. Calcd for C$_{12}$H$_{16}$N$_2$O$_2$S: C, 57.12%; H, 6.39%; N, 11.10%; Found: C, 57.33%; H, 6.10%; N, 10.84%.

3-[(2,5-Dimethylphenyl)(4-oxo-4,5-dihydro-1,3-thiazol-2-yl)amino]propanoic acid (**2**). A mixture of thioureido acid **1** (1.26 g, 5 mmol), 40 mL of aqueous 10% potassium carbonate and chloroacetic acid (0.57 g, 6 mmol) was stirred at room temperature for 24 h. Then, the mixture was acidified with acetic acid to pH 6. Obtained the precipitate was filtered off, washed with water, and crystallized. Yield 0.88 g, 60%; m.p. 159–160 °C (from 2-propanol and water mixture 1:1).
IR (KBr): ν 1581 (C=N), 1674, 1725 (2C=O), 3290 (OH) cm^{-1}.
^{1}H NMR (700 MHz, DMSO-d$_6$): δ 2.16 (s, 3H, CH$_3$), 2.30 (s, 3H, CH$_3$), 2.57 (t, 2H, J = 7.5 Hz, CH$_2$CO), 3.72–3.81 (m, 1H, NCH$_2$), 3.91 (s, 2H, SCH$_2$), 4.24–4.39 (m, 1H, NCH$_2$), 7.16 (s,1H, H$_{Ar}$), 7.22 (d, J = 7.8 Hz, 1H, H$_{Ar}$), 7.29 (d, J = 7.7 Hz, 1H, H$_{Ar}$), 11.07 (br. s, 1H, OH) ppm.
^{13}C NMR (176 MHz, DMSO-d$_6$): δ 16.5 (CH$_3$), 20.3 (CH$_3$), 32.3 (CH$_2$CO), 40.5 (SCH$_2$), 49.5 (NCH$_2$), 129.2, 130.6, 131.4, 132.7, 136.9, 138.7 (C$_{Ar}$), 172.2 (COOH), 183.2 (C=O), 187.0 (C=N) ppm.
Anal. Calcd for C$_{14}$H$_{16}$N$_2$O$_3$S: C, 57.52%; H, 5.52%; N, 9.58%; Found: C, 57.27%; H, 4.28%; N, 9.39%.

3-[(2,5-Dimethylphenyl)(1,3-thiazol-2-yl)amino]propanoic acid (**3a**). A mixture of the thioureido acid **1** (0.5 g, 2 mmol), aqueous 50% chloroacetaldehyde solution (0.79 g, 10 mmol) and acetone (20 mL) was refluxed for 12 h. After that, the formed precipitate was filtered, washed with acetone and dried. Purification was performed by dissolving the crystals in aqueous 10% sodium carbonate (75 mL), filtering, and acidifying the filtrate with acetic acid to pH 6 (the procedure was repeated 2 times). Yield 0.35 g, 64%, m.p. 112–113 °C.
IR (KBr): ν 3076 (OH), 1717 (CO), 1514 (CN) cm^{-1}.
^{1}H NMR (700 MHz, DMSO-d$_6$): δ 2.10 (s, 3H, CH$_3$), 2.29 (s, 3H, CH$_3$), 2.62 (t, J = 7.3 Hz, 2H, CH$_2$CO), 3.98 (br. s, 2H, NCH$_2$), 6.66, 7.16 (2d, 2H, J = 3.6 Hz, SCH, NCH), 7.11 (s, 1H, H$_{Ar}$), 7.13–7.16 (m, 1H, H$_{Ar}$), 7.26 (d, 1H, J = 7.8 Hz, H$_{Ar}$), 12.29 (s, 1H, OH) ppm.
^{13}C NMR (176 MHz, DMSO-d$_6$): δ 16.7 (CH$_3$), 20.4 (CH$_3$), 32.4 (CH$_2$CO), 48.1 (NCH$_2$), 108.0, 129.1, 129.2, 131.6, 133.0, 137.2, 139.3, 143.0 (C$_{Ar}$ + SCH + NCH), 170.1 (C=N), 172.7 (COOH) ppm.
Anal. Calcd for C$_{14}$H$_{16}$N$_2$O$_2$S: C, 60.85%; H, 5.48%; N, 10.14%; Found: C, 60.67%; H, 5.62%; N, 9.87%.

3-[(2,5-Dimethylphenyl)(4-methyl-1,3-thiazol-2-yl)amino]propanoic acid (**3b**). A mixture of thioureido acid **1** (1.26 g, 5 mmol), chloroacetone (0.64 g, 7 mmol) and water (20 mL) was stirred at room temperature for 24 h. Then, sodium acetate (0.82 g, 10 mmol) was added and the reaction mixture was brought to reflux. After cooling, the formed precipitate was filtered off and washed with water. Obtained organic salt was transformed to free-base by dissolving the crystals in 10% aqueous sodium carbonate (75 mL), filtering, and acidifying the filtrate with acetic acid to pH 6 (the purification procedure was repeated 2 times). Yield 0.88 g, 67%, m.p. 155–156 °C.
IR (KBr): ν 1527 (C=N), 1706 (C=O), 3392 (OH) cm^{-1}.
^{1}H NMR (700 MHz, DMSO-d$_6$): δ 2.09 (s, 3H, CH$_3$), 2.15 (s, 3H, CH$_3$), 2.28 (s, 3H, CH$_3$), 2.60 (t, 2H, J = 7.3 Hz, CH$_2$CO), 3.96 (br. s, 2H, NCH$_2$), 6.20 (d, 1H, J = 1.1 Hz, SCH), 7.09 (d, 1H, J = 1.2 Hz, H$_{Ar}$), 7.12 (dd, 1H, J = 7.9, 1.3 Hz, H$_{Ar}$), 7.25 (d, 1H, J = 7.8 Hz, H$_{Ar}$), 12.35 (s, 1H, OH) ppm.

^{13}C NMR (176 MHz, DMSO-d_6): δ 16.8 (CH$_3$), 17.6 (CH$_3$), 20.4 (CH$_3$), 32.4 (CH$_2$CO), 47.9 (NCH$_2$), 102.1 (SCH), 129.2, 129.4, 131.6, 133.1, 137.1, 142.8, 148.5 (C$_{Ar}$ + NC), 169.3 (C=N), 172.8 (COOH) ppm.

Anal. Calcd for C$_{15}$H$_{18}$N$_2$O$_2$S: C, 62.04%; H, 6.25%; N, 9.65%; Found: C, 62.02%; H, 6.28%; N, 9.40%.

General procedure for the synthesis of compounds **3c–k**. A mixture of the thioureido acid **1** (0.5 g, 2 mmol), the appropriate α-bromoacetophenone (2.2 mmol) and acetone (20 mL) was refluxed for 2–5 h and cooled down. The precipitate was filtered off, washed with acetone and dried. Obtained organic salts were transformed to free-base by dissolving the crystals in 10% aqueous sodium carbonate (75 mL), filtering and acidifying the filtrate with acetic acid to pH 6 (the purification procedure was repeated 2 times).

3-[(2,5-Dimethylphenyl)(4-phenyl-1,3-thiazol-2-yl)amino]propanoic acid (**3c**)
Yield 0.47 g, 67%, m.p. 104–105 °C.
IR (KBr): ν 1537 (C=N), 1710 (C=O), 3390 (OH) cm^{-1}.
^{1}H NMR (700 MHz, DMSO-d_6): δ 2.14 (s, 3H, CH$_3$), 2.29 (s, 3H, CH$_3$), 2.63 (t, 2H, J = 7.3 Hz, CH$_2$CO), 4.07 (br. s, 2H, NCH$_2$), 7.08 (s, 1H, SCH), 7.11–7.17 (m, 2H, H$_{Ar}$), 7.25–7.30 (m, 2H, H$_{Ar}$), 7.39 (t, 2H, J = 7.7 Hz, H$_{Ar}$) ppm.
^{13}C NMR (176 MHz, DMSO-d_6): δ 16.8 (CH$_3$), 20.4 (CH$_3$), 33.1 (CH$_2$CO), 48.5 (NCH$_2$), 102.6 (SCH), 125.7, 127.4, 128.5, 129.2, 129.3, 131.5, 133.1, 134.8, 137.2, 142.7, 150.5 (C$_{Ar}$ + NC), 169.3, (C=N), 173.1 (COOH) ppm.

Anal. Calcd for C$_{20}$H$_{20}$N$_2$O$_2$S: C, 68.16%; H, 5.72%; N, 7.95%; Found: C, 68.08%; H, 5.66%; N, 7.73%.

3-{(2,5-Dimethylphenyl)[4-(4-fluorophenyl)-1,3-thiazol-2-yl]amino}propanoic acid (**3d**)
Yield 0.56 g, 75%, m.p. 91–92 °C.
IR (KBr): ν 1223 (C-F), 1540 (C=N), 1711 (C=O), 3384 (OH) cm^{-1}.
^{1}H NMR (700 MHz, DMSO-d_6): δ 2.14 (s, 3H, CH$_3$), 2.30 (s, 3H, 2CH$_3$), 2.68 (t, 2H, J = 7.2 Hz, CH$_2$CO), 4.07 (br. s, 2H, NCH$_2$), 7.07 (s, 1H, SCH), 7.12–7.17 (m, 2H, H$_{Ar}$), 7.22 (t, 2H, J = 8.8 Hz, H$_{Ar}$), 7.28 (d, 2H, J = 8.2 Hz, H$_{Ar}$), 7.85–7.95 (m, 2H, H$_{Ar}$) ppm.
^{13}C NMR (176 MHz, DMSO-d_6): δ 16.8 (CH$_3$), 20.4 (CH$_3$), 32.6 (CH$_2$CO), 48.2 (NCH$_2$), 102.5 (SCH), 115.3, 115.4, 127.7, 129.3, 129.4, 131.3, 131.6, 133.0, 137.2, 142.7, 149.4, 160.9, 162.3 (C$_{Ar}$ + NC), 169.4 (C=N), 172.8 (COOH) ppm.

Anal. Calcd for C$_{20}$H$_{19}$FN$_2$O$_2$S: C, 64.85%; H, 5.17%; N, 7.56%; Found: C, 64.87%; H, 5.20%; N, 7.18%.

3-{[4-(4-Cyanophenyl)-1,3-thiazol-2-yl](2,5-dimethylphenyl)amino}propanoic acid (**3e**)
Yield 0.60 g, 80%, m.p. 132–133 °C.
IR (KBr): ν 1536 (C=N), 1737 (C=O), 2223 (C≡N), 3261 (OH) cm^{-1}.
^{1}H NMR (700 MHz, DMSO-d_6): δ 2.15 (2s, 3H, CH$_3$), 2.30 (2s, 3H, CH$_3$), 2.65–2.75 (m, 2H, CH$_2$CO), 3.86–4.28 (m, 2H, NCH$_2$), 7.12–7.21 (m, 2H, H$_{Ar}$ + SCH), 7.25–7.32 (m, 1H, H$_{Ar}$), 7.41 (d, 1H, J = 8.0 Hz, H$_{Ar}$), 7.85 (dd, 2H, J = 8.0, 4.9 Hz, H$_{Ar}$), 8.05 (m, 2H, J = 8.3 Hz, H$_{Ar}$) ppm.
^{13}C NMR (176 MHz, DMSO-d_6): δ 16.6 (CH$_3$), 20.4 (CH$_3$), 32.2 (CH$_2$CO), 47.4 (NCH$_2$), 91.8 (SCH), 109.5, 119.0, 126.3, 129.5, 131.7, 132.61, 132.63, 133.0, 137.3, 138.8, 142.5, 148.7 (C$_{Ar}$ + C≡N + NC), 169.6 (N=C), 172.7 (COOH) ppm.

Anal. Calcd for C$_{21}$H$_{19}$N$_3$O$_2$S: C, 66.82%; H, 5.07%; N, 11.13%; Found: C, 66.63%; H, 5.04%; N, 11.06%.

3-{[4-(4-Chlorophenyl)-1,3-thiazol-2-yl](2,5-dimethylphenyl)amino}propanoic acid (**3f**)
Yield 0.64 g, 83%, m.p. 94–95 °C.
IR (KBr): ν 835 (C-Cl), 1536 (C=N), 1710 (C=O), 3391 (OH) cm^{-1}.
^{1}H NMR (700 MHz, DMSO-d_6): δ 2.14, 2.16 (s, 3H, CH$_3$), 2.30 (s, 3H, CH$_3$), 2.57–2.75 (m, 2H, CH$_2$CO), 4.10 (br. s, 2H, NCH$_2$), 7.18 (d, 2H, J = 7.5 Hz, H$_{Ar}$ + SCH), 7.30 (d, 1H, J = 7.6 Hz, H$_{Ar}$), 7.47, 7.54 (2d, 2H, J = 8.4 Hz, H$_{Ar}$), 7.80–8.01 (m, 2H, H$_{Ar}$) ppm.
^{13}C NMR (176 MHz, DMSO-d_6): δ 16.8 (CH$_3$), 20.4 (CH$_3$), 32.4 (CH$_2$CO), 48.1 (NCH$_2$), 103.7 (SCH), 127.4, 128.4, 128.6, 129.3, 129.4, 129.7, 131.7, 131.9, 133.0, 133.5, 137.3, 142.6, 149.1 (C$_{Ar}$ + NC), 169.5 (C=N), 172.7 (COOH) ppm.

Anal. Calcd for $C_{20}H_{19}ClN_2O_2S$: C, 62.09%; H, 4.95%; N, 7.24%; Found: C, 62.27%; H, 4.91%; N, 7.03%.

3-{(2,5-Dimethylphenyl)[4-(4-nitrophenyl)-1,3-thiazol-2-yl]amino}propanoic acid (3g)
Yield 0.63 g, 79%, m.p. 136–137 °C.
IR (KBr): ν 1334, 1509 (NO_2), 1540 (C=N), 1712 (C=O); 3430 (OH) cm^{-1}.
^1H NMR (700 MHz, DMSO-d_6): δ 2.13 (s, 3H, CH_3), 2.28 (s, 3H, CH_3), 2.46–2.61 (m, 2H, CH_2CO), 3.85–4.22 (m, 2H, NCH_2), 7.08–7.18 (m, 2H, H_{Ar} + SCH), 7.26 (d, 1H, J = 8.2 Hz, H_{Ar}), 7.45 (s, 1H, H_{Ar}), 8.10 (d, 2H, J = 8.8 Hz, H_{Ar}), 8.24 (d, 2H, J = 8.9 Hz, H_{Ar}) ppm. ^{13}C NMR (176 MHz, DMSO-d_6): δ 16.8 (CH_3), 20.4 (CH_3), 34.1 ($\underline{C}H_2CO$), 49.2 (NCH_2), 107.3 (SCH), 124.0, 126.4, 129.3, 129.4, 131.6, 133.0, 137.2, 140.8, 142.5, 146.1, 148.5 (C_{Ar} + NC), 169.7 (C=N), 173.8 (COOH) ppm.
Anal. Calcd for $C_{20}H_{19}N_3O_4S$: C, 60.44%; H, 4.82%; N, 10.57%; Found: C, 60.50%; H, 4.64%; N, 10.35%.

3-{[4-(3,4-Dichlorophenyl)-1,3-thiazol-2-yl](2,5-dimethylphenyl)amino}propanoic acid (3h)
Yield 0.71 g, 84%, m.p. 114–115 °C.
IR (KBr): ν 1535 (C=N), 1710 (C=O), 3320 (OH) cm^{-1}.
^1H NMR (400 MHz, DMSO-d_6): δ 2.11, 2.27 (2s, 6H, $2CH_3$), 2.46–2.61 (m, 2H, CH_2CO), 3.85–4.22 (m, 2H, NCH_2), 7.04–7.19 (m, 2H, H_{Ar} + SCH), 7.20–7.38 (m, 2H, H_{Ar}), 7.61 (d, 1H, J = 8.4 Hz, H_{Ar}), 7.83 (dd, 1H, J = 8.2, 1.4 Hz, H_{Ar}), 8.06 (s, 1H, H_{Ar}) ppm.
^{13}C NMR (101 MHz, DMSO-d_6): δ 16.8, 20.4 ($2CH_3$), 33.8 ($\underline{C}H_2CO$), 48.9 (NCH_2), 103.8 (SCH), 125.8, 127.1, 129.3, 129.4, 129.6, 130.8, 131.4, 131.6, 133.0, 135.3, 137.3, 142.5, 147.9 (C_{Ar}, N–C), 169.5 (C=N), 171.7 (COOH) ppm.
Anal. Calcd for $C_{20}H_{18}Cl_2N_2O_2S$: C, 57.01%; H, 4.31% N, 6.65%; Found: C, 57.25%; H, 4.42%; N, 6.73%.

3-{[4-(4-Bromophenyl)-1,3-thiazol-2-yl](2,5-dimethylphenyl)amino}propanoic acid (3i)
Yield 0.64 g, 76%, m.p. 127–128 °C.
IR (KBr): ν 1539 (C=N), 1710 (C=O), 3310 (OH) cm^{-1}.
^1H NMR (400 MHz, DMSO-d_6): δ 2.12 (s, 3H, CH_3), 2.28 (s, 3H, CH_3), 2.50–2.62 (m, 2H, $\underline{C}H_2CO$), 4.02 (br. s, 2H, NCH_2), 7.06–7.30 (m, 4H, H_{Ar} + SCH), 7.56 (d, 2H, J = 8.5 Hz, H_{Ar}), 7.81 (d, 2H, J = 8.6 Hz, H_{Ar}) ppm.
^{13}C NMR (101 MHz, DMSO-d_6): δ 16.8 (CH_3), 20.4 (CH_3), 33.7 ($\underline{C}H_2CO$), 49.0 (NCH_2), 103.4 (SCH), 120.4, 127.7, 129.3, 129.4, 131.5, 131.6, 133.1, 134.0, 137.2, 142.7, 149.3 (C_{Ar}, N–C), 169.5 (C=N); 173.7 (COOH) ppm.
Anal. Calcd for $C_{20}H_{19}BrN_2O_2S$: C, 55.69%; H, 4.44%; N, 6.49%; Found: C, 55.93%; H, 4.46%; N, 6.28%.

3-{(2,5-Dimethylphenyl)[4-(naphthalen-2-yl)thiazol-2-yl]amino}propanoic acid (3j)
Yield 0.68 g, 84%, m.p. 121–122 °C.
IR (KBr): ν 1536 (C=N), 1707 (C=O), 3363 (OH) cm^{-1}.
^1H NMR (700 MHz, DMSO-d_6): δ 2.16 (s, 3H, CH_3), 2.29 (s, 3H, CH_3), 2.48–2.54 (m, 2H, CH_2CO), 4.09 (br. s, 2H, NCH_2), 7.06–7.18 (m, 2H, H_{Ar} + SCH), 7.21 (s, 1H, H_{Ar}), 7.27 (d, 1H, J = 7.7 Hz, H_{Ar}), 7.36–7.61 (m, 2H, H_{Ar}), 7.88, 7.95 (2d, 2H, J = 7.7 Hz, H_{Ar}), 7.90 (d, 1H, J = 8.6 Hz, H_{Ar}), 8.00 (d, 1H, J = 8.5 Hz, H_{Ar}), ppm.
^{13}C NMR (176 MHz, DMSO-d_6): δ 16.8 (CH_3), 20.4 (CH_3), 34.6 ($\underline{C}H_2CO$), 49.3 (NCH_2), 103.1 (SCH), 124.1, 124.2, 125.8, 126.3, 127.5, 128.0, 128.1, 129.2, 129.4, 131.5, 132.3, 132.4, 133.1, 133.2, 137.1, 142.7, 150.5 (C_{Ar}, N–C), 170.0 (C=N), 174.3 (COOH) ppm.
Anal. Calcd for $C_{24}H_{22}N_2O_2S$: C, 71.62%; H, 5.51%; N, 6.96%; Found: C, 71.79%; H, 5.57%; N, 6.91%.

3-{(2,5-Dimethylphenyl)[4-(2-oxo-2H-chromen-3-yl)thiazol-2-yl]amino}propanoic acid (3k)
Yield 0.72 g, 86%, m.p. 164–165 °C.
IR (KBr): ν 1540 (C=N), 1711, 1736 (2C=O), 3510 (OH) cm^{-1}.
^1H NMR (400 MHz, DMSO-d_6): δ 2.15 (s, 3H, CH_3), 2.31 (s, 3H, CH_3), 2.70 (t, 2H, J = 7.0 Hz, CH_2CO), 3.95–4.35 (m, 2H, NCH_2), 7.13–7.23 (m, 2H, H_{Ar} + SCH), 7.30 (d, 1H, J = 7.9 Hz, H_{Ar}), 7.39 (t, 1H, J = 7.5 Hz, H_{Ar}), 7.44 (d, 1H, J = 8.3 Hz, H_{Ar}), 7.57 (s, 1H,

H$_{Ar}$), 7.62 (t, 1H, J = 7.8 Hz, H$_{Ar}$), 7.90 (d, 1H, J = 7.7 Hz, H$_{Ar}$), 8.67 (s, 1H, H$_{Ar}$), 12.30 (s, 1H, OH) ppm.

^{13}C NMR (101 MHz, DMSO-d_6): δ 16.7 (CH$_3$), 20.4 (CH$_3$), 32.4 (CH$_2$CO), 47.7 (NCH$_2$), 110.0, 115.9, 119.3, 120.5, 124.8, 128.9, 129.4, 129.6, 131.6, 131.7, 133.1, 137.3, 138.5, 142.4, 144.0, 152.3 (C$_{Ar}$, N–C, SCH), 158.8 (O–C=O), 168.8 (C=N), 172.8 (COOH) ppm.

Anal. Calcd for C$_{23}$H$_{20}$N$_2$O$_4$S: C, 65.70%; H, 4.79%; N, 6.66%; Found: C, 65.89%; H, 4.89%; N, 6.75%.

General procedure for the synthesis of compounds 4i–k. A mixture of the corresponding compound **3i–k** (2 mmol) and polyphosphoric acid (15 g) was stirred at 120 °C for 2–3 h; then, the reaction mixture was cooled down and crushed ice (150 g) was added. The precipitate was filtered off, washed with water and dried. Purification was performed by recrystallization from 2-propanol.

1-[4-(4-Bromophenyl)-1,3-thiazol-2-yl]-5,8-dimethyl-2,3-dihydroquinolin-4(1H)-one (**4i**)
Yield 0.73 g, 88%, m.p. 145–146 °C.
IR (KBr): ν 1507 (C=N), 1673 (C=O) cm^{-1}.
^{1}H NMR (400 MHz, DMSO-d_6): δ 2.21 (s, 3H, CH$_3$), 2.53 (s, 3H, CH$_3$), 2.79 (t, 2H, J = 6.1 Hz, CH$_2$CO), 4.28 (t, 2H, J = 6.0 Hz, NCH$_2$), 7.18 (d, 1H, J = 7.9 Hz, H$_{Ar}$), 7.42–7.49 (m, 2H, H$_{Ar}$ + SCH), 7.57, 7.78 (2d, 4H, J = 8.5 Hz, H$_{Ar}$) ppm.
^{13}C NMR (101 MHz, DMSO-d_6): δ 18.1 (CH$_3$), 22.4 (CH$_3$), 39.3 (CH$_2$CO), 49.8 (NCH$_2$), 106.8, 121.3, 127.3, 128.2, 130.7, 131.9, 132.0, 133.9, 136.1, 139.1, 146.7, 149.9 (C$_{Ar}$, SCN, N-C), 168.5 (C=N), 196.7 (C=O) ppm.
Anal. Calcd for C$_{20}$H$_{17}$BrN$_2$OS: C, 58.12%; H, 4.15%; N, 6.78%; Found: C, 58.32%; H, 4.23%; N, 6.80%.

5,8-Dimethyl-1-[4-(naphthalen-2-yl)-1,3-thiazol-2-yl]-2,3-dihydroquinolin-4(1H)-one (**4j**)
Yield 0.62 g, 81%, m.p. 141–142 °C.
IR (KBr): ν 1547 (C=N), 1740 (C=O) cm^{-1}.
^{1}H NMR (400 MHz, (CDCl$_3$): δ 2.34 (s, 3H, CH$_3$), 2.66 (s, 3H, CH$_3$), 2.91 (t, 2H, J = 6.1 Hz, CH$_2$CO), 4.48 (t, 2H, J = 6.0 Hz, NCH$_2$), 6.96 (s, 1H, SCH), 7.12, 7.36 (2d, 2H, J = 7.8 Hz, H$_{Ar}$), 7.39–7.56 (m, 2H, H$_{Ar}$), 7.74–7.98 (m, 4H, H$_{Ar}$), 8.38 (s, 1H, H$_{Ar}$) ppm.
^{13}C NMR (101 MHz, (CDCl$_3$): δ 18.2 (CH$_3$), 22.9 (CH$_3$), 39.4 (CH$_2$CO), 49.9 (NCH$_2$), 104.6 (SCH), 124.1, 125.2, 126.1, 126.4, 127.2, 127.8, 128.4, 128.5, 130.7, 132.0, 132.1, 133.2, 133.8, 136.1, 140.3, 147.0, 152.1 (C$_{Ar}$, N–C), 169.0 (C=N), 196.9 (C=O) ppm.
Anal. Calcd for C$_{24}$H$_{20}$N$_2$OS: C, 74.97%; H, 5.24%; N, 7.29%; Found: C, 75.01%; H, 5.20%; N, 7.35%.

5,8-Dimethyl-1-[4-(2-oxo-2H-1-benzopyran-3-yl)-1,3-thiazol-2-yl]-2,3-dihydroquinolin-4(1H)-one (**4k**)
Yield 0.57 g, 71%, m.p. 205–206 °C.
IR (KBr): ν 1518 (C=N), 1681, 1716 (2C=O) cm^{-1}.
^{1}H NMR (400 MHz, DMSO-d_6): δ 2.23 (s, 3H, CH$_3$), 2.54 (s, 3H, CH$_3$), 2.81 (t, 2H, J = 6.2 Hz, CH$_2$CO,), 4.37 (t, 2H, J = 6.1 Hz, NCH$_2$), 7.21 (d, 1H, J = 7.9 Hz, H$_{Ar}$), 7.34–7.54 (m, 3H, H$_{Ar}$), 7.56–7.65 (m, 1H, H$_{Ar}$), 7.79 (s, 1H, SCH), 7.86 (d, 1H, J = 6.9 Hz, H$_{Ar}$), 8.63 (s, 1H, H$_{Chrom}$) ppm.
^{13}C NMR (101 MHz, DMSO-d_6): δ 17.5 (CH$_3$), 22.0 (CH$_3$), 38.9 (CH$_2$CO), 49.2 (NCH$_2$), 112.0, 115.9, 119.2, 120.2, 124.7, 126.9, 128.9, 130.5, 131.3, 131.8, 135.8, 138.8, 139.1, 144.1, 146.2, 152.4 (C$_{Ar}$, SCN, N-C), 158.7 (O-C=O), 167.6 (C=N), 196.2 (CH$_2$C=O) ppm.
Anal. Calcd for C$_{23}$H$_{18}$N$_2$O$_3$S: C, 68.64%; H, 4.51%; N, 6.96%; Found: C, 68.49%; H, 4.53%; N, 6.99%.

3-[(5-Acetyl-4-methyl-1,3-thiazol-2-yl)(2,5-dimethylphenyl)amino]propanoic acid (**5**). A mixture of the thioureido acid **1** (0.5 g, 2 mmol), 3-chloropentane-2,4-dione (0.29 g, 2.2 mmol) and acetone (20 mL) was refluxed for 2 h and cooled down. The formed precipitate was filtered off, washed with acetone and dried. Purification was performed by dissolving the crystals in 10% aqueous sodium carbonate, filtering and acidifying the filtrate with acetic acid to pH 6 (the procedure was repeated 2 times).
Yield 0.50 g, 75%, m.p. 172–173 °C.

IR (KBr): ν 1521 (C=N), 1656, 1717 (2C=O), 3631 (OH) cm^{-1}.

^{1}H NMR (700 MHz, DMSO-d_6): δ 2.11 (s, 3H, CH$_3$), 2.29 (s, 3H, CH$_3$), 2.30 (s, 3H, CH$_3$), 2.50 (s, 3H, CH$_3$), 2.57–2.65 (m, 2H, CH$_2$CO), 3.79–3.93 (m, 1H, NCH$_2$), 4.13–4.32 (m, 1H, NCH$_2$), 7.13 (s, 1H, H$_{Ar}$), 7.20 (d, 1H, J = 7.8 Hz, H$_{Ar}$), 7.30 (d, 1H, J = 7.8 Hz, H$_{Ar}$),12.36 (s, 1H, OH) ppm.

^{13}C NMR (176 MHz, DMSO-d_6): δ 16.5 (CH$_3$), 18.6 (CH$_3$), 20.4 (CH$_3$), 29.5 (CH$_3$), 32.1 (CH$_2$CO), 47.5 (NCH$_2$), 122.8, 128.8, 130.0, 131.8, 132.5, 137.5, 141.5, 157.5 (C$_{Ar}$ + SC + NC), 170.5 (C=N), 172.3 (COOH), 188.6 (CH$_3$C=O) ppm.

Anal. Calcd for C$_{17}$H$_{20}$N$_2$O$_3$S: C, 61.42%; H, 6.06%; N, 8.43%; Found: C, 61.19%; H, 6.20%; N, 8.53%.

General procedure for the preparation of compounds 6 and 7. A mixture of thioureido acid **1** (1.26 g, 5 mmol), 2,3-dichloroquinoxaline (**6**) (1 g, 5 mmol) or 2,3-dichloro-1,4-naphthoquinone (1.18 g, 5 mmol), sodium acetate (1.64 g, 20 mmol) and glacial acetic acid (20 mL) was stirred at room temperature for 24 h. Then, the temperature was raised to 70–80 °C and the reaction was continued for another 10 h. After the completion of the rection, the mixture was diluted with water (30 mL), the precipitate was filtered off, washed with water and dried. Purification was performed by dissolving the crystals in 10% aqueous sodium carbonate, filtering and acidifying the filtrate with acetic acid to pH 6 (the procedure was repeated 2 times).

3-[(2,5-Dimethylphenyl)([1,3]thiazolo [4,5-b]quinoxalin-2-yl)amino]propanoic acid (**6**)
Yield 1.30 g, 70%, m.p. 132–133 °C.

IR (KBr): ν 1520, 1562, 1591 (3C=N), 1724 (C=O), 2922 (OH) cm^{-1}.

^{1}H NMR (400 MHz, DMSO-d_6): δ 2.20 (s, 3H, CH$_3$), 2.33 (s, 3H, CH$_3$), 2.50–2.61 (m, 2H, CH$_2$CO), 3.91–4.00 (m, 1H, NCH$_2$), 4.34–4.54 (m, 1H, NCH$_2$), 7.06–7.37 (m, 3H, H$_{Ar}$), 7.58, 7.67 (2t, 2H, J = 7.3 Hz, H$_{Ar}$), 7.86 (t, 2H, J = 6.9 Hz, H$_{Ar}$)ppm.

^{13}C NMR (101 MHz, DMSO-d_6): δ 16.6, 20.4 (2CH$_3$), 34.2 (CH$_2$CO), 49.6 (NCH$_2$), 126.9, 127.9, 129.0, 129.4, 130.7, 131.8, 132.8, 137.6, 137.9, 140.0, 140.6, 154.2, 158.7, 169.5 (C$_{Ar}$ + 3C=N), 175.3 (COOH) ppm.

Anal. Calcd for C$_{20}$H$_{18}$N$_4$O$_2$S: C, 63.47%; H, 4.79%; N, 14.80%; Found: C, 63.63%; H, 4.69%; N, 14.24%.

3-[(2,5-Dimethylphenyl)(4,9-dioxo-4,9-dihydronaphtho [2,3-d][1,3]thiazol-2-yl)amino]propanoic acid (**7**)
Yield 1.32 g, 65%, m.p. 194–195 °C.

IR (KBr): ν 1530 (C=N), 1627, 1642, 1720 (3C=O), 3550 (OH) cm^{-1}.

^{1}H NMR (400 MHz, CDCl$_3$): δ 2.21 (s, 3H, CH$_3$), 2.35 (s, 3H, CH$_3$), 2.75–3.01 (m, 2H, CH$_2$CO), 3.93–4.14 (m, 1H, NCH$_2$), 4.30–4.92 (m, 1H, NCH$_2$), 7.04, 7.06 (2s, 1H, H$_{Ar}$), 7.20, 7.27 (2d, 2H, J = 7.8 Hz, H$_{Ar}$), 7.42, 7.61 (2t, 2H, J = 7.4 Hz, H$_{Ar}$), 7.99 (d, 1H, J = 7.5 Hz, H$_{Ar}$), 8.04 (d, 1H, J = 6.3 Hz, H$_{Ar}$) ppm.

^{13}C NMR (101 MHz, CDCl$_3$): δ 17.1, 21.0 (2CH$_3$), 32.5 (CH$_2$CO), 48.4 (NCH$_2$), 122.30, 126.5, 127.4, 128.6, 129.7, 130.7, 130.8, 131.1, 132.3, 132.5, 132.6, 132.7, 133.5, 135.2, 138.5, 141.1, 162.0, 170.7 (C$_{Ar}$), 176.2 (COOH), 177.3, 181.1 (2C=O) ppm.

Anal. Calcd for C$_{22}$H$_{18}$N$_2$O$_4$S: C, 65.01%; H, 4.46%; N, 6.89%; Found: C, 64.88%; H, 4.57%; N, 6.74%.

Methyl 3-[[4-(4-chlorophenyl)-1,3-thiazol-2-yl](2,5-dimethylphenyl)amino]propanoate (**8f**). A mixture of acid **3f** (1.94 g, 5 mmol), methanol (50 mL) and H$_2$SO$_4$ (0.5 mL) was refluxed for 4 h. Then, the mixture was cooled down and the solvent was evaporated. Sodium bicarbonate solution (5%) was used to neutralize the residues, which was then extracted with diethyl ether (3 × 100 mL). Afterwards, the ether was evaporated to give the title compound **8f** (brown resin, 1.84 g, 92%), R_f = 0.57 (ethyl acetate: hexane (1:10)).

IR (KBr): ν 1174 (C-O), 1733 (C=O) cm^{-1}.

^{1}H NMR (400 MHz, DMSO-d_6): δ 2.13 (s, 3H, CH$_3$), 2.30 (s, 3H, CH$_3$), 2.78 (t, J = 6.9 Hz, CH$_2$CO), 3.53 (s, 3H, OCH$_3$), 4.12 (br. s, 2H, NCH$_2$), 7.07–7.22 (m, 3H, H$_{Ar}$), 7.28 (d, 1H, J = 7.7 Hz, H$_{Ar}$), 7.45 (d, 2H, J = 8.3 Hz, H$_{Ar}$), 7.88 (d, 2H, J = 8.3 Hz, H$_{Ar}$) ppm.

^{13}C NMR (101 MHz, DMSO-d_6): δ 16.7 (CH$_3$), 20.4 (CH$_3$), 32.3 (CH$_2$CO), 48.0 (NCH$_2$), 51.4 (OCH$_3$), 103.7 (SCH), 127.3, 128.5, 129.2, 129.5, 131.6, 131.9, 133.0, 133.5, 137.2, 142.4, 149.2 (C$_{Ar}$), 169.4 (C=N), 171.6 (C=O) ppm.

Anal. Calcd for C$_{21}$H$_{21}$ClN$_2$O$_2$S: C, 62.91%; H, 5.28%; N, 6.99%. Found: C, 62.99%; H, 5.14%; N, 7.07%.

3-{[4-(4-Chlorophenyl)-1,3-thiazol-2-yl](2,5-dimethylphenyl)amino}propanehydrazide (9f). A mixture of ester **8f** (1.20 g, 1 mmol), hydrazine monohydrate (0,45 g, 9 mmol) and 1,4-dioxane (20 mL) was refluxed in for 5 h. Then, the reaction mixture was cooled down, the formed precipitate was filtered off, washed with 2-propanol and dried. Purification was performed by recrystallization from 2-propanol.

Yield 1.02 g, 85%, m.p. 136–137 °C.

IR (KBr): ν 1538 (C=N), 1662 (C=O), 3046 (NH), 3248 (NH$_2$) cm^{-1}.

^{1}H NMR (400 MHz, DMSO-d_6): δ 2.13 (s, 3H, CH$_3$), 2.30 (s, 3H, CH$_3$), 2.51–2.55 (m, 2H, CH$_2$CO), 4.07 (br. s, 2H, NH$_2$), 4.24 (br. s, 2H, NCH$_2$), 7.08–7.24 (m, 3H, H$_{Ar}$), 7.28 (d, 1H, J = 7.7 Hz, H$_{Ar}$), 7.45 (d, 2H, J = 8.6 Hz, H$_{Ar}$), 7.90 (d, 2H, J = 8.5 Hz, H$_{Ar}$), 9.11 (s, 1H, NH) ppm.

^{13}C NMR (101 MHz, DMSO-d_6): δ 16.8 (CH$_3$), 20.4 (CH$_3$), 31.9 (CH$_2$CO), 48.7 (NCH$_2$), 103.5 (SCH), 127.4, 128.5, 129.3, 129.4, 131.6, 131.8, 133.0, 133.6, 137.2, 142.7, 149.3 (C$_{Ar}$, NC), 169.35 (C=N), 169.4 (C=O) ppm.

Anal. Calcd for C$_{20}$H$_{21}$ClN$_4$OS: C, 59.92%, H, 5.28%; N, 13.97%; Found: C, 59.75%; H, 5.36%; N, 13.91%.

General procedure for the synthesis of hydrazones **10–12f**. A mixture of compound **8f** (0.40 g, 1 mmol), corresponding carbaldehyde (1.1 mmol), glacial acetic acid (2 drops) and 1,4-dioxane (20 mL) was heated at reflux for 2–12 h. Then, the reaction mixture was cooled down, the formed precipitate was filtered off, washed with 2-propanol and dried. Purification was performed by recrystallization from 2-propanol.

(Z/E)-3-{[4-(4-Chlorophenyl)thiazol-2-yl](2,5-dimethylphenyl)amino}-N'-[(5-nitrothiophen-2-yl)methylene]propanehydrazide (**10f**)

Yield 0.43 g, 79%, m.p. 102–103 °C.

IR (KBr): ν 1534 (C=N), 1679 (C=O), 3121 (NH) cm^{-1}.

^{1}H NMR (400 MHz, DMSO-d_6): δ 2.15, 2.16 (2s, 3H, CH$_3$), 2.28, 2.29 (2s, 3H, CH$_3$), 2.75 (t, 0.8H, J = 7.0 Hz, CH$_2$CO), 3.08 (t, 1.2H, J = 7.0 Hz, CH$_2$CO), 4.18 (br. s, 2H, NCH$_2$), 6.96–7.35 (m, 6H, H$_{Ar}$), 7.41, 7.44 (2d, 2H, J = 8.6 Hz, H$_{Ar}$), 7.74, 7.77 (2d, 1H, J = 3.9 Hz, H$_{Ar}$), 7.86–7.90 (m, 1H, H$_{Ar}$), 7.91 (s, 0.6H, N=CH), 8.12 (s, 0.4H, N=CH), 11.78 (s, 0.6H, NH), 11.88 (s, 0.4H, NH) ppm.

^{13}C NMR (101 MHz, DMSO-d_6): δ 16.8 (CH$_3$), 20.4 (CH$_3$), 20.5 (CH$_3$), 30.5 (CH$_2$CO), 33.1 (CH$_2$CO), 47.7 (NCH$_2$), 48.2 (NCH$_2$), 103.5 (SCH), 103.6 (SCH), 114.4, 114.6, 115.1, 127.3, 127.4, 128.5, 129.3, 129.4, 130.9, 131.6, 131.8, 133.0, 133.1, 133.5, 133.6, 134.0, 137.2, 142., 142.7, 149.2, 149.3, 151.6, 151.7 (C$_{Ar}$, N-C$_{thiaz}$), 167.4 (N-C=N), 169,4 (C=N), 169,5 (C=N), 172,9 (C=O) ppm.

Anal. Calcd for C$_{20}$H$_{21}$ClN$_4$OS: C, 55.60%; H, 4.11%; N, 12.97%; Found: C, 55.63%; H, 3.97%; N, 13.06%.

(Z/E)-3-((4-Chlorophenyl)thiazol-2-yl)(2,5-dimethylphenyl)amino)-N'-((5-nitrofuran-2-yl)-methylene)propanehydrazide (**11f**)

Yield 0.45 g, 85%, m.p. 78–79 °C.

IR (KBr): ν 1535 (C=N), 1679 (C=O), 3108 (NH) cm^{-1}.

^{1}H NMR (400 MHz, DMSO-d_6): δ 2.15, 2.16 (2s, 3H, CH$_3$), 2.28, 2.30 (2s, 3H, CH$_3$), 2.73 (t, 0.8H, J = 7.0 Hz, CH$_2$CO), 3.08 (t, 1.2H, J = 7.0 Hz, CH$_2$CO), 4.15 (br. s, 2H, NCH$_2$), 7.07–7.23 (m, 3H, H$_{Ar}$ + SCH), 7.28 (d, 1H, J = 7.7 Hz, H$_{Ar}$), 7.32–7.44 (m, 2H, H$_{Ar}$), 7.46, 7.50 (2d, 1H, J = 4.2 Hz, H$_{Ar}$), 8.12, 8.41 (2s, 1H, N=CH), 11.79 (s, 0.6H, NH), 11.83 (s, 0.4H, NH) ppm.

^{13}C NMR (101 MHz, DMSO-d_6): δ 16.7 (CH$_3$), 16.8 (CH$_3$), 20.4 (CH$_3$), 30.7 (CH$_2$CO), 33.1 (CH$_2$CO), 47.9 (NCH$_2$), 48.3 (NCH$_2$), 103.5 (SCH), 103.6 (SCH), 127.3, 127.4, 128.4, 128.5, 128.8, 129.4, 129.5, 130.4, 130.5, 131.7, 131.8, 132.9, 133.0, 133.5, 133.6, 136.1, 137.2,

139.7, 142.4, 142.6, 146.8, 146.9, 149.3, 150.3, 150.64 (C$_{Ar}$, N-C$_{thiaz}$), 167.3 (N-C=N), 169.4 (C=N), 169.5 (C=N), 172.7 (C=O) ppm.

Anal. Calcd for C$_{25}$H$_{22}$ClN$_5$O$_4$S: C, 57.31%; H, 4.23%; N, 13.37%; Found: C, 57.11%; H, 4.15%; N, 13.33%.

(Z/E)-N'-((1H-Indol-3-yl)methylene)-3-((4-(4-chlorophenyl)thiazol-2-yl)(2,5-dimethylphenyl)-amino)propanehydrazide **(12f)**

Yield 0.40 g, 75%, m.p. 72–73 °C.

IR (KBr): ν 1534, 1612 (C=N), 1660 (C=O), 3108, 3178 (2NH) cm^{-1}.

^{1}H NMR (400 MHz, DMSO-d_6): δ 2.16, 2.21, (2s, 3H, CH$_3$), 2.27 (s, 3H, CH$_3$), 2.69 (t, 0.8H, J = 7.2 Hz, CH$_2$CO), 3.13 (s, 1.2H, CH$_2$CO), 4.28 (br. s, 2H, NCH$_2$), 6.92 (t, 1H, J = 7.5 Hz, H$_{Ar}$), 7.10–7.45 (m, 8H, H$_{Ar}$), 7.74, 7.76 (2d, 1H, J = 2.5 Hz, H$_{Ar}$), 7.89, 7.92 (2d, 2.7H, J = 8.5 Hz, H$_{Ar}$), 8.16, 8.32 (2s, 1H, N=CH), 8.21 (d, 0.3H, J = 7.8 Hz, H$_{Ar}$), 11.06 (s, 0.6H, NH$_{ind}$), 11.13 (s, 0.4H, NH$_{ind}$), 11.50 (s, 0.6H, NH), 11.53 (s, 0.4H, NH) ppm.

^{13}C NMR (101 MHz, DMSO-d_6): δ 16.80 (CH$_3$), 16.83 (CH$_3$), 20.4 (CH$_3$), 20.5 (CH$_3$), 30.6 (CH$_2$CO), 33.0 (CH$_2$CO), 47.9 (NCH$_2$), 48.7 (NCH$_2$), 103.4 (SCH), 103.5 (SCH), 111.5, 111.6, 111.7, 111.8, 120.3, 121.3, 121.9, 122.5, 122.6, 124.0, 124.3, 127.3, 127.4, 128.5, 128.6, 129.3. 129.4, 129.5, 130.0, 130.2, 131.6, 131.8, 131.9, 133.0, 133.1, 133.6, 133.7, 137.0, 137.1, 137.2, 140.3, 142.6, 142.7, 143.3, 149.3 (C$_{Ar}$, N-C$_{thiaz}$), 165.7 (N-C=N), 169.5 (C=N), 169.6 (C=N), 171.5 (C=O) ppm.

Anal. Calcd for C$_{29}$H$_{26}$ClN$_5$OS: C, 65.96%; H, 4.96%; N, 13.26%; Found: C, 66.17%; H, 4.91%; N, 13.02%.

3-{[4-(4-Chlorophenyl)thiazol-2-yl](2,5-dimethylphenyl)amino}-N'-cyclopentylidenepropanehydrazide **(13f)**

A mixture of compound **8f** (0.40 g, 1 mmol), cyclopentanone (0.092 g, 1.1 mmol), a few drops of glacial acetic acid and 1,4-dioxane (20 mL) was refluxed for 3 h. Then, the reaction mixture was cooled, and the precipitate was filtered, washed with 2-propanol and dried. Purification was performed by recrystallization from 1,4-dioxane.

Yield 0.34 g (73 %), m.p. 117–118 °C;

IR (KBr): ν (cm^{-1}) 1540 (C=N), 1662 (C=O), 3187 (NH) cm^{-1};

^{1}H NMR (400 MHz, DMSO-d_6): δ 1.55–1.79 (m, 4H, CH$_2$), 2.14 (s, 3H, CH$_3$), 2.17–2.26 (m, 4H, CH$_2$), 2.29 (s, 3H, CH$_3$), 2.68 (t, 0.9H, J = 7.3 Hz, CH$_2$CO), 2.97 (t, 1.1H, J = 7.3 Hz, CH$_2$CO), 4.13 (br. s, 2H, NCH$_2$), 7.13–7.18 (m, 3H, H$_{Ar}$ + SCH), 7.25–7.30 (m, 1H, H$_{Ar}$), 7.41–7.46 (m, 2H, H$_{Ar}$), 7.88, 7.90 (2d, 2H, J = 6.0 Hz, H$_{Ar}$), 9.93 (s, 0.45H, NH), 9.97 (s, 0.55H, NH);

^{13}C NMR (101 MHz, DMSO-d_6): δ 16.8 (CH$_3$), 20.4 (CH$_3$), 24.2, 24.3, 24.4, 24.5, 28.0, 28.3, 32.3,32.8 (4CH$_2$), 30.8 (CH$_2$CO), 32.9 (CH$_2$CO), 48.1 (NCH$_2$), 48.5 (NCH$_2$), 103.38 (SCH), 103.43 (SCH), 127.3, 127.4, 128.5, 129.29, 129.33, 131.6 131.8, 132.96, 133.02, 133.58, 133.62, 137.09, 137.14, 142.6 142.7, 149.21, 149.24, (C$_{Ar}$, N-C$_{thiaz}$), 162.2 (N-C=N), 165.7, 166.4 (N-C=N), 169.38 (C=N), 169.43 (C=N), 172.3 (C=O);

Anal. Calcd for C$_{25}$H$_{27}$ClN$_4$OS: C, 65.96%; H, 4.96%; N, 13.26%; Found: C, 66.17%; H, 4.91%; N, 13.02%.

General procedure for the synthesis of compounds **14f** *and* **15f**. A mixture of compound **8f** (0.40 g, 1 mmol), the corresponding ketone (1.1 mmol), 1,4-dioxane (20 mL) and glacial acetic acid (2 drops) was refluxed for 4–8 h. Then, the reaction mixture was cooled down, the obtained precipitate was filtered off, washed with 2-propanol and dried. Purification was performed by recrystallization from 1,4-dioxane.

(Z/E)-N'-(Butan-2-ylidene)-3-{[4-(4-chlorophenyl)thiazol-2-yl](2,5-dimethylphenyl)amino}propanehydrazide **(14f)**

Yield 0.35 g, 77%, m.p. 86–87 °C.

IR (KBr): ν 1514, 1537 (2C=N), 1669 (C=O), 3187 (NH) cm^{-1}.

^{1}H NMR (400 MHz, DMSO-d_6): δ 1.69 (m, 5H, CH$_3$ and CH$_2$), 2.14 (s, 3H, CH$_3$), 2.29 (s, 3H, CH$_3$), 2.50 (s, 3H, CH$_3$), 2.68 (t, 1H, J = 7.3 Hz, CH$_2$CO), 2.98 (t, 1H, J = 7.3 Hz, CH$_2$CO), 4.12 (br. s, 2H, NCH$_2$), 7.13–7.18 (m, 3H, H$_{Ar}$ + SCH), 7.28 (d, 1H, J = 7.6 Hz, H$_{Ar}$), 7.44 (d,

2H, *J* = 8.3 Hz, H$_{Ar}$), 7.89 (dd, 2H, *J* = 8.0, 6.1 Hz, H$_{Ar}$), 10.03 (s, 0.5H, NH), 10.08 (s, 0.5H, NH) ppm.

^{13}C NMR (101 MHz, DMSO-d_6): δ 16.8 (CH$_3$), 17.0 (CH$_3$), 17.5 (CH$_3$), 20.4 (CH$_3$), 24.9 (CH$_2$), 25.1 (CH$_2$), 30.9 (CH$_2$CO), 32.4 (CH$_2$CO), 48.1 (NCH$_2$), 48.5 (NCH$_2$), 103.4 (SCH), 103.5 (SCH), 127.3, 127.4, 128.5, 129.3, 131.6, 131.8, 132.9, 133.0, 133.58, 133.62, 137.1, 137.2, 142.6, 142.7 149.2, 150.1, 154.7, (C$_{Ar}$, N-C$_{thiaz}$), 166.5 (N-C=N), 169.38 (C=N), 169.44 (C=N), 172.4 (C=O) ppm.

Anal. Calcd for C$_{24}$H$_{27}$ClN$_4$OS: C, 63.35%; H, 5.98%; N, 12.31%; Found: C, 63.41%; 5.92%; N, 12.09%.

(Z/E)-3-{[4-(4-Chlorophenyl)thiazol-2-yl](2,5-dimethylphenyl)amino}-N'-(octan-2-ylidene)pr-opanehydrazide (**15f**)

Yield 0.38 g, 75%, m.p. 70–71 °C.

IR (KBr): ν 1538 (C=N), 1669 (C=O), 3178 (NH) cm^{-1}.

^{1}H NMR (400 MHz, DMSO-d_6): δ 0.72–0.83 (m, 3H, CH$_3$), 1.10–1.45 (m, 8H, 4CH$_2$), 1.78, 1.81, 1.87 (3s, 3H, CH$_3$), 2.01–2.25 (m, 5H, CH$_2$ and CH$_3$), 2.29 (2s, 3H, CH$_3$), 2.69 (t, 0.8H, *J* = 7.3 Hz, CH$_2$CO), 3.00 (t, 1.2H, *J* = 7.3 Hz, CH$_2$CO), 4.12 (br. s, 2H, NCH$_2$), 7.01–7.22 (m, 3H, H$_{Ar}$ + SCH), 7.23–7.31 (m, 1H, H$_{Ar}$), 7.36–7.51 (m, 2H, H$_{Ar}$), 7.89 (t, 2H, *J* = 8.0 Hz, H$_{Ar}$), 10.00 (s, 0.3H, NH), 10.08 (s, 0.1H, NH), 10.10 (s, 0.5H, NH), 10.22 (s, 0.1H, NH) ppm.

^{13}C NMR (101 MHz, DMSO-d_6): δ 13.88 (CH$_3$), 13.92 (CH$_3$), 15.9 (CH$_3$), 16.0 (CH$_3$), 16.75 (CH$_3$), 16.79 (CH$_3$), 20.4 (CH$_3$), 20.4 (CH$_3$), 22.0 (CH$_2$), 25.0 (CH$_2$), 25.3 (CH$_2$), 26.0 (CH$_2$), 28.2 (CH$_2$), 28.4 (CH$_2$), 28.7 (CH$_2$), 30.0 (CH$_2$CO), 31.05 (CH$_2$CO), 31.09 (CH$_2$CO), 32.5 (CH$_2$CO), 38.3 (CH$_2$CO), 48.2 (NCH$_2$), 48.5 (NCH$_2$), 103.3 (SCH), 103.4 (SCH), 127.3, 127.4, 128.5, 129.27, 129.31, 131.5, 131.6, 131.7, 131.8, 132.95, 133.02, 133.6, 133.6, 137.1, 137.12, 142.6, 142.7, 149.2, 152.6, 157.5 (C$_{Ar}$, N-C$_{thiaz}$), 166.5 (N-C=N), 169.3 (C=N), 169.4 (C=N), 172.5 (C=O), 172.6 (C=O) ppm.

Anal. Calcd for C$_{24}$H$_{27}$ClN$_4$OS: C, 65.80%; H, 6.90%; N, 10.96%; Found: C, 65.94%; H, 6.86%; N, 11.15%.

General procedure for the synthesis of compounds **16c, f, h**. A mixture of the corresponding compound **3c, f, h** (2 mmol), *o*-phenylenediamine (0.32 g, 3 mmol) and 15% hydrochloric acid (30 mL) was refluxed for 72 h. Then, the reaction mixture was cooled down, diluted with water (150 mL), and the obtained precipitate was filtered off, washed with water and dried. Then, the crystals were dissolved in 2-propanol and diluted with an aqueous 10% potassium carbonate solution. The formed precipitate was filtered off, washed with water and dried. Purification was performed by recrystallization from a mixture of toluene with hexane (1:1).

N-[2-(1H-Benzo[d]imidazol-2-yl)ethyl]-N-(2,5-dimethylphenyl)-4-phenylthiazol-2-amine (**16c**)

Yield 0.55 g (65 %), m.p. 95–97 °C;

IR (KBr): ν 1538, 1621 (C=N), 3055 (NH) cm^{-1};

^{1}H NMR (400 MHz, CDCl$_3$): δ 2.12 (s, 3H, CH$_3$), 2.34 (s, 3H, CH$_3$), 3.40–3.59 (m, 2H, CH$_2$), 4.53, 4.67 (2br. s, 2H, NCH$_2$), 6.72 (s, 1H, H$_{Ar}$), 7.01 (s, 1H, SCH), 7.14–7.47 (m, 7H, H$_{Ar}$), 7.54 (t, 2H, *J* = 7.5 Hz, H$_{Ar}$), 8.00 (d, 2H, *J* = 7.7 Hz, H$_{Ar}$), 12.39 (br. s, 1H, NH) ppm;

^{13}C NMR (101 MHz, CDCl$_3$): δ 17.1 (CH$_3$), 21.0 (CH$_3$), 29.2 (CH$_2$), 49.8 (NCH$_2$), 102.5 (SCH), 122.1, 126.0, 128.3, 129.1, 129.6, 130.27, 132.3, 133.6, 134.6, 138.3, 141.8, 150.7, 153.2 (C$_{Ar}$, C$_{benzimid}$.), 172.4 (N-C=N) ppm;

Anal. Calcd for C$_{26}$H$_{24}$N$_4$S: C, 73.55%; H, 5.70%; N, 13.20%; Found: C, 73.71%; H, 5.93%; N, 13.37%.

N-[2-(1H-Benzo[d]imidazol-2-yl)ethyl]-4-(4-chlorophenyl)-N-(2,5-dimethylphenyl)thiazol-2-amine (**16f**)

Yield 0.59 g (64 %), m.p. 85–86 °C;

IR (KBr): ν 1537, 1620 (2C=N), 3051 (NH) cm^{-1};

^{1}H NMR (400 MHz, CDCl$_3$): δ 2.04 (s, 3H, CH$_3$), 2.11 (s, 3H, CH$_3$), 3.36 (s, 2H, CH$_2$), 4.16, 4.45 (2br. s, 2H, NCH$_2$), 6.79 (s, 1H, 1H, H$_{Ar}$), 7.08–7.27 (m, 5H, H$_{Ar}$ + SCH), 7.39, 7.52

(2d, 2H, J = 6.1 Hz, H$_{Ar}$), 7.45 (d, 2H, J = 8.1 Hz, H$_{Ar}$), 7.91 (d, 2H, J = 7.8 Hz, H$_{Ar}$), 12.30 (s, 1H, NH) ppm;
^{13}C NMR (101 MHz, CDCl$_3$) δ 16.7 (CH$_3$), 20.1 (CH$_3$), 27.2 (CH$_2$), 50.8 (NCH$_2$), 103.6 (SCH), 110.8, 118.2, 120.9, 121.6, 127.4, 128.5, 129.3, 129.3, 131.5, 131.8, 132.8, 133.6, 134.2, 137.1, 142.8, 143.3, 149.4, 152.4 (C$_{Ar}$, C$_{benzimid}$.), 169.3 (N-C=N) ppm;
Anal. Calcd for C$_{26}$H$_{23}$ClN$_4$S: C, 68.03%; H, 5.05%; N, 12.21%; Found: C, 68.22%; H, 5.29%; N, 12.39%.

N-[2-(1H-Benzo[d]imidazol-2-yl)ethyl]-4-(3,4-dichlorophenyl)-N-(2,5-dimethylphenyl)thiazol-2-amine (**16h**)
Yield 0.61 g (62 %), m.p. 100–101 °C;
IR (KBr): ν 1533 (2C=N), 1621, 3051 (NH) cm^{-1};
^{1}H NMR (400 MHz, DMSO-d_6): δ 2.04 (s, 3H, CH$_3$), 2.10 (s, 3H, CH$_3$), 3.30–3.34 (m, 2H, CH$_2$), 4.13, 4.50 (br. s, 2H, NCH$_2$), 6.78 (s, 1H, 1H, H$_{Ar}$), 7.05–7.15 (m, 3H, H$_{Ar}$ + SCH), 7.25 (d, 1H, J = 7.8 Hz, H$_{Ar}$), 7.32 (s, 1H, H$_{Ar}$), 7.39 (d, 1H, J = 6.7 Hz, H$_{Ar}$), 7.52 (d, 1H, J = 7.9 Hz, H$_{Ar}$), 7.65 (d, 1H, J = 8.4 Hz, H$_{Ar}$), 7.87 (dd, 1H, J = 8.4, 1.8 Hz, H$_{Ar}$), 8.13 (d, 1H, J = 1.8 Hz, H$_{Ar}$), 12.30 (s, 1H, NH) ppm;
^{13}C NMR (101 MHz, DMSO-d_6): δ 16.6 (CH$_3$), 20.1 (CH$_3$), 27.2 (CH$_2$), 50.8 (NCH$_2$), 105.0 (SCH), 110.7, 118.2, 120.9, 121.6, 125.8, 127.2, 129.3, 129.4, 129.6, 130.7, 131.4, 131.6, 132.8, 134.2, 135.3, 137.1, 142.7, 143.3, 148.0, 152.4 (C$_{Ar}$, C$_{benzimid}$.), 169.4 (N-C=N) ppm;
Anal. Calcd for C$_{26}$H$_{22}$Cl$_2$N$_4$S: C, 63.29%; H, 4.49%; N, 11.35%; Found: C, 63.10%; H, 4.55%; N, 11.47%.

General procedure for the synthesis of compounds **17c, f, h**. A mixture of the corresponding compound **3c, f, h** (1 mmol), sulfanilamide (0.19 g, 1.1 mmol), triethylamine (0.30 g, 3 mmol) and DMF (5 mL) was stirred at room temperature for 0.5 h. HBTU (0.57 g, 1.5 mmol) was dissolved in DMF (3 mL) at room temperature in an inert atmosphere and then added to the reaction mixture over 15 min. The reaction mixture was stirred at room temperature for 72 h, then diluted with an aqueous 10% potassium carbonate (50 mL) solution. The obtained precipitate was filtered off, washed with water and dried. Purification was performed by column chromatography using hexane: ethyl acetate (1:2) as eluent.

3-[(2,5-Dimethylphenyl)(4-phenylthiazol-2-yl)amino]-N-(4-sulfamoylphenyl)propanamide (**17c**)
Yield 0.43 g, 85%, R_f = 0.62 (hexane: ethyl acetate (1:2)), m.p. 78–79 °C.
IR (KBr): ν (cm^{-1}) 1538 (C=N), 1681 (C=O), 3253 (NH), 3600 (NH$_2$) cm^{-1}.
^{1}H NMR (400 MHz, DMSO-d_6): δ 2.15 (s, 3H, CH$_3$), 2.22 (s, 3H, CH$_3$), 2.71–2.93 (m, 3H, COCH$_2$), 4.11 (br. s, 2H, NCH$_2$), 7.11, 7.15 (2s, 3H, H$_{Ar}$, SCH), 7.24 (s, 2H, NH$_2$), 7.25, 7.29 (2d, 2H, J = 6.9 Hz, H$_{Ar}$), 7.38, 7.89 (t, 4H, J = 7.5 Hz, H$_{Ar}$), 7.70, 7.74 (2d, 4H, J = 8.9 Hz, H$_{Ar}$), 10.35 (s, 1H, NH) ppm.
^{13}C NMR (101 MHz, DMSO-d_6): δ 16.5 (CH$_3$), 16.6 (CH$_3$), 20.2 (CH$_3$), 34.9 (CH$_2$CO), 48.1 (NCH$_2$), 102.6 (SCH), 118.4, 125.5, 126.4, 127.3, 128.3, 128.6, 129.0, 129.1, 131.4, 132.8, 134.5, 134.6, 136.9, 138.0, 141.8, 142.6, 150.3 (C$_{Ar}$, N-C$_{thiaz}$), 169.0 (N-C=N), 169.1 (N-C=N), 169.6 (C=O) ppm.
Anal. Calcd for C$_{26}$H$_{22}$Cl$_2$N$_4$S: C, 61.64%; H, 5.17%; N, 11.06%; Found: C, 61.37%; H, 5.05%; N, 10.98%.

3-[(4-(4-Chlorophenyl)thiazol-2-yl)(2,5-dimethylphenyl)amino]-N-(4-sulfamoylphenyl)propanamide (**17f**)
Yield 0.44 g, 81%, R_f = 0.63 (hexane: ethyl acetate (1:2)), m.p. 126–127 °C.
IR (KBr): ν 1533 (C=N), 1667 (C=O), 3248 (NH), 3600 (NH$_2$) cm^{-1}.
^{1}H NMR (400 MHz, DMSO-d_6): δ 2.14 (s, 3H, CH$_3$), 2.22 (s, 3H, CH$_3$), 2.74–2.89 (m, 2H, COCH$_2$), 4.19 (br. s, 2H, NCH$_2$), 7.14 (s, 2H, H$_{Ar}$), 7.18 (s, 1H, SCH), 7.25–7.29 (m, H, H$_{Ar}$), 7.44, 7.90 (2d, 4H, J = 8.4 Hz, H$_{Ar}$), 7.61, 7.66 (2d, 4H, J = 8.6 Hz, H$_{Ar}$), 8.76 (br. s, 2H, NH$_2$) ppm.
^{13}C NMR (101 MHz, DMSO-d_6): δ 16.7 (CH$_3$), 20.4 (CH$_3$), 34.9 (CH$_2$CO), 48.4 (NCH$_2$), 103.6 (SCH), 118.3, 126.2, 127.4, 128.5, 129.3, 129.4, 131.6, 131.8, 133.0, 133.6, 137.2, 140.7, 141.8, 142.7, 149.3 (C$_{Ar}$, N-C$_{thiaz}$), 169.5 (N-C=N), 169.6 (C=O) ppm.

Anal. Calcd for $C_{26}H_{25}ClN_4O_3S_2$: C, 57.72%; H, 4.66%; N, 10.35%; Found: C, 57.86%; H, 4.79%; N, 10.51%.

3-((4-(3,4-Dichlorophenyl)thiazol-2-yl)(2,5-dimethylphenyl)amino)-N-(4-sulfamoylphenyl)propanamide (**17h**)

Yield 0.45 g, 78%, R_f = 0.62 (hexane: ethyl acetate (1:2)), m.p. 98–99 °C.

IR (KBr): ν 1532 (C=N), 1682 (C=O), 3253 (NH), 3653 (NH$_2$) cm^{-1}.

^{1}H NMR (400 MHz, DMSO-d_6): δ 2.14 (s, 3H, CH$_3$), 2.22 (s, 3H, CH$_3$), 2.84 (t, 2H, J = 6.9 Hz, COCH$_2$), 4.21 (br. s, 2H, NCH$_2$), 7.14, 7.15 (2s, 2H, H$_{Ar}$, SCH), 7.24 (s, 2H, NH$_2$), 7.28 (d, 1H, J = 8.2 Hz, H$_{Ar}$), 7.33 (s, 1H, H$_{Ar}$), 7.64 (d, 1H, J = 8.4 Hz, H$_{Ar}$), 7.70, 7.74 (2d, 4H, J = 8.9 Hz, H$_{Ar}$), 7.87 (dd, 1H, J = 8.4, 1.5 Hz, H$_{Ar}$), 8.12 (s, 1H, H$_{Ar}$), 10.35 (s, 1H, NH) ppm.

^{13}C NMR (101 MHz, DMSO-d_6): δ 16.7 (CH$_3$), 20.4 (CH$_3$), 35.0 (CH$_2$CO), 48.3 (NCH$_2$), 105.0 (SCH), 118.6, 125.7, 126.6, 127.2, 129.2, 129.5, 129.6, 130.7, 131.4, 131.6, 132.9, 135.3, 137.2, 138.2, 141.9, 142.6, 147.9 (C$_{Ar}$, N-C$_{thiaz}$), 169.6 (N-C=N), 169.8 (C=O) ppm.

Anal. Calcd for $C_{26}H_{24}Cl_2N_4O_3S_2$: C, 54.26%; H, 4.20%; N, 9.74%; Found: C, 54.08%; H, 4.12%; N, 9.83%.

3.2. Bacterial Strains and Culture Conditions

The multidrug-resistant and genetically defined isolates were obtained from the AR isolate bank at the Centre for Disease Control (CDC, United States). *S. aureus* TCH 1516 (USA300) was obtained from the American Type Culture Collection. Prior to the study, all strains were maintained in commercial cryopreservation systems at −80 °C. Bacterial strains were subcultured on Columbia Sheep Blood agar or Tryptic-Soy agar (Becton Dickenson, Franklin Lakes, NJ, USA). Fungal strains were cultured on Saburoud-Dextrose agar. Unless otherwise specified, all antimicrobial susceptibility studies with bacterial pathogens were performed in Cation-Adjusted Mueller–Hinton broth (CAMBH) for liquid cultures (Liofilchem, Italy). Antifungal studies were conducted using RPMI/MOPS broth.

3.3. Minimal Inhibitory Concentration Determination

3.3.1. Antibacterial Activity Characterization

The minimal inhibitory concentrations (MICs) of compounds **1–17** as well as various antibiotics were determined according to the recommendations of the Clinical and Laboratory Standards Institute (CLSI). The MICs for the compounds and comparator antibiotics were determined according to the testing standard broth microdilution methods described in CLSI document M07-A8 against the libraries of Gram-positive and Gram-negative pathogens. Compounds and antibiotics that were used as a control were dissolved in dimethyl sulfoxide (DMSO) to achieve a final concentration of 15–30 mg/mL. A series of compound dilutions were prepared in deep, polypropylene 96-well microplates to achieve 2× of concentrations (0.5–64 µg/mL) and were then transferred to the assay single-use, flat bottom plates. The prepared microplates were stored at −80 °C until the day of the experiment.

A standardized bacterial inoculum was prepared using the colony suspension method. The inoculum suspension was diluted in sterile CAMBH to achieve final concentrations of approximately 5×10^5 CFU/mL (range, 2×10^5 to 8×10^5 CFU/mL) in each well. The inoculum was transferred to the assay plates to achieve 1× assay concentration. Inoculated microdilution plates were incubated at 35 °C for 16 to 20 h in an ambient-air incubator within 15 min of the addition of the inoculum.

3.3.2. Antifungal Activity Characterization

The MIC of compounds **1–17** as well as clinically approved antifungal drugs was determined by CLSI recommendations, described in document M27-A3 [84,85]. Briefly, before the experiments, multidrug-resistant *Candida* spp., strains were sub-cultured on Saburoud-Dextrose agar for 24 h at 35 °C. The colonies were suspended in sterile saline to reach approximately 5×10^6 CFU/mL. Then, the fungal suspension is diluted in RPMI/MOPS broth to reach 5×10^5 CFU/mL and microplates containing test compounds, prepared as described above are inoculated using a multichannel pipette. Inoculated microdilution plates were incubated at 35 °C for 16 to 20 h in an ambient-air incubator within 15 min of the addition of the inoculum.

3.4. Cell Lines and Culture Conditions

The non-small-cell human lung carcinoma A549 cells were obtained from American Type Culture Collection (Rockville, MD, USA). Caco-2 human corectal adenocarcinoma cells were obtained from Dr. Iliyan Iliev's laboratory (Institute for Research in IBD, Weill Cornell Medicine of Cornell University). Cells were maintained in Dulbecco's Modified Eagle Medium/Nutrient Mixture F-12 (DMEM/F-12) (Gibco, Waltham, MA, USA) supplemented with 10% fetal bovine serum (10% FBS) (Gibco, Waltham, MA, USA) and 100 U/mL penicillin and 100 µg/mL streptomycin (P/S). Cells were cultured at 37 °C humidified atmosphere containing 5% of CO_2. Cells were fed every 2–3 days and subculture upon reaching 70–80% confluence.

3.5. In Vitro Cytotoxic Activity Determination

The viability of A549 and Caco-2 cells after the treatment with compounds or cisplatin that served as cytotoxicity control was evaluated by using commercial MTT (3-[4,5-methylthiazol-2-yl]-2,5-diphenyltetrazolium bromide) assay (ThermoFisher Scientific, United States). Briefly, cells were plated in the flat-bottomed 96-well microplates (1×10^4 cells/well) and incubated overnight to facilitate the attachment. The test compounds were dissolved in hybridoma-grade DMSO (Sigma-Aldrich, St. Louis, MO, USA) and then further serially diluted in cell culture media containing 0.25 % DMSO to achieve 100 µM of each compound.

Subsequently, the media from the cells was aspirated and the compounds were added to the microplates. The cells were incubated at 37 °C, 5% CO_2 for 24 h. After incubation, a 10 µL of Vybrant® MTT Cell Proliferation Reagent (ThermoFisher Scientific) was added, and cells were further incubated for 4 h. After incubation, the media was aspirated, and the resulting formazan was solubilized by the addition of 100 µL of DMSO. The absorbance was then measured at 570 nm by using a microplate reader (Multiscan, ThermoFisher Scientific). The following formula was used to calculate the % of A549 viability: ([AE-AB]/[AC-AB]) × 100%. AE, AC, and AB were defined as the absorbance of experimental samples, untreated samples, and blank controls, respectively. The experiments were performed in triplicates.

3.6. Statistical Analysis

The results are expressed as mean ± standard deviation (SD). Statistical analyses were performed with Prism (GraphPad Software, San Diego, CA, USA), using Kruskal–Wallis test and two-way ANOVA. $p < 0.05$ was accepted as significant.

4. Conclusions

In the present study, a series of 2-aminothiazole derivatives containing N-2,5-dimethyl phenyl and β-alanine moieties in the molecules were synthesized and evaluated for their in vitro antimicrobial activity using a panel of multidrug-resistant bacterial and fungal pathogens with emerging and genetically defined resistance mechanisms. In addition, we characterized the cytotoxic and anticancer properties using A549 and Caco-2 pulmonary and corectal adenocarcinoma models.

The results revealed that thiazoles with the 4-aryl substituted showed profound and selective antimicrobial activity against Gram-positive pathogens. Compound **3j** possessed the most potent activity against tested strains multidrug-resistant *S. aureus* and *E. faecium* (MIC 1–2 µg/mL). Strikingly, compounds **3h, 3j** and **7** showed antibacterial activity against especially clinically challenging tedizolid/linezolid-resistant *S. aureus* strains.

On the other hand, the modified carboxyl group in thiazoles **8f**, **9f** and **14f** provided promising antifungal properties against drug-resistant *Candida* strains, including *C. glabrata*, *C. parapsilosis* and *C. hemulonii*. Moreover, ester **8f** was found to have broader antifungal activity on multiple *Candida* species (1–8 μg/mL) including the emerging fungal pathogen *C. auris*.

During the anticancer activity study, a structure-dependent anticancer activity against A549 and Caco-2 cells was observed. Structure–activity relation analysis revealed naphthoquinone-fused thiazole **7** structure and 2,4-diCl-C_6H_3 moiety **3j** to provide broad-spectrum anticancer against both A549 and Caco-2 cells.

Compounds based on 2-aminothiazole derivatives containing *N*-2,5-dimethyl phenyl and β-alanine moieties could be further explored as novel scaffolds for the development of novel and highly active compounds targeting multidrug-resistant pathogens, including tedizolid/linezolid-resistant *S. aureus* as well as vancomycin-resistant *Enterococcus*. Furthermore, a series of novel compounds based on **8f** could be further explored as novel antifungals targeting challenging and multidrug-resistant *Candida auris*. Further studies are needed to better understand the safety, pharmacological properties as well as cellular targets of 2-aminothiazole derivatives **1–17**.

Supplementary Materials: The following supporting information can be downloaded at: https://www.mdpi.com/article/10.3390/antibiotics12020220/s1, Figure S1: ^{1}H-NMR of compound **1**, Figure S2: ^{13}C-NMR of compound **1**, Figure S3: ^{1}H-NMR of compound **2**, Figure S4: ^{13}C-NMR of compound **2**, Figure S5: ^{1}H-NMR of compound **3a**, Figure S6: ^{13}C-NMR of compound **3a**, Figure S7: ^{1}H-NMR of compound **3b**, Figure S8: ^{13}C-NMR of compound **3b**, Figure S9: ^{1}H-NMR of compound **3c**, Figure S10: ^{13}C-NMR of compound **3c**, Figure S11: ^{1}H-NMR of compound **3d**, Figure S12: ^{13}C-NMR of compound **3d**, Figure S13: ^{1}H-NMR of compound **3e**, Figure S14: ^{13}C-NMR of compound **3e**, Figure S15: ^{1}H-NMR of compound **3f**, Figure S16: ^{13}C-NMR of compound **3f**, Figure S17: ^{1}H-NMR of compound **3g**, Figure S18: ^{13}C-NMR of compound **3g**, Figure S19: ^{1}H-NMR of compound **3h**, Figure S20: ^{13}C-NMR of compound **3h**, Figure S21: ^{1}H-NMR of compound **3i**, Figure S22: ^{13}C-NMR of compound **3i**, Figure S23: ^{1}H-NMR of compound **3j**, Figure S24: ^{13}C-NMR of compound **3j**, Figure S25: ^{1}H-NMR of compound **3k**, Figure S26: ^{13}C-NMR of compound **3k**, Figure S27: ^{1}H-NMR of compound **4i**, Figure S28: ^{13}C-NMR of compound **4i**, Figure S29: ^{1}H-NMR of compound **4j**, Figure S30: ^{13}C-NMR of compound **4j**, Figure S31: ^{1}H-NMR of compound **4k**, Figure S32: ^{13}C-NMR of compound **4k**, Figure S33: ^{1}H-NMR of compound **5**, Figure S34: ^{13}C-NMR of compound **5**, Figure S35: ^{1}H-NMR of compound **6**, Figure S36: ^{13}C-NMR of compound **6**, Figure S37: ^{1}H-NMR of compound **7**, Figure S38: ^{13}C-NMR of compound **7**, Figure S39: ^{1}H-NMR of compound **8f**, Figure S40: ^{13}C-NMR of compound **8f**, Figure S41: ^{1}H-NMR of compound **9f**, Figure S42: 13C-NMR of compound **9f**, Figure S43: ^{1}H-NMR of compound **10f**, Figure S44: ^{13}C-NMR of compound **10f**, Figure S45: ^{1}H-NMR of compound **11f**, Figure S46: ^{13}C-NMR of compound **11f**, Figure S47: ^{1}H-NMR of compound **12f**, Figure S48: ^{13}C-NMR of compound **12f**, Figure S49: ^{1}H-NMR of compound **13f**, Figure S50: ^{13}C-NMR of compound **13f**, Figure S51: ^{1}H-NMR of compound **14f**, Figure S52: ^{13}C-NMR of compound **14f**, Figure S53: ^{1}H-NMR of compound **15f**, Figure S54: ^{13}C-NMR of compound **15f**, Figure S55: ^{1}H-NMR of compound **16c**, Figure S56: ^{13}C-NMR of compound **16c**, Figure S57: ^{1}H-NMR of compound **16f**, Figure S58: ^{13}C-NMR of compound **16f**, Figure S59: ^{1}H-NMR of compound **16h**, Figure S60: ^{13}C-NMR of compound **16h**, Figure S61: ^{1}H-NMR of compound **17c**, Figure S62: ^{13}C-NMR of compound **17c**, Figure S63: ^{1}H-NMR of compound **17f**, Figure S64: ^{13}C-NMR of compound **17f**, Figure S65: ^{1}H-NMR of compound **17h**, Figure S66: ^{13}C-NMR of compound **17h**. References [86,87] are cited in the supplementary materials.

Author Contributions: Conceptualization, V.M.; Data curation, B.G., B.S.-B., K.A., A.K., G.S., V.P., R.P., E.N. and A.G.; Formal analysis, P.K., R.V., E.N. and A.G.; Funding acquisition, V.M.; Investigation, P.K., B.G., R.V., B.S.-B., K.A., A.K. and G.S.; Methodology, B.G., R.V., B.S.-B., A.K., G.S. and K.A.; Project administration, B.S.-B. and V.M.; Resources, P.K. and K.A.; Software, P.K., K.A. and A.G.; Supervision, V.M.; Validation, P.K., V.P. and R.P.; Visualization, P.K., K.A. and R.V.; Writing—original draft, R.V., K.A., A.K., G.S. and P.K.; Writing—review and editing, B.G., R.V., V.P., R.P. and V.M. All authors have read and agreed to the published version of the manuscript.

Funding: This research received no external funding.

Institutional Review Board Statement: Not applicable.

Informed Consent Statement: Not applicable.

Data Availability Statement: Not applicable.

Conflicts of Interest: The authors declare no conflict of interest.

References

1. Petraitis, V.; Petraitiene, R.; Kavaliauskas, P.; Naing, E.; Garcia, A.; Sutherland, C.; Kau, A.Y.; Goldner, N.; Bulow, C.; Nicolau, D.P.; et al. Pharmacokinetics, Tissue Distribution, and Efficacy of VIO-001 (Meropenem/Piperacillin/Tazobactam) for Treatment of Methicillin-Resistant Staphylococcus Aureus Bacteremia in Immunocompetent Rabbits with Chronic Indwelling Vascular Catheters. *Antimicrob. Agents Chemother.* **2021**, *65*, e0116821. [CrossRef] [PubMed]
2. Holubar, M.; Meng, L.; Deresinski, S. Bacteremia Due to Methicillin-Resistant Staphylococcus Aureus. *Infect. Dis. Clin. N. Am.* **2016**, *30*, 491–507. [CrossRef] [PubMed]
3. Hashem, Y.A.; Amin, H.M.; Essam, T.M.; Yassin, A.S.; Aziz, R.K. Biofilm Formation in Enterococci: Genotype-Phenotype Correlations and Inhibition by Vancomycin. *Sci. Rep.* **2017**, *7*, 5733–5745. [CrossRef] [PubMed]
4. Navarro, S.; Sherman, E.; Colmer-Hamood, J.A.; Nelius, T.; Myntti, M.; Hamood, A.N. Urinary Catheters Coated with a Novel Biofilm Preventative Agent Inhibit Biofilm Development by Diverse Bacterial Uropathogens. *Antibiotics* **2022**, *11*, 1514. [CrossRef] [PubMed]
5. Kean, R.; Rajendran, R.; Haggarty, J.; Townsend, E.M.; Short, B.; Burgess, K.E.; Lang, S.; Millington, O.; Mackay, W.G.; Williams, C.; et al. Candida Albicans Mycofilms Support Staphylococcus Aureus Colonization and Enhances Miconazole Resistance in Dual-Species Interactions. *Front. Microbiol.* **2017**, *8*, 258. [CrossRef] [PubMed]
6. Kong, E.F.; Tsui, C.; Kuchaříková, S.; Andes, D.; Van Dijck, P.; Jabra-Rizk, M.A. Commensal Protection of Staphylococcus Aureus against Antimicrobials by Candida Albicans Biofilm Matrix. *MBio* **2016**, *7*, e01365-16. [CrossRef]
7. Jacobs, S.E.; Jacobs, J.L.; Dennis, E.K.; Taimur, S.; Rana, M.; Patel, D.; Gitman, M.; Patel, G.; Schaefer, S.; Iyer, K.; et al. Candida Auris Pan-Drug-Resistant to Four Classes of Antifungal Agents. *Antimicrob. Agents Chemother.* **2022**, *66*, e0005322. [CrossRef]
8. Thatchanamoorthy, N.; Rukumani Devi, V.; Chandramathi, S.; Tay, S.T. Candida Auris: A Mini Review on Epidemiology in Healthcare Facilities in Asia. *J. Fungi* **2022**, *8*, 1126. [CrossRef]
9. Rybak, J.M.; Cuomo, C.A.; David Rogers, P. The Molecular and Genetic Basis of Antifungal Resistance in the Emerging Fungal Pathogen Candida Auris. *Curr. Opin. Microbiol.* **2022**, *70*, 102208–102216. [CrossRef]
10. Short, F.L.; Lee, V.; Mamun, R.; Malmberg, R.; Li, L.; Espinosa, M.I.; Venkatesan, K.; Paulsen, I.T. Benzalkonium Chloride Antagonises Aminoglycoside Antibiotics and Promotes Evolution of Resistance. *EBioMedicine* **2021**, *73*, 103653–103659. [CrossRef]
11. Liu, G.; Stokes, J.M. A Brief Guide to Machine Learning for Antibiotic Discovery. *Curr. Opin. Microbiol.* **2022**, *69*, 102190–102197. [CrossRef] [PubMed]
12. Evren, A.E.; Dawbaa, S.; Nuha, D.; Yavuz, Ş.A.; Gül, Ü.D.; Yurttaş, L. Design and Synthesis of New 4-Methylthiazole Derivatives: In Vitro and in Silico Studies of Antimicrobial Activity. *J. Mol. Struct.* **2021**, *1241*, 130692–130706. [CrossRef]
13. Moreira, J.; Durães, F.; Freitas-Silva, J.; Szemerédi, N.; Resende, D.I.S.P.; Pinto, E.; da Costa, P.M.; Pinto, M.; Spengler, G.; Cidade, H.; et al. New Diarylpentanoids and Chalcones as Potential Antimicrobial Adjuvants. *Bioorg. Med. Chem. Lett.* **2022**, *67*, 128743–128752. [CrossRef] [PubMed]
14. Dinesh Kumar, S.; Park, J.H.; Kim, H.S.; Seo, C.D.; Ajish, C.; Kim, E.Y.; Lim, H.S.; Shin, S.Y. Cationic, Amphipathic Small Molecules Based on a Triazine-Piperazine-Triazine Scaffold as a New Class of Antimicrobial Agents. *Eur. J. Med. Chem.* **2022**, *243*, 114747–114763. [CrossRef] [PubMed]
15. Zhang, M.; Wang, Y.; Wang, S.; Wu, H. Synthesis and Biological Evaluation of Novel Pyrimidine Amine Derivatives Bearing Bicyclic Monoterpene Moieties. *Molecules* **2022**, *27*, 8104. [CrossRef] [PubMed]
16. Hosny, Y.; Abutaleb, N.S.; Omara, M.; Alhashimi, M.; Elsebaei, M.M.; Elzahabi, H.S.; Seleem, M.N.; Mayhoub, A.S. Modifying the Lipophilic Part of Phenylthiazole Antibiotics to Control Their Drug-Likeness. *Eur. J. Med. Chem.* **2020**, *185*, 111830–111847. [CrossRef]
17. AboulMagd, A.M.; Abdelwahab, N.S.; Abdelrahman, M.M.; Abdel-Rahman, H.M.; Farid, N.F. Lipophilicity Study of Different Cephalosporins: Computational Prediction of Minimum Inhibitory Concentration Using Salting-out Chromatography. *J. Pharm. Biomed. Anal.* **2021**, *206*, 114358–114368. [CrossRef]
18. Sadowski, E.; Bercot, B.; Chauffour, A.; Gomez, C.; Varon, E.; Mainardis, M.; Sougakoff, W.; Mayer, C.; Sachon, E.; Anquetin, G.; et al. Lipophilic Quinolone Derivatives: Synthesis and in Vitro Antibacterial Evaluation. *Bioorg. Med. Chem. Lett.* **2022**, *55*, 128450–128456. [CrossRef]
19. Mohanty, P.; Behera, S.; Behura, R.; Shubhadarshinee, L.; Mohapatra, P.; Barick, A.K.; Jali, B.R. Antibacterial Activity of Thiazole and Its Derivatives: A Review. *Biointerface Res. Appl. Chem.* **2022**, *12*, 2171–2195. [CrossRef]
20. Constantinescu, T.; Lungu, C.N.; Lung, I. Lipophilicity as a Central Component of Drug-like Properties of Chalchones and Flavonoid Derivatives. *Molecules* **2019**, *24*, 1505. [CrossRef]

21. Pivovarova, E.; Climova, A.; Świątkowski, M.; Staszewski, M.; Walczyński, K.; Dzięgielewski, M.; Bauer, M.; Kamysz, W.; Krześlak, A.; Jóźwiak, P.; et al. Synthesis and Biological Evaluation of Thiazole-Based Derivatives with Potential against Breast Cancer and Antimicrobial Agents. *Int. J. Mol. Sci.* **2022**, *23*, 9844. [CrossRef] [PubMed]
22. Arshad, M.F.; Alam, A.; Alshammari, A.A.; Alhazza, M.B.; Alzimam, I.M.; Alam, M.A.; Mustafa, G.; Ansari, M.S.; Alotaibi, A.M.; Alotaibi, A.A.; et al. Thiazole: A Versatile Standalone Moiety Contributing to the Development of Various Drugs and Biologically Active Agents. *Molecules* **2022**, *27*, 3994. [CrossRef] [PubMed]
23. Kamat, V.; Santosh, R.; Poojary, B.; Nayak, S.P.; Kumar, B.K.; Sankaranarayanan, M.; Faheem; Khanapure, S.; Barretto, D.A.; Vootla, S.K. Pyridine- And Thiazole-Based Hydrazides with Promising Anti-Inflammatory and Antimicrobial Activities along with Their in Silico Studies. *ACS Omega* **2020**, *5*, 25228–25239. [CrossRef]
24. Othman, I.M.M.; Alamshany, Z.M.; Tashkandi, N.Y.; Gad-Elkareem, M.A.M.; Abd El-Karim, S.S.; Nossier, E.S. Synthesis and Biological Evaluation of New Derivatives of Thieno-Thiazole and Dihydrothiazolo-Thiazole Scaffolds Integrated with a Pyrazoline Nucleus as Anticancer and Multi-Targeting Kinase Inhibitors. *RSC Adv.* **2022**, *12*, 561–577. [CrossRef]
25. Yurttaş, L.; Özkay, Y.; Karaca Gençer, H.; Acar, U. Synthesis of Some New Thiazole Derivatives and Their Biological Activity Evaluation. *J. Chem.* **2015**, *2015*, 464379. [CrossRef]
26. Elsebaei, M.M.; Mohammad, H.; Abouf, M.; Abutaleb, N.S.; Hegazy, Y.A.; Ghiaty, A.; Chen, L.; Zhang, J.; Malwal, S.R.; Oldfield, E.; et al. Alkynyl-Containing Phenylthiazoles: Systemically Active Antibacterial Agents Effective against Methicillin-Resistant Staphylococcus Aureus (MRSA). *Eur. J. Med. Chem.* **2018**, *148*, 195–209. [CrossRef] [PubMed]
27. Gao, H.D.; Liu, P.; Yang, Y.; Gao, F. Sulfonamide-1,3,5-Triazine-Thiazoles: Discovery of a Novel Class of Antidiabetic Agents: Via Inhibition of DPP-4. *RSC Adv.* **2016**, *6*, 83438–83447. [CrossRef]
28. Santosh, R.; Selvam, M.K.; Kanekar, S.U.; Nagaraja, G.K.; Kumar, M. Design, Synthesis, DNA Binding, and Docking Studies of Thiazoles and Thiazole-Containing Triazoles as Antibacterials. *ChemistrySelect* **2018**, *3*, 3892–3898. [CrossRef]
29. Cheng, K.; Xue, J.Y.; Zhu, H.L. Design, Synthesis and Antibacterial Activity Studies of Thiazole Derivatives as Potent EcKAS III Inhibitors. *Bioorg. Med. Chem. Lett.* **2013**, *23*, 4235–4238. [CrossRef]
30. Parašotas, I.; Anusevičius, K.; Jonuškiene, I.; Mickevičius, V. Synthesis and Antibacterial Activity of N-Carboxyethyl-N-(4-Hydroxyphenyl)- 2-Aminothiazoles and Dihydrothiazolones. *Chemija* **2014**, *25*, 107–114.
31. Prusiner, S.B. Molecular Biology of Prion Diseases. *Science* **1991**, *252*, 1515–1522. [CrossRef] [PubMed]
32. Al-Humaidi, J.Y.; Badrey, M.G.; Aly, A.A.; Nayl, A.E.A.A.; Zayed, M.E.M.; Jefri, O.A.; Gomha, S.M. Evaluation of the Binding Relationship of the RdRp Enzyme to Novel Thiazole/Acid Hydrazone Hybrids Obtainable through Green Synthetic Procedure. *Polymers* **2022**, *14*, 3160. [CrossRef] [PubMed]
33. Almalki, S.A.; Bawazeer, T.M.; Asghar, B.; Alharbi, A.; Aljohani, M.M.; Khalifa, M.E.; El-Metwaly, N. Synthesis and Characterization of New Thiazole-Based Co(II) and Cu(II) Complexes; Therapeutic Function of Thiazole towards COVID-19 in Comparing to Current Antivirals in Treatment Protocol. *J. Mol. Struct.* **2021**, *1244*, 130961–130973. [CrossRef] [PubMed]
34. Gürsoy, E.; Dincel, E.D.; Naesens, L.; Ulusoy Güzeldemirci, N. Design and Synthesis of Novel Imidazo[2,1-b]Thiazole Derivatives as Potent Antiviral and Antimycobacterial Agents. *Bioorg. Chem.* **2020**, *95*, 103496–103505. [CrossRef]
35. Pacca, C.C.; Marques, R.E.; Espindola, J.W.P.; Filho, G.B.O.O.; Leite, A.C.L.; Teixeira, M.M.; Nogueira, M.L. Thiosemicarbazones and Phthalyl-Thiazoles Compounds Exert Antiviral Activity against Yellow Fever Virus and Saint Louis Encephalitis Virus. *Biomed. Pharmacother.* **2017**, *87*, 381–387. [CrossRef]
36. Abdel-Sattar, N.E.A.; El-Naggar, A.M.; Abdel-Mottaleb, M.S.A. Novel Thiazole Derivatives of Medicinal Potential: Synthesis and Modeling. *J. Chem.* **2017**, *2017*, 4102796. [CrossRef]
37. Raghunatha, P.; Inamdar, M.N.; Asdaq, S.M.B.; Almuqbil, M.; Alzahrani, A.R.; Alaqel, S.I.; Kamal, M.; Alsubaie, F.H.; Alsanie, W.F.; Alamri, A.S.; et al. New Thiazole Acetic Acid Derivatives: A Study to Screen Cardiovascular Activity Using Isolated Rat Hearts and Blood Vessels. *Molecules* **2022**, *27*, 6138. [CrossRef]
38. Bagheri, M.; Shekarchi, M.; Jorjani, M.; Ghahremani, M.H.; Vosooghi, M.; Shafiee, A. Synthesis and Antihypertensive Activity of 1-(2-Thiazolyl)-3,5-Disubstituted -2-Pyrazolines. *Arch. Pharm.* **2004**, *337*, 25–34. [CrossRef]
39. Pember, S.O.; Mejia, G.L.; Price, T.J.; Pasteris, R.J. Piperidinyl Thiazole Isoxazolines: A New Series of Highly Potent, Slowly Reversible FAAH Inhibitors with Analgesic Properties. *Bioorg. Med. Chem. Lett.* **2016**, *26*, 2965–2973. [CrossRef]
40. Kumar, G.; Singh, N.P. Synthesis, Anti-Inflammatory and Analgesic Evaluation of Thiazole/Oxazole Substituted Benzothiazole Derivatives. *Bioorg. Chem.* **2021**, *107*, 104608. [CrossRef]
41. Kalkhambkar, R.G.; Kulkarni, G.M.; Shivkumar, H.; Rao, R.N. Synthesis of Novel Triheterocyclic Thiazoles as Anti-Inflammatory and Analgesic Agents. *Eur. J. Med. Chem.* **2007**, *42*, 1272–1276. [CrossRef] [PubMed]
42. Gao, J.; Wells, J.A. Identification of Specific Tethered Inhibitors for Caspase-5. *Chem. Biol. Drug Des.* **2012**, *79*, 209–215. [CrossRef] [PubMed]
43. Maghraby, M.T.E.; Abou-Ghadir, O.M.F.; Abdel-Moty, S.G.; Ali, A.Y.; Salem, O.I.A. Novel Class of Benzimidazole-Thiazole Hybrids: The Privileged Scaffolds of Potent Anti-Inflammatory Activity with Dual Inhibition of Cyclooxygenase and 15-Lipoxygenase Enzymes. *Bioorganic Med. Chem.* **2020**, *28*, 115403–115422. [CrossRef] [PubMed]
44. Neelam; Khatkar, A.; Sharma, K.K. Phenylpropanoids and Its Derivatives: Biological Activities and Its Role in Food, Pharmaceutical and Cosmetic Industries. *Crit. Rev. Food Sci. Nutr.* **2020**, *60*, 2655–2675. [CrossRef]
45. Sahu, S.; Sahu, T.; Kalyani, G.; Gidwani, B. Synthesis and Evaluation of Antimicrobial Activity of 1, 3, 4-Thiadiazole Analogues for Potential Scaffold. *J. Pharmacopuncture* **2021**, *24*, 32–40. [CrossRef]

46. Coluccia, A.; Bufano, M.; La Regina, G.; Puxeddu, M.; Toto, A.; Paone, A.; Bouzidi, A.; Musto, G.; Badolati, N.; Orlando, V.; et al. Anticancer Activity of (S)-5-Chloro-3-((3,5-Dimethylphenyl) Sulfonyl)-N-(1-Oxo-1-((Pyridin-4-Ylmethyl)Amino)Propan-2-Yl)-1H-Indole-2-Carboxamide (RS4690), a New Dishevelled 1 Inhibitor. *Cancers* **2022**, *14*, 1358. [CrossRef]
47. Moore, B.P.; Chung, D.H.; Matharu, D.S.; Golden, J.E.; Maddox, C.; Rasmussen, L.; Noah, J.W.; Sosa, M.I.; Ananthan, S.; Tower, N.A.; et al. (S)-N-(2,5-Dimethylphenyl)-1-(Quinoline-8-Ylsulfonyl)Pyrrolidine-2-Carboxamide as a Small Molecule Inhibitor Probe for the Study of Respiratory Syncytial Virus Infection. *J. Med. Chem.* **2012**, *55*, 8582–8587. [CrossRef]
48. Abbasi, M.A.; Irshad, M.; Aziz-Ur-Rehman; Siddiqui, S.Z.; Nazir, M.; Ali Shah, S.A.; Shahid, M. Synthesis of Promising Antibacterial and Antifungal Agents: 2-[[(4-Chlorophenyl)Sulfonyl](2,3-Dihydro-1,4-Benzodioxin-6-Yl)Amino]-N(Un/Substituted-Phenyl)Acetamides. *Pak. J. Pharm. Sci.* **2020**, *33*, 2161–2170. [CrossRef]
49. Minickaitė, R.; Grybaitė, B.; Vaickelionienė, R.; Kavaliauskas, P.; Petraitis, V.; Petraitienė, R.; Tumosienė, I.; Jonuškienė, I.; Mickevičius, V. Synthesis of Novel Aminothiazole Derivatives as Promising Antiviral, Antioxidant and Antibacterial Candidates. *Int. J. Mol. Sci.* **2022**, *23*, 7688. [CrossRef]
50. Anusevicius, K.; Vaickelioniene, R.; Mickevicius, V. Unexpected Cyclization of N-Aryl-N-Carboxy-Ethyl-β-Alanines to 5,6-Dihydrouracils. *Chem. Heterocycl. Compd.* **2012**, *48*, 1105–1107. [CrossRef]
51. Bouherrou, H.; Saidoun, A.; Abderrahmani, A.; Abdellaziz, L.; Rachedi, Y.; Dumas, F.; Demenceau, A. Synthesis and Biological Evaluation of New Substituted Hantzsch Thiazole Derivatives from Environmentally Benign One-Pot Synthesis Using Silica Supported Tungstosilisic Acid as Reusable Catalyst. *Molecules* **2017**, *22*, 757. [CrossRef] [PubMed]
52. Anusevicius, K.; Jonuskiene, I.; Mickevičius, V. Synthesis and Antimicrobial Activity of N-(4-Chlorophenyl)-β-Alanine Derivatives with an Azole Moiety. *Mon. Chem.* **2013**, *144*, 1883–1891. [CrossRef]
53. Vaickelioniene, R.; Mickeviciene, K.; Anusevicius, K.; Siugzdaite, J.; Kantminiene, K.; Mickevicius, V. Synthesis and Antibacterial Activity of Novel N-Carboxyalkyl-N-Phenyl-2-Aminothia(Oxa)Zole Derivatives. *Heterocycles* **2015**, *91*, 747–763. [CrossRef]
54. Vaickelioniene, R.; Mickevičus, V.; Vaickelionis, G.; Stasevych, M.; Komarovska-Porokhnyavets, O.; Novikov, V. Synthesis and Antibacterial and Antifungal Activity of N-(4-Fluorophenyl)-N-Carboxyethylaminothiazole Derivatives. *Arkivoc* **2015**, *2015*, 303–318. [CrossRef]
55. Pham, T.D.M.; Ziora, Z.M.; Blaskovich, M.A.T. Quinolone Antibiotics. *Medchemcomm* **2019**, *10*, 1719–1739. [CrossRef] [PubMed]
56. Grybaite, B.; Jonuškiene, I.; Vaickelioniene, R.; Mickevičius, V. Synthesis, Transformation and Antibacterial Activity of New N,N-Disubstituted 2-Aminothiazole Derivatives. *Chemija* **2017**, *28*, 64–73.
57. Parašotas, I.; Urbonavičiute, E.; Anusevičius, K.; Tumosiene, I.; Jonuškiene, I.; Kantminiene, K.; Vaickelioniene, R.; Mickevičius, V. Synthesis and Biological Evaluation of Novel DI- and Trisubstituted Thiazole Derivatives. *Heterocycles* **2017**, *94*, 1074–1097. [CrossRef]
58. Parašotas, I.; Anusevičius, K.; Vaickelioniene, R.; Jonuškiene, I.; Stasevych, M.; Zvarych, V.; Olena, K.P.; Novikov, V.; Belyakov, S.; Mickevičius, V. Synthesis and Evaluation of the Antibacterial, Antioxidant Activities of Novel Functionalized Thiazole and Bis(Thiazol-5-Yl)Methane Derivatives. *Arkivoc* **2018**, *2018*, 240–256. [CrossRef]
59. Kappe, T.; Karem, A.S.; Stadlbauer, W. Synthesis of Benzo-Halogenated 4-Hydroxy-2(1H)-Quinolones. *J. Heterocycl. Chem.* **1988**, *25*, 857–862. [CrossRef]
60. Zaki, Y.H.; Al-Gendey, M.S.; Abdelhamid, A.O. A Facile Synthesis, and Antimicrobial and Anticancer Activities of Some Pyridines, Thioamides, Thiazole, Urea, Quinazoline, β-Naphthyl Carbamate, and Pyrano[2,3-d]Thiazole Derivatives. *Chem. Cent. J.* **2018**, *12*, 70–84. [CrossRef]
61. Omar, A.M.; Ihmaid, S.; Habib, E.-S.E.; Althagfan, S.S.; Ahmed, S.; Abulkhair, H.S.; Ahmed, H.E.A. The Rational Design, Synthesis, and Antimicrobial Investigation of 2-Amino-4-Methylthiazole Analogues Inhibitors of GlcN-6-P Synthase. *Bioorg. Chem.* **2020**, *99*, 103781–103793. [CrossRef] [PubMed]
62. Muluk, M.B.; Dhumal, S.T.; Rehman, N.N.M.A.; Dixit, P.P.; Kharat, K.R.; Haval, K.P. Synthesis, Anticancer and Antimicrobial Evaluation of New (E)-N'-Benzylidene-2-(2-ethylpyridin-4-yl)-4-methylthiazole-5-carbohydrazides. *ChemistrySelect* **2019**, *4*, 8993–8997. [CrossRef]
63. Mickevičius, V.; Voskiene, A.; Jonuškiene, I.; Kolosej, R.; Šiugždaite, J.; Venskutonis, P.R.; Kazernavičiute, R.; Braziene, Z.; Jakiene, E. Synthesis and Biological Activity of 3-[Phenyl(1,3-Thiazol-2-Yl)-Amino] Propanoic Acids and Their Derivatives. *Molecules* **2013**, *18*, 15000–15018. [CrossRef]
64. Vaickelioniene, R.; Mickevicius, V.; Mikulskiene, G. Molecules Synthesis and Cyclizations of N-(2,3-,3,4- and 3,5-Dimethylphenyl)-β-Alanines. *Molecules* **2005**, *10*, 407–416. [CrossRef] [PubMed]
65. Matsuoka, M.; Iwamoto, A.; Kitao, T. Reaction of 2,3-dichloro-1,4-naphthoquinone with Dithiooxamide. Synthesis of Dibenzo[b,i]Thianthrene-5,7,12,14-tetrone. *J. Heterocycl. Chem.* **1991**, *28*, 1445–1447. [CrossRef]
66. Matsuoka, M.; Iwamoto, A.; Furukawa, N.; Kitao, T. Syntheses of Polycyclic-1,4-dithiines and Related Heterocycles. *J. Heterocycl. Chem.* **1992**, *29*, 439–443. [CrossRef]
67. Katritzky, A.R.; Fan, W.-Q. A Reexamination of the Reactions of 2,3-dichloro-1,4-naphthoquinone with Thioamides. *J. Heterocycl. Chem.* **1993**, *30*, 1679–1681. [CrossRef]
68. Ballatore, C.; Huryn, D.M.; Smith, A.B. Carboxylic Acid (Bio)Isosteres in Drug Design. *ChemMedChem* **2013**, *8*, 385–395. [CrossRef]
69. Grybaitė, B.; Vaickelionienė, R.; Stasevych, M.; Komarovska-Porokhnyavets, O.; Novikov, V.; Mickevičius, V. Synthesis, Transformation of 3-[(4-Arylthiazol-2-Yl)-(p-Tolyl)Amino]Propanoic Acids, Bis(Thiazol-5-Yl)Phenyl-, Bis(Thiazol-5-Yl)Methane Derivatives, and Their Antimicrobial Activity. *Heterocycles* **2018**, *96*, 86–105. [CrossRef]

70. Grybaitė, B.; Vaickelionienė, R.; Stasevych, M.; Komarovska-Porokhnyavets, O.; Kantminienė, K.; Novikov, V.; Mickevičius, V. Synthesis and Antimicrobial Activity of Novel Thiazoles with Reactive Functional Groups. *ChemistrySelect* **2019**, *4*, 6965–6970. [CrossRef]
71. Malūkaitė, D.; Grybaitė, B.; Vaickelionienė, R.; Vaickelionis, G.; Sapijanskaitė-Banevič, B.; Kavaliauskas, P.; Mickevičius, V. Synthesis of Novel Thiazole Derivatives Bearing β-Amino Acid and Aromatic Moieties as Promising Scaffolds for the Development of New Antibacterial and Antifungal Candidates Targeting Multidrug-Resistant Pathogens. *Molecules* **2022**, *27*, 74. [CrossRef]
72. Anusevičius, K.; Mickevičius, V.; Mikulskiene, G. Synthesis and Structure of N-(4-Bromophenyl)-N-Carboxyethyl-β-Alanine Derivatives. *Chemija* **2010**, *21*, 127–134.
73. De Oliveira, D.M.P.; Forde, B.M.; Kidd, T.J.; Harris, P.N.A.; Schembri, M.A.; Beatson, S.A.; Paterson, D.L.; Walker, M.J. Antimicrobial Resistance in ESKAPE Pathogens. *Clin. Microbiol. Rev.* **2020**, *33*, e00181. [CrossRef] [PubMed]
74. Allen, D.; Wilson, D.; Drew, R.; Perfect, J. Azole Antifungals: 35 Years of Invasive Fungal Infection Management. *Expert Rev. Anti. Infect. Ther.* **2015**, *13*, 787–798. [CrossRef] [PubMed]
75. Arendrup, M.C.; Patterson, T.F. Multidrug-Resistant Candida: Epidemiology, Molecular Mechanisms, and Treatment. *J. Infect. Dis.* **2017**, *216*, S445–S451. [CrossRef] [PubMed]
76. Nastasă, C.; Tiperciuc, B.; Duma, M.; Benedec, D.; Oniga, O. New Hydrazones Bearing Thiazole Scaffold: Synthesis, Characterization, Antimicrobial, and Antioxidant Investigation. *Molecules* **2015**, *20*, 17325–17338. [CrossRef] [PubMed]
77. Zha, G.-F.; Leng, J.; Darshini, N.; Shubhavathi, T.; Vivek, H.K.; Asiri, A.M.; Marwani, H.M.; Rakesh, K.P.; Mallesha, N.; Qin, H.-L. Synthesis, SAR and Molecular Docking Studies of Benzo[d]Thiazole-Hydrazones as Potential Antibacterial and Antifungal Agents. *Bioorg. Med. Chem. Lett.* **2017**, *27*, 3148–3155. [CrossRef]
78. Kauthale, S.; Tekale, S.; Damale, M.; Sangshetti, J.; Pawar, R. Synthesis, Antioxidant, Antifungal, Molecular Docking and ADMET Studies of Some Thiazolyl Hydrazones. *Bioorg. Med. Chem. Lett.* **2017**, *27*, 3891–3896. [CrossRef]
79. Sahil; Kaur, K.; Jaitak, V. Thiazole and Related Heterocyclic Systems as Anticancer Agents: A Review on Synthetic Strategies, Mechanisms of Action and SAR Studies. *Curr. Med. Chem.* **2022**, *29*, 4958–5009. [CrossRef]
80. Pawar, S.; Kumar, K.; Gupta, M.K.; Rawal, R.K. Synthetic and Medicinal Perspective of Fused-Thiazoles as Anticancer Agents. *Anticancer. Agents Med. Chem.* **2020**, *21*, 1379–1402. [CrossRef]
81. Sharma, P.C.; Bansal, K.K.; Sharma, A.; Sharma, D.; Deep, A. Thiazole-Containing Compounds as Therapeutic Targets for Cancer Therapy. *Eur. J. Med. Chem.* **2020**, *188*, 112016–112063. [CrossRef] [PubMed]
82. Swain, R.J.; Kemp, S.J.; Goldstraw, P.; Tetley, T.D.; Stevens, M.M. Assessment of Cell Line Models of Primary Human Cells by Raman Spectral Phenotyping. *Biophys. J.* **2010**, *98*, 1703–1711. [CrossRef] [PubMed]
83. Sun, H.; Chow, E.C.Y.; Liu, S.; Du, Y.; Pang, K.S. The Caco-2 Cell Monolayer: Usefulness and Limitations. *Expert Opin. Drug Metab. Toxicol.* **2008**, *4*, 395–411. [CrossRef] [PubMed]
84. Pfaller, M.A.; Espinel-Ingroff, A.; Bustamante, B.; Canton, E.; Diekema, D.J.; Fothergill, A.; Fuller, J.; Gonzalez, G.M.; Guarro, J.; Lass-Flörl, C.; et al. Multicenter Study of Anidulafungin and Micafungin MIC Distributions and Epidemiological Cutoff Values for Eight Candida Species and the CLSI M27-A3 Broth Microdilution Method. *Antimicrob. Agents Chemother.* **2014**, *58*, 916–922. [CrossRef] [PubMed]
85. Peano, A.; Beccati, M.; Chiavassa, E.; Pasquetti, M. Evaluation of the Antifungal Susceptibility of Malassezia Pachydermatis to Clotrimazole, Miconazole and Thiabendazole Using a Modified CLSI M27-A3 Microdilution Method. *Vet. Dermatol.* **2012**, *23*, 131-e29. [CrossRef]
86. Fulmer, G.R.; Miller, A.J.M.; Sherden, N.H.; Gottlieb, H.E.; Nudelman, A.; Stoltz, B.M.; Bercaw, J.E.; Goldberg, K.I. NMR Chemical Shifts of Trace Impurities: Common Laboratory Solvents, Organics, and Gases in Deuterated Solvents Relevant to the Organometallic Chemist. *Organometallics* **2010**, *29*, 2176–2179. [CrossRef]
87. Babij, N.R.; McCusker, E.O.; Whiteker, G.T.; Canturk, B.; Choy, N.; Creemer, L.C.; De Amicis, C.V.; Hewlett, N.M.; Johnson, P.L.; Knobelsdorf, J.A.; et al. NMR Chemical Shifts of Trace Impurities: Industrially Preferred Solvents Used in Process and Green Chemistry. *Org. Process Res. Dev.* **2016**, *20*, 661–667. [CrossRef]

Disclaimer/Publisher's Note: The statements, opinions and data contained in all publications are solely those of the individual author(s) and contributor(s) and not of MDPI and/or the editor(s). MDPI and/or the editor(s) disclaim responsibility for any injury to people or property resulting from any ideas, methods, instructions or products referred to in the content.

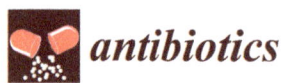

Article

Development of 4-[4-(Anilinomethyl)-3-phenyl-pyrazol-1-yl] Benzoic Acid Derivatives as Potent Anti-Staphylococci and Anti-Enterococci Agents

Hansa Raj KC [1], David F. Gilmore [2] and Mohammad A. Alam [1,*]

[1] Department of Chemistry and Physics, The College of Sciences and Mathematics, Arkansas State University, Jonesboro, AR 72401, USA; hansa.kc@smail.astate.edu
[2] Department of Biological Sciences, The College of Sciences and Mathematics, Arkansas State University, Jonesboro, AR 72401, USA; dgilmore@astate.edu
* Correspondence: malam@astate.edu

Abstract: From a library of compounds, 11 hit antibacterial agents have been identified as potent anti-Gram-positive bacterial agents. These pyrazole derivatives are active against two groups of pathogens, staphylococci and enterococci, with minimum inhibitory concentration (MIC) values as low as 0.78 µg/mL. These potent compounds showed bactericidal action, and some were effective at inhibiting and eradicating *Staphylococcus aureus* and *Enterococcus faecalis* biofilms. Real-time biofilm inhibition by the potent compounds was studied, by using Bioscreen C. These lead compounds were also very potent against *S. aureus* persisters as compared to controls, gentamycin and vancomycin. In multiple passage studies, bacteria developed little resistance to these compounds (no more than $2 \times$ MIC). The plausible mode of action of the lead compounds is the permeabilization of the cell membrane determined by flow cytometry and protein leakage assays. With the detailed antimicrobial studies, both in planktonic and biofilm contexts, some of these potent compounds have the potential for further antimicrobial drug development.

Keywords: pyrazole; persisters; *Staphylococcus aureus*; *Enterococcus faecalis*; resistance

Citation: Raj KC, H.; Gilmore, D.F.; Alam, M.A. Development of 4-[4-(Anilinomethyl)-3-phenyl-pyrazol-1-yl] Benzoic Acid Derivatives as Potent Anti-Staphylococci and Anti-Enterococci Agents. *Antibiotics* **2022**, *11*, 939. https://doi.org/10.3390/antibiotics11070939

Academic Editor: Charlotte A. Huber

Received: 28 June 2022
Accepted: 10 July 2022
Published: 13 July 2022

Publisher's Note: MDPI stays neutral with regard to jurisdictional claims in published maps and institutional affiliations.

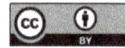

Copyright: © 2022 by the authors. Licensee MDPI, Basel, Switzerland. This article is an open access article distributed under the terms and conditions of the Creative Commons Attribution (CC BY) license (https://creativecommons.org/licenses/by/4.0/).

1. Introduction

Antimicrobial resistance (AMR) poses one of the greatest threats to human health around the world and it has been argued that AMR could kill 10 million people per year by 2050 [1]. The six pathogens, SPEAKS (*Staphylococcus aureus*, *Pseudomonas aeruginosa*, *Escherichia coli*, *Acinetobacter baumannii*, *Klebsiella pneumoniae*, and *Streptococcus pneumoniae*) are the leading causes of AMR deaths. *S. aureus* and its methicillin-resistant variant (MRSA) caused more than 100,000 deaths worldwide in 2019. On the other hand, ESKAPE pathogens (*Enterococcus faecium*, *S. aureus*, *K. pneumoniae*, *A. baumannii*, *P. aeruginosa*, and *Enterobacter* spp.) cause the majority of nosocomial infections and these bacteria have the ability to evade the existing treatments [2]. *S. aureus* infection is a major problem in the United States, which causes almost 100,000 infections and 20,000 deaths every year [3]. *S. aureus* infections are caused by different strains, including methicillin-sensitive *S. aureus* (MSSA), MRSA, vancomycin-intermediate *S. aureus* (VISA), and vancomycin-resistant *S. aureus* (VRSA). While most staphylococcal infections are due to MRSA, any *S. aureus* infection can be dangerous and lethal [4]. Hospitals are the major places for highly drug-resistant pathogens, such as MRSA, increasing the menace of hospitalization kills instead of cures [5–8]. MRSA has emerged as a multidrug-resistant pathogen in nosocomial infections and this pathogen is bypassing HIV in terms of fatality rate [9].

Enterococcus faecium, a Gram-positive bacterium, is a normal microbiota of the gastrointestinal tract (GI) and female genital tracts of humans and most other animals, including insects. This bacterium can cause a variety of problems when introduced into other parts of the body. Endocarditis and bacteremia are the most serious and life-threatening diseases caused by *E. faecium* [10]. *E. faecium* readily acquires antibiotic resistance genes and has become 80% vancomycin and 90% ampicillin-resistant [11,12]. About 30% of all healthcare-associated enterococcal infections are caused by vancomycin-resistant (VRE) strains, and these resistant strains are increasingly becoming resistant to other antibiotics. In 2017, VRE caused 54,500 patient hospitalizations and 5400 deaths in the United States. According to the CDC's National Healthcare Safety Network, solid organ transplant units reported vancomycin-resistant *E. faecium* as the most common cause of central line-associated bloodstream infections [13]. Furthermore, enterococci biofilms contribute to 25% of all catheter-associated urinary tract infections [14].

Pyrazole nucleus has widely been found in approved drugs, such as apixaban (Eliquis®), celecoxib (Celecox®), and several others (https://go.drugbank.com/categories/DBCAT000650 accessed on 8 July 2022). A myriad number of synthetic derivatives of this azole have been reported for their a nticancer [15,16], antibacterial [17], antiviral [18], and several other therapeutic properties [19]. In our research on azole derivatives as potent antibacterial [20–22] and antineoplastic agents [23–25], we found pyrazole-derived hydrazones are potent growth inhibitors of *A. baumannii* [21,26] and the aniline derivatives of pyrazoles are potent growth inhibitors of Gram-positive bacteria [22,27]. In this article, we report data on the antimicrobial activities, and the modes of action, of a series of hit compounds (Figure 1) [28,29]. The featured compounds (MIC ≤ 32 µg/mL) were selected for further studies following screening for antimicrobial activity, low toxicity against human embryonic kidney cell lines (HEK293) and their low lipophilicity, compared to other compounds [28,29].

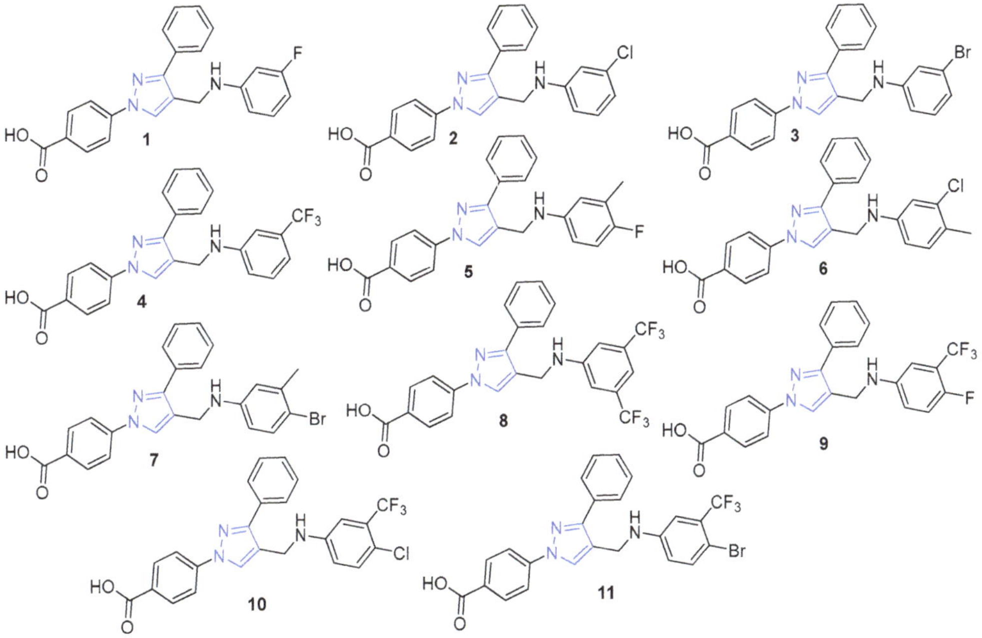

Figure 1. Structure of the hit compounds.

2. Results and Discussion

2.1. MIC Studies

The identified hit compounds (**1–11**) were tested against 13 Gram-positive bacterial strains (Table 1). The mono-substituted compounds were moderate growth inhibitors of these bacterial strains. 3-Fluorophenyl aniline (**1**) is a weak inhibitor of tested bacterial strains. The 3-chlorophenyl derivative (**2**) showed better activity than the fluoro derivative

(1), with MIC values in the range of 50 to 6.25 µg/mL. 3-Bromo (3) and 3-trifluoromethyl (4) derivatives showed similar antimicrobial properties. Overall, disubstituted compounds, except the 4-fluoro-3-methyl substituted derivative (5), showed better activity than those of the mono-substituted compounds (1–4). The 4-fluoro-3-methyl aniline derivative (5) showed moderate growth inhibition activity, with MIC values as low as 12.5 µg/mL against *Bacillus subtilis*. The 3-chloro-4-methyl derivative (6) was a potent growth inhibitor of the tested strains. This compound (6) inhibited the growth of *S. aureus* strains, with MIC values in the range of 3.12–6.25 µg/mL. This compound was also potent against enterococci, *B. subtilis*, and *Staphylococcus epidermidis* bacteria. The 4-bromo-3-methyl aniline derivative (7) showed similar activities as its chloro analogue (6). Bis(trifluoromethyl)aniline (8) was the best compound in the series, with potent activity across the tested strains. This disubstituted aniline derivative (8) was very active in inhibiting the growth of *S. aureus* strains, with MIC values as low as 0.78 µg/mL. *Enterococcus faecalis* and *E. faecium* strains were inhibited effectively, with an MIC value of 3.12 µg/mL, by this compound (8). *B. subtilis* and *S. epidermidis* strains were inhibited, with MIC values 0.78 and 6.25 µg/mL, respectively. 4-Fluoro-3-trifluoromethyl-substituted derivative (9) showed varied activity against different strains, with MIC values as low as 3.12 µg/mL against *S. aureus* Newman and *B. subtilis* strains. Chloro and bromo analogues (10 and 11) were very potent across the *S. aureus* strains, with an MIC value of 3.12 µg/mL. These compounds were also effective against the enterococci and *B. subtilis* strains.

Table 1. MIC values of the lead compounds (µg/mL): antibiotic susceptible *S. aureus* ATCC 25923 (Sa23), antibiotic-resistant *S. aureus* ATCC 700699 (Sa99), *S. aureus* BAA-2312 (Sa12), *S. aureus* ATCC 33592 (Sa92), *S. aureus* ATCC 33591 (Sa91), *S. aureus* Newman (SaN), *S. aureus* USA300 (Sa00), *S. aureus* UAMS-1 (Sa1), vancomycin-resistant *E. faecium* ATCC 700221 (Ef21), antibiotic susceptible *E. faecalis* ATCC 29212 (Ef12), *E. faecalis* ATCC 51299 (Ef99), *Bacillus subtilis* ATCC 6623 (Bs), *S. epidermidis* ATCC 700296 (Se). Vancomycin (Van), and Daptomycin (Dap) were used as positive control. DMSO (2.5%) and growth media were used as negative controls.

Comp	Sa23	Sa99	Sa12	Sa92	Sa91	SaN	Sa00	Sa1	Ef12	Ef21	Ef99	Bs	Se
1	25	25	25	50	25	>50	>50	>50	>50	50	>50	25	50
2	12.5	12.5	12.5	25	12.5	12.5	12.5	12.5	12.5	50	25	6.25	25
3	12.5	12.5	12.5	25	12.5	12.5	12.5	12.5	>50	50	25	6.25	25
4	12.5	12.5	12.5	12.5	12.5	6.25	12.5	12.5	12.5	25	25	6.25	25
5	25	25	50	50	25	>50	>50	>50	50	>50	25	12.5	50
6	6.25	3.12	6.25	6.25	3.12	3.12	6.25	6.25	6.25	12.5	6.25	3.12	12.5
7	3.12	6.25	6.25	12.5	6.25	3.12	6.25	6.25	6.25	12.5	6.25	3.12	12.5
8	1.56	1.56	0.78	3.12	0.78	1.56	1.56	1.56	3.12	3.12	3.12	0.78	6.25
9	6.25	12.5	12.5	12.5	6.25	3.12	12.5	12.5	6.25	25	25	3.12	25
10	3.12	3.12	3.12	3.12	3.12	3.12	3.12	3.12	3.12	6.25	6.25	1.56	6.25
11	3.12	3.12	3.12	3.12	3.12	3.12	3.12	3.12	3.12	6.25	6.25	1.56	6.25
Van	0.78	3.12	0.78	1.56	1.56	0.78	0.78	0.78	3.12	>50	>50	0.19	3.12
Dap	1.56	6.25	0.78	3.12	6.25	3.12	3.12	3.12	12.5	12.5	12.5	0.78	0.78

2.2. Bactericidal Properties and Time-Kill Assay

The minimum bactericidal concentration (MBC) is the minimum concentration that kills > 99.9% of a bacterial species within 18–24 h of treatment. If the MBC value of an antibacterial agent is not more than four times the MIC value, then the antibacterial agent is considered to be bactericidal. If the MBC/MIC value is more than four, then the antibacterial agent is considered to be bacteriostatic. Generally, the bacteriostatic agents inhibit protein synthesis and the bactericidal agents target the cell wall of bacteria [30]. As Table 2 shows, the hit compounds (6–10) were bactericidal for the *B. subtilis* strain, except for compound 11, which is a bacteriostatic agent. These compounds were bactericidal for the *S. epidermidis* strain. Compound 6 was bactericidal or bacteriostatic, based on the strain of *S. aureus* bacteria. Compounds 7–11 were bactericidal for the tested *S. aureus* strains.

The bactericidal action was consistent with the compounds being membrane disruptors. We performed the time kill assay at 4 × MIC concentration to determine the bactericidal properties of our hit compounds. As can be seen in Figure 2, potent compounds **8**, **10**, and **11** killed the bacteria within 6 h. Compound **6** did not kill the bacterial cells even after 24 h. Vancomycin eliminated bacteria up to the level of the detection limit within 8 h. These observations corresponded to the bacteriostatic nature of compound **6** and bactericidal properties of compounds **8**, **10** and **11**. These observations agreed with the MBC values (Table 2) of the compounds and the positive control, vancomycin. Since bactericidal activity was determined from bacteria exposed to compounds for 20 h, it cannot be completely ruled out that low colony counts could have arisen from a failure of a subpopulation to recover from a viable non-culturable state brought on by antibiotic exposure [31].

Table 2. MBC values of the potent compounds against susceptible bacteria.

Comp	Bs	Sa12	Sa23	Sa99	Sa91	Sa92	Se
6	12.5	50	50	50	12.5	50	50
7	12.5	50	25	25	12.5	50	50
8	3.12	3.12	12.5	6.25	3.12	12.5	12.5
10	6.25	12.5	25	12.5	12.5	25	25
11	12.5	25	12.5	12.5	12.5	25	25
Van	1.56	1.56	12.5	6.25	6.25	6.25	3.12

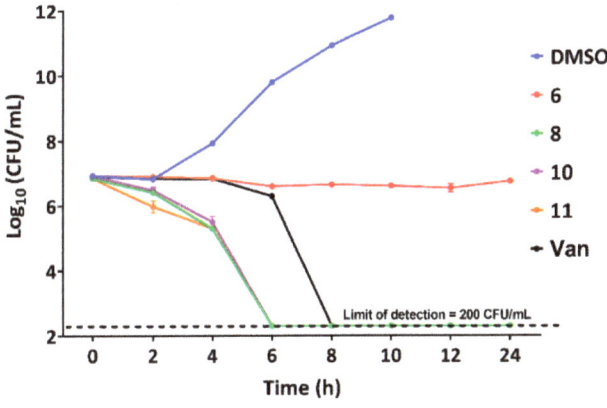

Figure 2. Time-kill assay (TKA) of *S. aureus* ATCC 700699 against the potent compounds treated at 4 × MIC concentration. Each data point represents the mean value of viable colony counts performed in triplicate and the error bars represent standard deviation values.

2.3. Activity against Biofilms

We studied the biofilm inhibition properties of three potent compounds against the *S. aureus* ATCC 25923 strain (Figure 3). Compound (**8**) was very effective at inhibiting the growth of *S. aureus* biofilm at 2 × MIC concentration but potency decreased at lower concentrations. Compounds **10** and **11** showed very strong biofilm inhibition properties at all the tested concentrations: 2×, 1×, and 0.5 × MIC values. The positive control, vancomycin (Van), showed good activity at 2×, and 1 × MIC values, but this approved drug inhibited only ~60% biofilm formation at 0.5 × MIC treatment. We studied the biofilm eradication properties of these potent compounds. Among these compounds, the bis(trifluoromethyl)aniline derivative (**8**) was a moderate biofilm eradicator of *S. aureus*, which eradicated ~80% biofilm at 2 × MIC. Decreasing the concentration of this compound reduced the biofilm elimination property significantly. Compound **10** eliminated the

S. aureus biofilm effectively in all three concentrations. Compound **11** showed good biofilm eradication properties at 2× and 1 × MIC values, albeit only ~55% biofilm eradication at 0.5 × MIC value. The positive control, vancomycin, showed weak biofilm elimination activity as compared to our lead compounds **10** and **11**. The ability of compounds **10** and **11** to significantly inhibit and eradicate biofilm at the concentration of 0.5 × MIC was particularly noteworthy, indicating that the observation was not just a side effect of the bacteriostatic or bactericidal properties of the compounds.

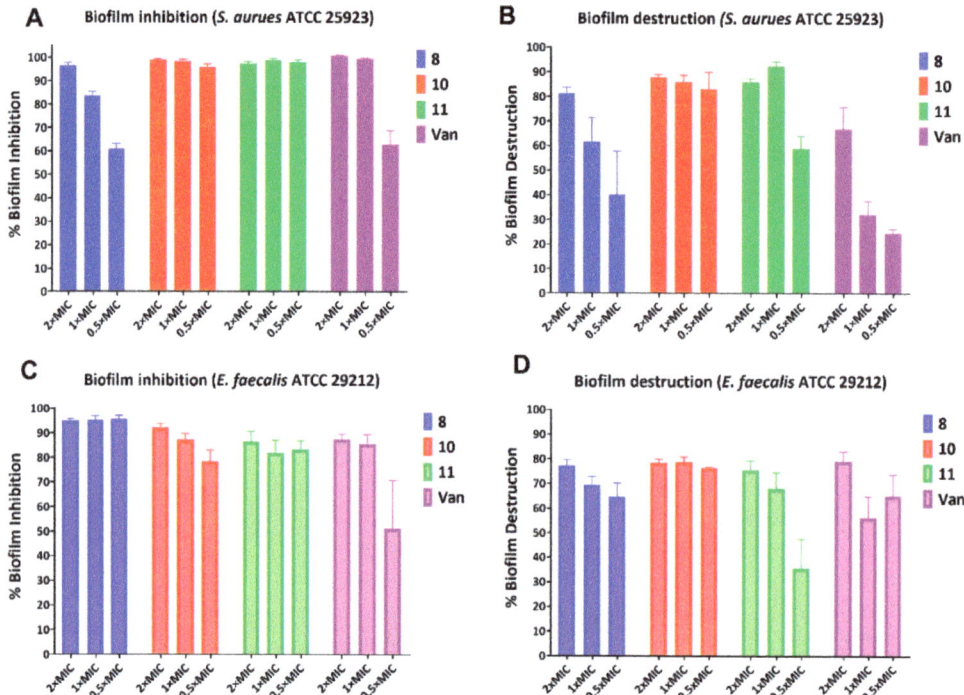

Figure 3. Biofilm inhibition of *S. aureus* (**A**) and *E. faecalis* (**C**) and biofilm destruction of *S. aureus* (**B**) and *E. faecalis* (**D**) by potent compounds (**8**, **10**, and **11**). Vancomycin (Van) is the positive control. Data based on retention of crystal violet by biofilm as compared to DMSO (the solvent of compound diluent as negative control). Error bars represent standard deviation values of the readings obtained in triplicates.

We also studied the biofilm inhibition properties of the molecules against *E. faecalis* ATCC 29212. Compound **8** inhibited >90% biofilm growth in all three tested concentrations. Compound **10** inhibited >90% biofilm formation at 2 × MIC value, but the inhibition potency decreased gradually at lower concentrations. The third potent lead compound (**11**) inhibited the biofilm formation of *E. faecalis*, at lower potency. Vancomycin showed similar potency at 2× and 1 × MIC values but, nevertheless, biofilm inhibition potency decreased significantly at the sub-MIC value. In the *E. faecalis* biofilm eradication studies of our hit compounds, we observed potent activity comparable to the positive control. In particular, compound **10** again showed moderate biofilm inhibition and eradication below the MIC and MBC concentrations.

We determined the minimal biofilm eradication concentration (MBEC), the lowest concentration of compound sufficient to prevent growth from a treated biofilm, to further determine the potency of the effective lead compounds. As shown in Table 3, compounds **8**, **10**, and **11** eradicated the established biofilms of *S. aureus* ATTCC 25923 and *E. faecalis* ATCC

29212 at concentrations 2× and 4 × MIC, respectively. Compounds were less effective at eradicating the biofilm of S. aureus USA300, with concentrations as high as 50 µg/mL (16 × MIC) needed to reach the MBEC (compound **10**). Our studies showed that the positive control used in MIC tests, vancomycin, was not effective in eradicating the tested biofilms. These studies are very significant, as S. aureus biofilms are very challenging to treat with the existing antibiotics [32]. Similarly, E. faecalis readily forms biofilms, which are recalcitrant to existing treatments [33].

Table 3. MIC and MBEC values of the three lead compounds against Sa23, Sa00 and EFs12 determined by Calgary Biofilm methods.

Comps	Sa23		Sa00		Efs12	
	MIC	MBEC	MIC	MBEC	MIC	MBEC
8	1.56	3.12	1.56	12.5	3.12	6.25
10	3.12	6.25	3.12	50	3.12	12.5
11	3.12	6.25	3.12	25	3.12	6.25
Van	0.78	>50	0.78	>50	3.12	>50

2.4. Real-Time Monitoring of S. aureus Biofilm

Bacteria within a biofilm matrix are better protected from host defenses and antibiotics. Regular doses of antibiotics can reduce the biofilm but rarely eliminate it [34,35]. We treated biofilms produced by two strains of S. aureus with the lead compounds at various concentrations, as well as with conventional antibiotics, and monitored real-time biofilm growth/inhibition using the Bioscreen C Pro. This test depends on the production of planktonic cells from the biofilm or any increase in the biofilm itself. The effects of various concentrations of compounds **8**, **11**, vancomycin and daptomycin on S. aureus ATCC 25923 and S. aureus USA300 biofilm, as compared to the DMSO treated negative control, are shown in Figures 4 and 5. The biofilm minimum inhibitory concentration (BMIC) is defined as the lowest concentration of the compound at which the optical density remains at baseline at the 24 h time point. The BMIC for compound **8** against S. aureus ATCC 25923, as measured kinetically using Bioscreen C Pro, was observed to be 4 × MIC of planktonic cells (6.25 µg/mL) (Figure 4A) and 4 × MIC (12.5 µg/mL) against S. aureus USA300 (Figure 4A). BMIC for compound **11** was 2 × MIC (6.25 µg/mL) for S. aureus ATCC 25923 and 4 × MIC for S. aureus USA300, while MPC against both the strains was 4 × MIC concentrations (Figure 4B and 5B). BMIC for vancomycin was observed to be 8 × MIC and 16 × MIC for S. aureus ATCC 25923 and S. aureus USA300, respectively. Daptomycin exhibited a BMIC value to be 16 × MIC, and an MPC value being >16 × MIC, against S. aureus ATCC 25923 biofilm (Figure 4D).

2.5. Activity against Persisters

Persisters are dormant phenotypic variants of bacteria that are recalcitrant to killing by antibiotics. Persisters are a chronic and continuous nidus of infection that can result in treatment failure [36]. Bacteria comparable to persisters can be produced by allowing a culture to grow until the stationary phase is well established. We tested our potent lead molecules (**8**, **10**, and **11**) for their ability to eliminate such persister cells of S. aureus ATCC 700699 (Figure 6). Cells were incubated in phosphate buffered saline (PBS), conditions, under which they do not resume growth. As can be seen (Figure 6A), our compounds (**8**, **10**, and **11**) reduced the persisters' viability after 4 h at 8 × MIC treatment. The positive controls, approved antibiotics (gentamicin and vancomycin), did not show any effectiveness against the persisters and showed similar viability as the negative control (2.5% DMSO). The lack of bactericidal activity by vancomycin is to be expected, since cell wall inhibiting antibiotics lack effectiveness against non-growing cells. To observe the persister elimination pattern with time, persister cells were incubated in PBS with various concentrations of compounds (**8**, **10** and **11**). Aliquots were drawn out every 2 h for a viable colony count for up to 8 h total time (Figure 6B–D). Compound **8** considerably reduced the concentration of persisters at 2 ×, 4 ×, and 8 × MIC values. *S. aureus* persisters were markedly reduced by 16 × MIC treatment. Compound **10** was more effective in decreasing persisters at similar concentrations. This compound (**10**) decreased *S. aureus* persisters up to the detection limit at 8 × MIC treatment in 8 h. The 16 × MIC treatment eliminated the persisters in 6 h. Although the hit compound **11** showed weak activity at 2 × MIC treatment, it showed comparable potency at higher treatment doses. It was found that 8 × MIC and 16 × MIC treatments eliminated persisters within 8 h and 6 h, respectively. Based on the anti-persister activity, we could conclude that our potent compounds were very effective at killing *S. aureus* persisters in vitro. This finding warrants further development of these compounds as antibiotics.

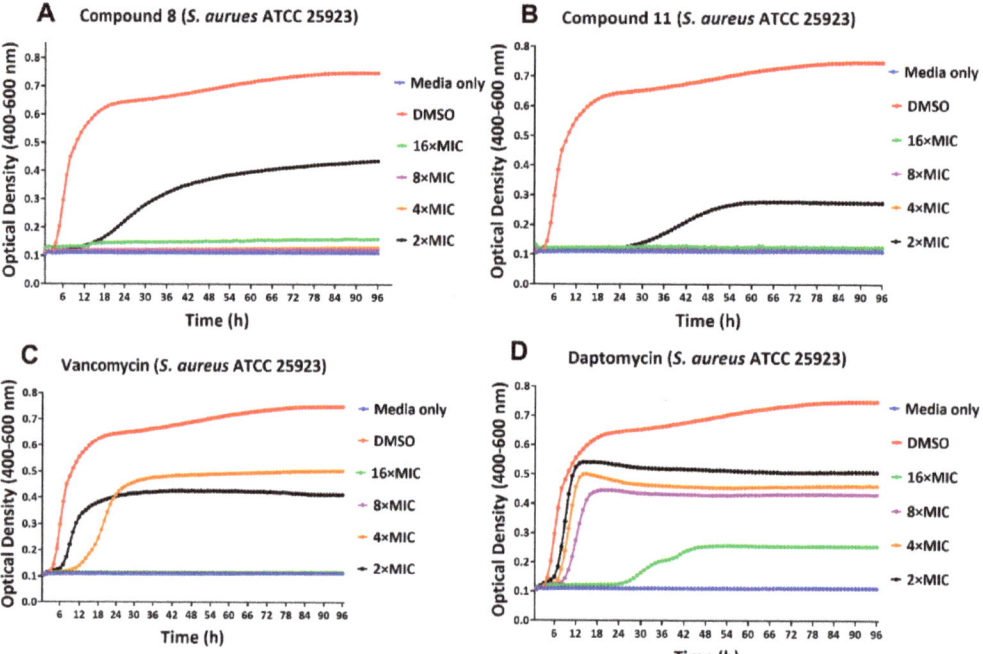

Figure 4. Real-Time monitoring of *S. aureus* ATCC 25923 biofilm. Effect of various concentrations of compound **8** (**A**), compound **11** (**B**), Vancomycin (**C**) and Daptomycin (**D**) against *S. aureus* ATCC 25923 biofilm growth, as monitored by Bioscreen C Pro up to 96 h. Legends indicate treatment of preformed biofilm with DMSO control and various MIC concentrations of each compound. An additional control consisted of growth medium with no pre-formed biofilm in the wells. Each data point represents the mean value of the optical density readings performed in triplicates.

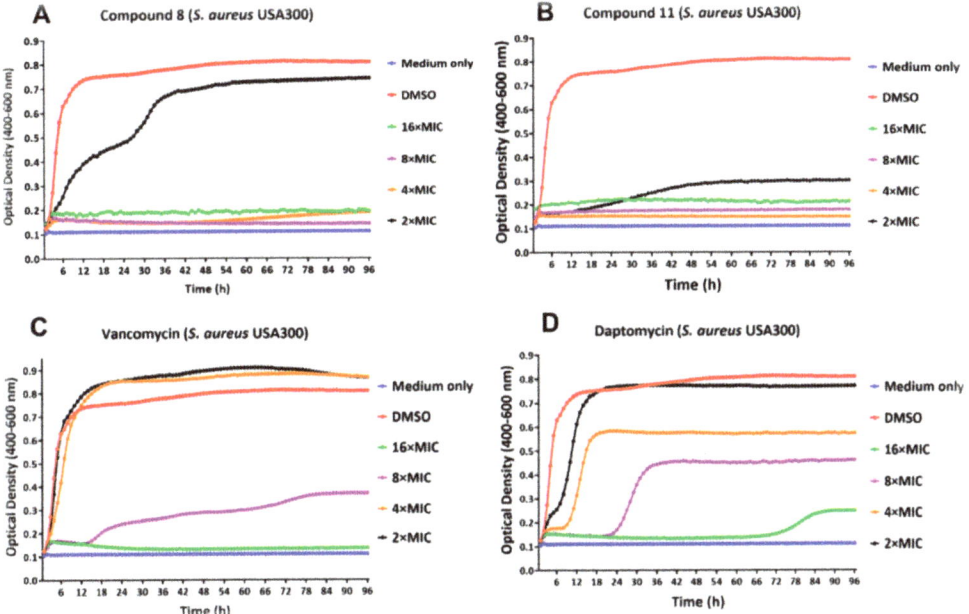

Figure 5. Real-time monitoring of *S. aureus* USA300 biofilms. Effect of various concentrations of compound **8** (**A**), compound **11** (**B**), Vancomycin (**C**) and Daptomycin (**D**) against *S. aureus* USA300 biofilm growth, as monitored by Bioscreen C Pro up to 96 h. Legends indicate treatment of preformed biofilm with DMSO control and various MIC concentrations of each compound. An additional control consisted of growth medium with no pre-formed biofilm in the wells. Each data point represents the mean value of the optical density readings performed in triplicates

2.6. Multistep Resistance Studies

The success of antibiotics over the years has been threatened by the evolution of antimicrobial resistance (AMR). Microbial pathogens have the ability to avoid or delay death upon exposure to antibiotics that were supposed to kill them [27,28]. We studied the ability of *S. aureus* and *E. faecalis* strains to develop resistance against our potent lead compounds (Figure 7). *S. aureus* ATCC 700699 was treated with lead compound **8** and the bacteria became slightly less susceptible by the third day (two-fold increase in MIC). However, no further resistance against this compound (**8**) was seen up to 14 days in our study. Lead compound **11** at 1 × MIC was effective against *S. aureus* up to 7 days, after which the MIC increased only to two-fold of the original. Bacteria developed resistance to vancomycin to two-fold on the sixth passage and four-fold after the ninth day of treatment. *E. faecalis* did not develop resistance to our compounds through all 14 days of the study, while the MIC of vancomycin increased two-fold on the 7th day. Based on these observations, *S. aureus* failed to develop resistance to our compounds easily, and *E. faecalis* did not develop resistance at all up to 14 days. While these studies show a failure to acquire resistance by mutations, they do not rule out the possibility of gaining resistance by horizontal gene transfer in natural environments if such resistance exists.

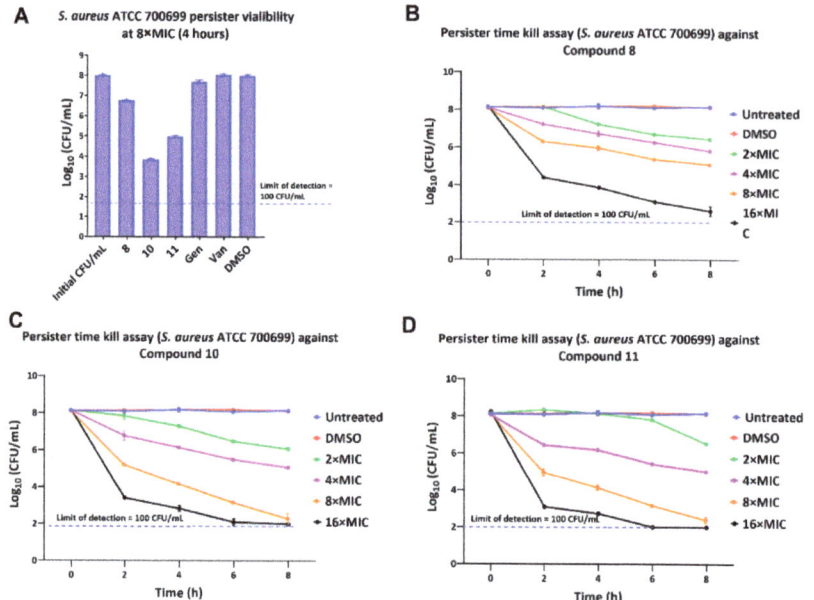

Figure 6. Effect of the lead compounds on the *S. aureus* ATCC 700699 persisters viability. (**A**) Effect of compounds (**8**, **10**, and **11**), positive controls (gentamicin and vancomycin), and DMSO on persisters. Effect of different concentrations of lead compounds **8** (**B**), **10** (**C**) and **11** (**D**) at different time points on *S. aureus* persisters. Each data point in all graphs represents the mean of viable colony counts performed in triplicates and error bars represent the standard deviation

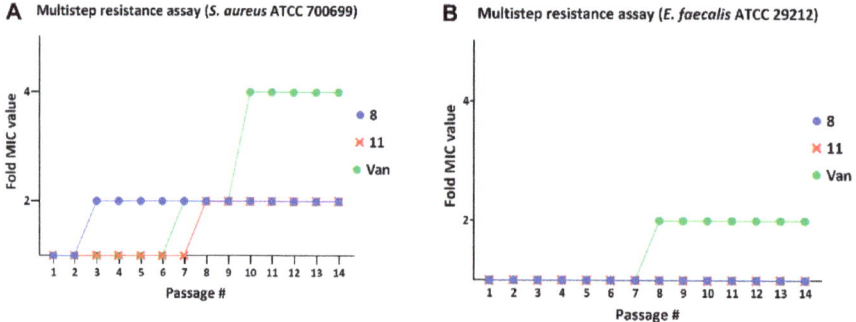

Figure 7. Multistep resistance assay of potent compounds against (**A**) *S. aureus* ATCC 700699 and (**B**) *E. faecalis* ATCC 29212. Vancomycin (van) is a positive control and resistance studies were done for 14 days.

2.7. Membrane Permeability Studies

Determination of the mode of action of antimicrobial compounds is crucial for the development of new drugs, as well as for new therapeutic applications for existing drugs [29]. To examine whether membrane permeabilization has a role in the mode of action, kinetic fluorescence measurement and flow cytometry analysis were performed in the presence of the fluorescent dye propidium iodide (PI) (Figure 8). PI fails to accumulate in cells with healthy membranes, but if the bacterium is unable to exclude this red fluorescent dye, it binds to DNA by intercalation increasing its fluorescence. If the test compound disrupts the permeability of the bacterial membrane, PI enters the cell and can be detected fluorometrically once it binds to DNA.

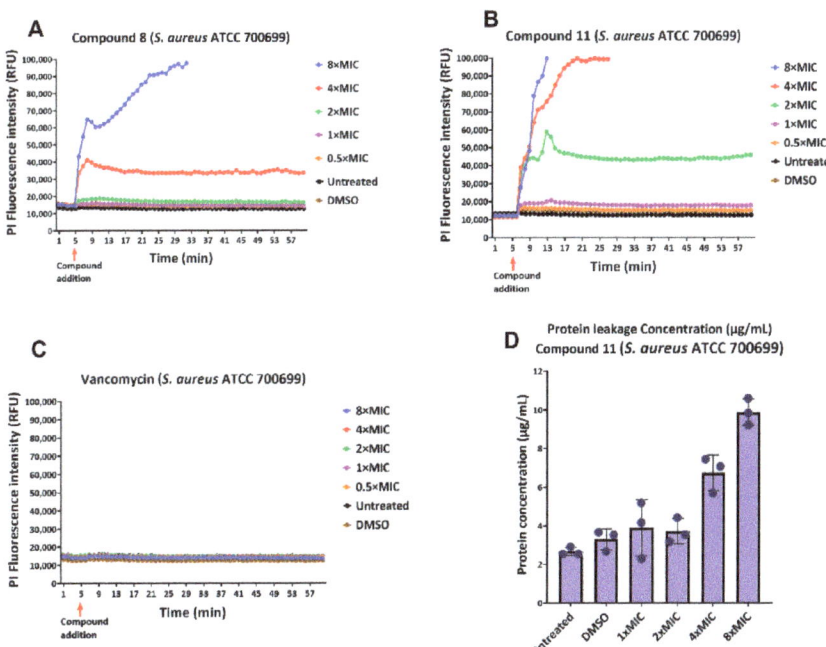

Figure 8. Kinetic fluorescence measurements to detect membrane permeabilization of *S. aureus* ATCC 700699 caused by compounds **8** (**A**), **11** (**B**) and Vancomycin (**C**) at various concentrations using propidium iodide. Each data point in the line graphs represents mean value of PI fluorescence performed in triplicates. Protein leakage concentration against compound **11** is shown in bar graph (**D**). Each value in the bar graph represents the mean of protein concentration measured in triplicates and error bars represent standard deviation.

For kinetic fluorescence measurement, *S. aureus* ATCC 700699 was incubated with the test compounds at various MIC concentrations in PBS containing 10 µg/mL Propidium Iodide (PI) at 37 °C in 96-well black microtiter plate. Figure 8A–C show kinetic fluorescence measurements of PI after treatment of bacterial cells with various MIC concentrations of the compounds. After the addition of the compound at 5 min (red arrow indicates compound addition), fluorescence was observed to increase rapidly at higher MIC concentrations for both test compounds **8** and **11**, while there was a slight increase in fluorescence at lower MIC values. For compound **8**, there was a rapid increase in fluorescence at 8 × MIC until 33 min, after which the fluorescence intensity was above the detectable limit (>100,000 RFU) for the device. At 4 × MIC, which is the MBC for this compound, there was a rapid increase in fluorescence up to the 9th minute, after which the fluorescence remained constant till the end of the experiment (Figure 8A). For compound **11**, there was a rapid increase in fluorescence at 8× and 4 × MIC concentrations up to the 13th and 29th minutes, after which fluorescence was above the detectable limit. A rapid increase was observed at 2 × MIC (below the MBC) up to the 13th minute, with a slight decrease followed by constant fluorescence till the end (Figure 8B). No increase in fluorescence was observed up to 8 × MIC concentration of vancomycin, indicating no membrane permeabilization for the tested highest concentration for this conventional drug.

Figure 8D shows a protein leakage assay that was performed to determine the leakage of cellular proteins. Once the bacterial cell membrane has been irreversibly disrupted, cellular contents, such as DNA, RNA, and proteins, will leak [30,31]. An increase in protein concentration with increasing MIC doses, in comparison to negative controls, untreated and DMSO treated samples, were observed, indicating the possibility of cell membrane damage and protein leakage.

Flow cytometry analysis was performed to determine the membrane-disrupting ability of the potent compounds. Various MIC concentrations of compounds **8** and **11** were treated with *S. aureus* ATCC 700699, and then stained with PI to measure PI permeabilization into the bacterium cells. As observed in Figure 9A, only 7.09% of the cells were stained in 1% DMSO treated cells, which was our negative control. Almost 96.11% of cells were stained in the positive control sample that was treated with 70% ethanol (Figure 9B). Vancomycin, which was used as technical control, showed cell staining similar to DMSO treated cells, indicating non-permeabilization of bacterial cells at 4 × MIC concentration (Figure 9C). Compound **8** treated cells showed higher PI intensity, with a good dose-response correlation. Treatment with 1×, 2×, and 4 × MIC concentrations showed 10.18%, 12.94%, and 67.82% PI-permeant cells, respectively (Figure 9D–F). Compound **11** demonstrated better PI permeability with dose-response in comparison to our lead compound **8**. For compound **11**, PI permeability was 12.63% and 34.93%, respectively, at 1 × MIC and 2 × MIC. Compound **11** at 4 × MIC treatment showed 91.23% PI-permeant cells. These results demonstrated that the compounds might have directly damaged or interfered with the membrane functions, as shown by the failure to exclude PI. However, it cannot be ruled out that membrane destabilization was a result of cell death, and not the direct cause.

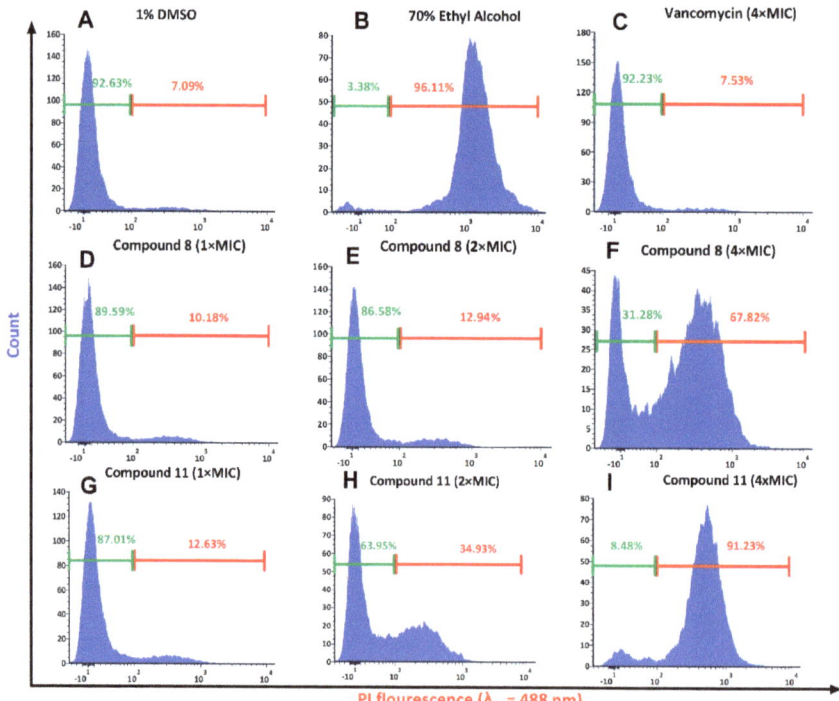

Figure 9. Flow cytometry analysis of bacteria treated with potent compounds. The membrane permeability of *S. aureus* ATCC 700699 treated by compounds at various concentrations and controls was measured by an increase of fluorescent intensity of propidium iodide at 4 °C for 30 min. (**A**) 1% DMSO; (**B**) 70% ethanol; (**C**) Vancomycin at 4 × MIC; (**D**) Compound **8** at 1 × MIC; (**E**) Compound **8** at 2 × MIC; (**F**) Compound **8** at 4 × MIC; (**G**) Compound **11** at 1 × MIC; (**H**) Compound **11** at 2 × MIC ; (**I**) Compound **11** at 4 × MIC3.

3. Materials and Methods

3.1. Antimicrobial Compounds (1–11)

The compounds (1–11) were synthesized as reported by us previously [28,29]. The purity of the compounds was determined by ^{1}H NMR before testing.

3.2. Minimum Inhibitory Concentration (MIC)

MIC for the compounds was determined using the standard microdilution technique recommended by the Clinical and Laboratory Standards Institute (CLSI). The starting concentration of the compounds was 32 µg/mL and a 2-fold dilution was performed along the 96-honeycomb well plate column to determine the MIC. MIC was confirmed in at least two occurrences of three replicates performed. A concentration was considered inhibitory when no visually detectable turbidity was present after about 20 h. Slow growth (up to 2 log increase over 20 h) could still fail to produce turbidity and would be considered inhibited.

3.3. Minimum Bactericidal Concentration (MBC)

MBC was determined for some compounds against various bacterial strains under study. After determination of MIC in 96-well columns, non-turbid well contents, including the MIC wells, were diluted 10-fold (10^0, 10^1 and 10^2) and then spot plated on TSA plates to quantify viable cells. The plates were incubated and colonies were counted to determine the percentage of viable cells, compared to the initial CFU/mL. The MBC was defined as the lowest concentration that reduced bacterial concentration by at least 99.9%.

3.4. Time-Kill Assay

Time-kill assay was performed following the methodology described earlier [22]. The exponential phase bacterial culture of *S. aureus* ATCC 700699 was diluted to ~5 × 10^6 CFU/mL in CAMHB, then treated with 4 × MIC of the test compounds and incubated at 35 °C. Every 2 h, the treated aliquot was diluted 10-fold in PBS and viable cells were quantified by viable colony count on TSA plates.

3.5. Biofilm Inhibition and Eradication Assays

Biofilm inhibition and eradication assays were performed as described previously [32]. In brief for biofilm inhibition assay, overnight bacterial culture was suspended to 0.5 McFarland standard in sterile PBS, which was then diluted 1:1000 in cation adjusted Muller Hilton Broth (CAMHB) supplemented with 1% glucose. Bacterial suspension, along with desired concentrations of the compound, were placed in triplicates into 96-well flat-bottom plates and incubated for 24 h at 35 °C. After incubation, each well was washed with PBS thrice to remove planktonic cells, then dried in the oven at 60 °C for 15 min. The wells were stained with crystal violet (0.1% w/v) for 15 min, then washed with deionized water to remove unstained dyes and dried in the oven for 15 min. Acetic acid (33%) was added to the stained wells to solubilize crystal violet, then optical density was measured using a Biotek Cytation 5 plate reader at 620 nm excitation wavelength.

For destruction assay, bacterial biofilm was first established in 96-well plates by culturing the overnight bacteria in CAMHB supplemented with 1% glucose and incubating 24 h at 35 °C. After incubation, the wells were washed thrice by PBS, then CAMHB, containing various concentrations of the compound, were added in triplicates to challenge the established biofilm in the wells. After an additional 24 h of incubation, washing, drying, staining by crystal violet, solubilizing stained biofilm, and measuring optical density were performed as described above. Percentage biofilm inhibition and destruction were calculated using the optical density of DMSO treated wells as negative control and media-only wells as a positive control.

3.6. Antibiofilm Studies Using Calgary Device

Calgary biofilm device was utilized to determine the minimum biofilm eradication concentration (MBEC) following the methodology described earlier [27]. Briefly, biofilm was established on the lid pegs of the device using overnight bacterial culture diluted in CAMHB supplemented with 1% glucose at 35 °C for 24 h. After incubation, the lid was removed, washed with PBS in a fresh 96-well plate, then transferred to the "challenge plate" which contained 2-fold serial diluted compounds in PBS. The challenge plate was incubated for 24 h, then the lid was transferred to the next 96-well plate containing fresh CAMHB with 1% glucose and further incubated for 24 h. Following the final incubation, the plates were observed for visible turbidity to determine MBEC, which was the lowest concentration of compound well that resulted in no turbidity. Each compound was tested in triplicates to confirm the MBEC value.

3.7. Real-Time Monitoring of S. aureus Biofilm

Real-time monitoring of biofilm growth/inhibition was performed following the methodology described by Elkhatib et al. [34] with few modifications. Overnight culture of *S. aureus* was diluted (1×10^6 CFU/mL) in CAMHB with 1% glucose and seeded (150 µL) into 100-well polystyrene honeycomb plates to establish biofilm. Several control wells received only culture medium and no cells so that no biofilm would be produced. The plate was incubated in the chamber of Bioscreen C Pro (Growth curves USA, Piscataway, NJ, USA) for 24 h at 37 °C without shaking. Following incubation, each well of the plate was washed thrice with sterile PBS to remove planktonic cells. CAMHB with 1% glucose, containing desired concentrations of the compound, were prepared and transferred to the biofilm established wells (200 µL). Control wells consisted of DMSO treated and wells without bacteria (medium only). The prepared honeycomb plate was placed in the preheated chamber of Bioscreen C Pro programmed to maintain the temperature of 37 °C for 96 h without shaking. A wide-band filter with a spectrum range of 400–600 nm was programmed to measure the optical densities every 1 h up to 96 h of real-time monitoring of biofilm growth/inhibition.

3.8. Persister Cell Killing Assay

Persister cell killing assay was performed following the methodology described earlier [22]. Briefly, *S. aureus* was grown in CAMHB for 24 h by shaking at 200 rpm at 35 °C to the stationary phase. The stationary phase cells were washed thrice in PBS and then diluted to around 10^8 CFU/mL in the same buffer. The diluted persister suspension was treated with the desired concentration of the compound in a sterile 10×75 mm plastic culture tube by shaking at 200 rpm at 35 °C. At a desired interval of time, aliquots were taken in microcentrifuge tubes, washed with PBS twice, 10-fold serially diluted, and spot plated in tryptic soy agar (TSA) plates for viable colony count to determine CFU/mL for each treatment.

3.9. Multi-Step Resistance Assay

The ability of *S. aureus* ATCC 700699 (MRSA) and *E. faecalis* ATCC 29212 to develop resistance to the test compounds was investigated by multi-step resistance assay. The minimum inhibitory concentration (MIC) was determined on the first day, which was the first passage of the assay. Sub-MIC well from the first passage 96-well plate was used as bacterial inoculum to determine MIC for second passage. The experiment was repeated similarly for further passages and MIC for each passage was recorded for up to 14 passages to investigate resistance development.

3.10. Kinetic Fluorescence Measurements to Detect Membrane Permeabilization Using Propidium Iodide

The kinetic fluorescence measurement to detect membrane permeabilization was conducted following the methodology described by Boix-Lemonche et. al. [35] with few modifications. Exponential phase *S. aureus* ATCC 700699 (MRSA) was harvested by centrifugation, washed and diluted in PBS (1×10^8 CFU/mL). Propidium iodide (PI) was added to a final concentration of 10 µg/mL, followed by incubation for 15 min in the dark. After incubation, the mixture was vortexed and 195 µL was transferred to wells of a black 96-well plate. The plate was placed in the chamber of the Biotek Cytation™ 5 plate reader at 37 °C and fluorescence was measured at excitation and emission wavelengths 535 nm and 617 nm, respectively, every minute for 5 min, or until readings were stabilized. After this, the plate was ejected and compounds at various concentrations (5 µL dissolved in DMSO) were added to pre-designated wells. The plate was further monitored with fluorescence reading parameters mentioned earlier every minute up to a total of 60 min, shaking continuously.

3.11. Protein Leakage Assay

Protein leakage from the bacterial cells, due to damage to the bacterial cell membrane, was determined using the methodology described by Xie et al. [36], with a few modifications. Exponential phase bacterial cells were collected by centrifugation at $5000 \times$ g for 10 min, followed by washing thrice with PBS and suspending in the same buffer. The bacterial suspension was treated with various MIC concentrations of compound **11** at 37 °C by shaking at 200 rpm for 2 h. The treatment sample was then centrifuged at $10,000 \times$ g for 5 min and the supernatant was used to estimate the protein concentration, using a standard Bradford assay. Untreated bacterial cell samples and DMSO-treated samples, which were negative control for this experiment, were also processed accordingly.

3.12. Flow Cytometry for Membrane Permeability

Membrane permeabilization using propidium iodide (PI) was further quantified using flow cytometry analysis as described previously [37]. Briefly, exponential phase *S. aureus* ATCC 700699 cells grown in CAMHB were harvested at 4000 rpm for 10 min, followed by washing twice with PBS, and then diluting to $\sim 10^5$ CFU/mL in the same buffer. The bacterial suspension was incubated with various desired MIC concentrations of compounds for 30 min at 35 °C, while shaking at 200 rpm. The cells were again harvested from the treatment by centrifugation, and washed with PBS to remove excess compounds. The washed cells were incubated for 30 min with 10 µg/mL of PI in PBS at 4 °C in the dark. The cells were then washed again to remove unbound dye, and, then, data were recorded with an excitation wavelength of 488 nm (Phycoerythrin-Texas Red A filter), using BD FASAria™ cell sorter (BD Biosciences, Franklin Lakes, NJ, USA). After that, 1% DMSO and 70% ethanol-treated cells were taken as the negative and positive controls, respectively. Conventional antibiotic vancomycin was used as technical control.

4. Conclusions

We studied the antimicrobial properties of 11 lead compounds and four of these compounds were potent growth inhibitors of different Gram-positive bacterial strains, with some MIC values at sub-µg/mL concentration against several of the tested strains. These potent compounds were very effective against bacteria, both in planktonic and biofilms contexts. Two potent compounds (**8** and **11**) were very potent biofilm inhibitors at $2 \times$ MIC doses, and were consistently better than the positive control, vancomycin. In the real-time effect of potent compounds on biofilm inhibition studies, hit compounds were several-fold more effective than the control antibiotics, vancomycin and daptomycin. *E. faecalis* bacteria failed to develop any resistance against two of our compounds over 14 days. The most potent compounds were bactericidal and directly, or indirectly, caused membrane damage, as shown by protein leakage assays and propidium iodide permeability assays using flow cytometry.

Author Contributions: Conceptualization, M.A.A.; methodology, H.R.K.; resources, M.A.A. and D.F.G.; writing—original draft preparation, M.A.A.; writing—review and editing, D.F.G. and H.R.K.; funding acquisition, M.A.A. All authors have read and agreed to the published version of the manuscript.

Funding: This research was funded by National Institute of General Medical Sciences (NIGMS), grant number P20 GM103429 for the INBRE summer research grant, ABI mini-200028 grant, and NSF MRI grant (Award Number: 2117138).

Acknowledgments: This publication was made possible by the Arkansas INBRE Summer Research Grant, supported by a grant from the National Institute of General Medical Sciences, (NIGMS), P20 GM103429 from the National Institutes of Health. ABI infrastructure and facilities help to achieve the results for this publication.

Conflicts of Interest: The authors declare no conflict of interest.

References

1. Murray, C.J.L.; Ikuta, K.S.; Sharara, F.; Swetschinski, L.; Aguilar, G.R.; Gray, A.; Han, C.; Bisignano, C.; Rao, P.; Wool, E.; et al. Global burden of bacterial antimicrobial resistance in 2019: A systematic analysis. *Lancet* **2022**, *399*, 629–655. [CrossRef]
2. Scholtz, V.; Vaňková, E.; Kašparová, P.; Premanath, R.; Karunasagar, I.; Julák, J. Non-thermal plasma treatment of ESKAPE pathogens: A review. *Front Microbiol.* **2021**, *12*, 737535. [CrossRef] [PubMed]
3. Kavanagh, K.T. Control of MSSA and MRSA in the United States: Protocols, policies, risk adjustment and excuses. *Antimicrob. Resist. Infect. Control* **2019**, *8*, 103. [CrossRef] [PubMed]
4. CDC General Information about Staphylococcus Aureus. Available online: https://www.cdc.gov/hai/organisms/staph.html (accessed on 15 June 2022).
5. Moisse, K. Antibiotic Resistance Could Bring "End of Modern Medicine". Available online: http://abcnews.go.com/blogs/health/2012/03/16/antibiotic-resistance-could-bring-end-of-modern-medicine/ (accessed on 1 May 2020).
6. Tal-Jasper, R.; Katz, D.E.; Amrami, N.; Ravid, D.; Avivi, D.; Zaidenstein, R.; Lazarovitch, T.; Dadon, M.; Kaye, K.S.; Marchaim, D. Clinical and epidemiological significance of carbapenem resistance in acinetobacter baumannii infections. *Antimicrob. Agents Chemother.* **2016**, *60*, 3127–3131. [CrossRef]
7. Marsit, H.; Koubaa, M.; Gargouri, M.; Ben Jemaa, T.; Gaddour, H.; Kotti, F.; Sammoudi, A.; Turki, M.; Ben Jemaa, M. Hospital-acquired infections due to multidrug resistant acinetobacter baumannii: How challenging is the management? *Fund Clin Pharmacol* **2016**, *30*, 87.
8. Farha, M.A.; Leung, A.; Sewell, E.W.; D'Elia, M.A.; Allison, S.E.; Ejim, L.; Pereira, P.M.; Pinho, M.G.; Wright, G.D.; Brown, E.D. Inhibition of WTA synthesis blocks the cooperative action of PBPs and sensitizes MRSA to beta-lactams. *ACS Chem. Biol.* **2013**, *8*, 226–233. [CrossRef]
9. Mistry, T.L.; Truong, L.; Ghosh, A.K.; Johnson, M.E.; Mehboob, S. Benzimidazole-based fabi inhibitors: A promising novel scaffold for anti-staphylococcal drug development. *ACS Infect. Dis.* **2017**, *3*, 54–61. [CrossRef]
10. Agudelo Higuita, N.I.; Huycke, M.M. Enterococcal disease, epidemiology, and implications for treatment. In *Enterococci: From Commensals to Leading Causes of Drug Resistant Infection*; Gilmore, M.S., Clewell, D.B., Ike, Y., Shankar, N., Eds.; Massachusetts Eye and Ear Infirmary: Boston, MA, USA, 2014.
11. García-Solache, M.; Rice, L.B. The enterococcus: A model of adaptability to its environment. *Clin. Microbiol. Rev.* **2019**, *32*, e00058-18. [CrossRef]
12. Said, M.S.; Tirthani, E.; Lesho, E. *Enterococcus Infections*; StatPearls: Treasure Island, FL, USA, 2022.
13. CDC Vancomycin-Resistant Enterococci (VRE). Available online: https://www.cdc.gov/drugresistance/pdf/threats-report/vre-508.pdf (accessed on 23 May 2020).
14. Ch'ng, J.-H.; Chong, K.K.L.; Lam, L.N.; Wong, J.J.; Kline, K.A. Biofilm-associated infection by enterococci. *Nat. Rev. Microbiol.* **2019**, *17*, 82–94. [CrossRef]
15. Alkhaibari, I.S.; Raj, K.C.H.; Alnufaie, R.; Gilmore, D.; Alam, M.A. Synthesis of chimeric thiazolo-nootkatone derivatives as potent antimicrobial agents. *ChemMedChem* **2021**, *16*, 2628–2637. [CrossRef]
16. Delancey, E.; Allison, D.; Kc, H.R.; Gilmore, D.F.; Fite, T.; Basnakian, A.G.; Alam, M.A. Synthesis of 4,4'-(4-formyl-1h-pyrazole-1,3-diyl) dibenzoic acid derivatives as narrow spectrum antibiotics for the potential treatment of acinetobacter baumannii infections. *Antibiotics* **2020**, *9*, 650. [CrossRef] [PubMed]
17. Allison, D.; Delancey, E.; Ramey, H.; Williams, C.; Alsharif, Z.A.; Al-khattabi, H.; Ontko, A.; Gilmore, D.; Alam, M.A. Synthesis and antimicrobial studies of novel derivatives of 4-(4-formyl-3-phenyl-1H-pyrazol-1-yl) benzoic acid as potent anti-Acinetobacter baumannii agents. *Bioorg. Med. Chem. Lett.* **2017**, *27*, 387–392. [CrossRef] [PubMed]
18. Brider, J.; Rowe, T.; Gibler, D.J.; Gottsponer, A.; Delancey, E.; Branscum, M.D.; Ontko, A.; Gilmore, D.; Alam, M.A. Synthesis and antimicrobial studies of azomethine and N-arylamine derivatives of 4-(4-formyl-3-phenyl-1H-pyrazol-1-yl) benzoic acid as potent anti-methicillin-resistant Staphylococcus aureus agents. *Med. Chem. Res.* **2016**, *25*, 2691–2697. [CrossRef]

19. Hansa, R.K.; Khan, M.M.K.; Frangie, M.M.; Gilmore, D.F.; Shelton, R.S.; Savenka, A.V.; Basnakian, A.G.; Shuttleworth, S.L.; Smeltzer, M.S.; Alam, M.A. 4–4-(Anilinomethyl)-3-[4-(trifluoromethyl)phenyl]-1H-pyrazol-1-ylbenzoic acid derivatives as potent anti-gram-positive bacterial agents. *Eur. J. Med. Chem.* **2021**, *219*, 113402. [CrossRef] [PubMed]
20. Pankey, G.A.; Sabath, L.D. Clinical relevance of bacteriostatic versus bactericidal mechanisms of action in the treatment of gram-positive bacterial infections. *Clin. Infect. Dis.* **2004**, *38*, 864–870. [CrossRef]
21. Ayrapetyan, M.; Williams, T.; Oliver, J.D. Relationship between the viable but nonculturable state and antibiotic persister cells. *J. Bacteriol.* **2018**, *200*, e00249-18. [CrossRef]
22. Bhattacharya, M.; Wozniak, D.J.; Stoodley, P.; Hall-Stoodley, L. Prevention and treatment of Staphylococcus aureus biofilms. *Expert Rev. Anti. Infect. Ther.* **2015**, *13*, 1499–1516. [CrossRef]
23. Zheng, J.-X.; Bai, B.; Lin, Z.-W.; Pu, Z.-Y.; Yao, W.-M.; Chen, Z.; Li, D.-Y.; Deng, X.-B.; Deng, Q.-W.; Yu, Z.-J. Characterization of biofilm formation by enterococcus faecalis isolates derived from urinary tract infections in China. *J. Med. Microbiol.* **2018**, *67*, 60–67. [CrossRef]
24. Costerton, W.; Veeh, R.; Shirtliff, M.; Pasmore, M.; Post, C.; Ehrlich, G. The application of biofilm science to the study and control of chronic bacterial infections. *J. Clin. Investig.* **2003**, *112*, 1466–1477. [CrossRef]
25. Hall-Stoodley, L.; Stoodley, P. Biofilm formation and dispersal and the transmission of human pathogens. *Trends Microbiol.* **2005**, *13*, 7–10. [CrossRef]
26. Conlon, B.P.; Rowe, S.E.; Gandt, A.B.; Nuxoll, A.S.; Donegan, N.P.; Zalis, E.A.; Clair, G.; Adkins, J.N.; Cheung, A.L.; Lewis, K. Persister formation in staphylococcus aureus is associated with ATP depletion. *Nat. Microbiol.* **2016**, *1*, 16051. [CrossRef] [PubMed]
27. Schrader, S.M.; Botella, H.; Jansen, R.; Ehrt, S.; Rhee, K.; Nathan, C.; Vaubourgeix, J. Multiform antimicrobial resistance from a metabolic mutation. *Sci. Adv.* **2021**, *7*, eabh2037. [CrossRef] [PubMed]
28. Igler, C.; Rolff, J.; Regoes, R. Multi-step vs. single-step resistance evolution under different drugs, pharmacokinetics, and treatment regimens. *eLife* **2021**, *10*, e64116. [CrossRef] [PubMed]
29. Terstappen, G.C.; Schlüpen, C.; Raggiaschi, R.; Gaviraghi, G. Target deconvolution strategies in drug discovery. *Nat. Rev. Drug Discov.* **2007**, *6*, 891–903. [CrossRef]
30. Shi, Y.-G.; Zhang, R.-R.; Zhu, C.-M.; Xu, M.-F.; Gu, Q.; Ettelaie, R.; Lin, S.; Wang, Y.-F.; Leng, X.-Y. Antimicrobial mechanism of alkyl gallates against escherichia coli and staphylococcus aureus and its combined effect with electrospun nanofibers on Chinese Taihu icefish preservation. *Food Chem.* **2021**, *346*, 128949. [CrossRef]
31. Sun, H.; Huang, S.-Y.; Jeyakkumar, P.; Cai, G.-X.; Fang, B.; Zhou, C.-H. Natural berberine-derived azolyl ethanols as new structural antibacterial agents against drug-resistant escherichia coli. *J. Med. Chem.* **2022**, *65*, 436–459. [CrossRef]
32. Saleh, I.; Kc, H.R.; Roy, S.; Abugazleh, M.K.; Ali, H.; Gilmore, D.; Alam, M.A. Design, synthesis, and antibacterial activity of N-(trifluoromethyl)phenyl substituted pyrazole derivatives. *RSC Med. Chem.* **2021**, *12*, 1690–1697. [CrossRef]
33. Alkhaibari, I.S.; Kc, H.R.; Roy, S.; Abu-gazleh, M.K.; Gilmore, D.F.; Alam, M.A. Synthesis of 3,5-Bis(trifluoromethyl)phenyl-substituted pyrazole derivatives as potent growth inhibitors of drug-resistant bacteria. *Molecules* **2021**, *26*, 5083. [CrossRef]
34. Elkhatib, W.; Noreddin, A. In vitro antibiofilm efficacies of different antibiotic combinations with zinc sulfate against pseudomonas aeruginosa recovered from hospitalized patients with urinary tract infection. *Antibiotics* **2014**, *3*, 64–84. [CrossRef]
35. Boix-Lemonche, G.; Lekka, M.; Skerlavaj, B. A rapid fluorescence-based microplate assay to investigate the interaction of membrane active antimicrobial peptides with whole gram-positive bacteria. *Antibiotics* **2020**, *9*, 92. [CrossRef]
36. Xie, Y.-P.; Sangaraiah, N.; Meng, J.-P.; Zhou, C.-H. Unique carbazole-oxadiazole derivatives as new potential antibiotics for combating gram-positive and negative bacteria. *J. Med. Chem.* **2022**, *65*, 6171–6190. [CrossRef] [PubMed]
37. Alkhaibari, I.; Kc, H.R.; Angappulige, D.H.; Gilmore, D.; Alam, M.A. Novel pyrazoles as potent growth inhibitors of staphylococci, enterococci and acinetobacter baumannii bacteria. *Future Med. Chem.* **2022**, *14*, 233–244. [CrossRef] [PubMed]

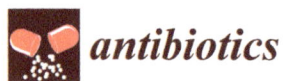

Article

Exploring the Antimicrobial Activity of Sodium Titanate Nanotube Biomaterials in Combating Bone Infections: An In Vitro and In Vivo Study

Atiah H. Almalki [1], Walid Hamdy Hassan [2], Amany Belal [1,*], Ahmed Farghali [3], Romissaa M. Saleh [3], Abeer Enaiet Allah [4], Abdalla Abdelwahab [3,5], Sangmin Lee [6,7,*], Ahmed H.E. Hassan [8,9], Mohammed M. Ghoneim [10,11], Omeima Abdullah [12], Rehab Mahmoud [4] and Fatma I. Abo El-Ela [13]

1. Department of Pharmaceutical Chemistry, College of Pharmacy, Taif University, Taif 21944, Saudi Arabia
2. Bacteriology, Immunology and Mycology Department, Faculty of Veterinary Medicine, Beni-Suef University, Beni-Suef 62511, Egypt
3. Materials Science and Nanotechnology Department, Faculty of Postgraduate Studies for Advanced Sciences, Beni-Suef University, Beni-Suef 62511, Egypt
4. Department of Chemistry, Faculty of Science, Beni-Suef University, Beni-Suef 62511, Egypt
5. Faculty of Science, Galala University, Sokhna, Suez 43511, Egypt
6. Department of Fundamental Pharmaceutical Science, Graduate School, Kyung Hee University, 26 Kyungheedae-ro, Dongdaemun-gu, Seoul 02447, Republic of Korea
7. Department of Regulatory Science, Graduated School, Kyung Hee University, 26 Kyungheedae-ro, Dongdaemun-gu, Seoul 02447, Republic of Korea
8. Department of Medicinal Chemistry, Faculty of Pharmacy, Mansoura University, Mansoura 35516, Egypt
9. Medicinal Chemistry Laboratory, College of Pharmacy, Kyung Hee University, 26 Kyungheedae-ro, Seoul 02447, Republic of Korea
10. Department of Pharmacy Practice, College of Pharmacy, AlMaarefa University, Ad Diriyah, Riyadh 13713, Saudi Arabia
11. Pharmacognosy and Medicinal Plants Department, Faculty of Pharmacy, Al-Azhar University, Cairo 11884, Egypt
12. Pharmaceutical Chemistry Department, College of pharmacy, Umm Al-Qura University, Makkah 21955, Saudi Arabia
13. Department of Pharmacology, Faculty of Veterinary Medicine, Beni-Suef University, Beni-Suef 62511, Egypt
* Correspondence: abilalmoh1@yahoo.com or a.belal@tu.edu.sa (A.B.); leesm@khu.ac.kr (S.L.)

Citation: Almalki, A.H.; Hassan, W.H.; Belal, A.; Farghali, A.; Saleh, R.M.; Allah, A.E.; Abdelwahab, A.; Lee, S.; Hassan, A.H.E.; Ghoneim, M.M.; et al. Exploring the Antimicrobial Activity of Sodium Titanate Nanotube Biomaterials in Combating Bone Infections: An In Vitro and In Vivo Study. *Antibiotics* **2023**, *12*, 799. https://doi.org/10.3390/antibiotics12050799

Academic Editor: Charlotte A. Huber

Received: 17 February 2023
Revised: 4 April 2023
Accepted: 19 April 2023
Published: 22 April 2023

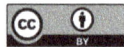

Copyright: © 2023 by the authors. Licensee MDPI, Basel, Switzerland. This article is an open access article distributed under the terms and conditions of the Creative Commons Attribution (CC BY) license (https:// creativecommons.org/licenses/by/ 4.0/).

Abstract: The majority of bone and joint infections are caused by Gram-positive organisms, specifically staphylococci. Additionally, gram-negative organisms such as *E. coli* can infect various organs through infected wounds. Fungal arthritis is a rare condition, with examples including Mucormycosis (*Mucor rhizopus*). These infections are difficult to treat, making the use of novel antibacterial materials for bone diseases crucial. Sodium titanate nanotubes (NaTNTs) were synthesized using the hydrothermal method and characterized using a Field Emission Scanning Electron Microscope (FESEM), High-Resolution Transmission Electron Microscope (HRTEM), X-ray diffraction (XRD), Fourier-transform infrared spectroscopy (FTIR), Brunauer–Emmett–Teller (BET), and Zeta sizer. The antibacterial and antifungal activity of the NaTNT framework nanostructure was evaluated using Minimum Inhibitory Concentration (MIC), Minimum Bactericidal Concentration (MBC), Disc Diffusion assays for bacterial activity, and Minimum Fungicidal Concentration (MFC) for antifungal investigation. In addition to examining in vivo antibacterial activity in rats through wound induction and infection, pathogen counts and histological examinations were also conducted. In vitro and in vivo tests revealed that NaTNT has substantial antifungal and antibacterial effects on various bone-infected pathogens. In conclusion, current research indicates that NaTNT is an efficient antibacterial agent against a variety of microbial pathogenic bone diseases.

Keywords: bone disorders; bone infections; sodium titanate nanotubes; anti-bacterial; anti-fungal; biomaterial; wound infections; rat model

1. Introduction

The vast majority of bone and joint infections are caused by Gram-positive germs. In areas with limited blood supply, bone infections can be difficult to treat and often require prolonged antibiotic therapy in combination with surgical drainage or debridement. Ineffective or delayed therapy can result in severe morbidities such as pain, loss of function, and the need for additional surgery and antibiotics. Therefore, when selecting the most appropriate systemic antibiotic therapy, consideration must be given to factors such as the organism(s) isolated and their sensitivity profile, pharmacokinetic factors such as penetration into bone, the presence of prosthetic material, vascular supply of the affected limb, and the patient's individual tolerance for the drugs [1].

Staphylococcus aureus is the most common bacterium responsible for osteomyelitis [2,3] and septic arthritis [4,5]. *Streptococcus pneumonia* and *Listeria monocytogenes* can also cause septic arthritis and raise concerns about underlying immune suppression [6–8]. Other microorganisms that may contribute to osteomyelitis in vasculopathic infections [9] include diabetic foot infections and septic arthritis caused by animal bites. Although certain patient populations are predisposed to Gram-negative infections, they account for a small proportion of bone and joint infections. Prior to the introduction of the Hib vaccine, *Haemophilus influenza* was a leading cause of septic arthritic joints in preschool children, but this is now less common [10].

Fungal infections are a rare but significant cause of osteomyelitis and arthritis. The most common fungal diseases that cause osteomyelitis are Candida, Aspergillosis, and Mucormycosis. Osteomyelitis and arthritis induced by mucormycetes are uncommon conditions that are among the most difficult consequences in orthopedic and trauma surgery [11]. The epidemiology of these musculoskeletal manifestations of fungal infections is a significant problem in both animals and humans. The Candida species are widespread yeasts. *Candida albicans* is a common human commensal, and other species can survive in non-living conditions such as soil. Aspergillus species infections of the bone and joints are characterized by a poor clinical prognosis and complex neurological consequences. Host-predisposing factors include immunosuppression, intravenous drug use, chronic underlying illnesses, and past surgical operations. Nosocomial diseases can be transmitted by polluted air ventilation systems or water pipes. *Aspergillus fumigatus* is the most common pathogen, followed by *Aspergillus flavus* and A. niger, but focused and customized antifungal medication is necessary [12]. Since the development of antibiotic therapy in the 1940s, particularly with the widespread use of immunosuppression and parenteral lines, candidiasis and mucormycosis have contributed to an increase in mucocutaneous and deep-organ infections [13].

Sodium titanate is an inorganic ion exchanger with a strong affinity for numerous metals. It acts effectively in mediums with different pH levels, either highly alkaline, neutral, or mildly acidic fluids. Titanate has been utilized in numerous applications [14]. Their electrophoretic deposition allows them to be supported on solid substrates [15]. Zhou and Yu developed super hydrophilic surfaces through the electrophoretic deposition of titanate [16]. They are also effective against Gram-positive and Gram-negative pathogens, such as *Staphylococcus aureus* and *Escherichia coli* [14]. These bacteria are among the most prevalent causes of nosocomial infections and are transmissible through contaminated surfaces [14]. Additionally, bacterial adherence to surfaces is an essential step in the creation of hazardous biofilms [17]. Inhibiting early bacterial adherence is therefore a promising antibacterial strategy [18].

Humans are often infected by microbes such as bacteria, fungi, and viruses throughout everyday life. The use of antimicrobial agents is crucial for imparting sterility (e.g., hospital trays) and preventing infection (e.g., wound dressing) one route from a bone infection. Antibacterial compounds incorporating diverse natural and inorganic substrates have been thoroughly studied [19]. In comparison to other antimicrobial compounds, TiO_2 has garnered greater attention owing to its favorable qualities, such as excellent stability, environmental friendliness, safety, and broad-spectrum antibiosis [20]. Using fine TiO_2

particles in antibacterial formulations has been the subject of a great deal of research. Yet, the powder TiO_2 catalyst has the disadvantage of slurry post-application separation [20]. Therefore, surface-immobilized TiO_2 with a large specific surface area is more promising for antibacterial applications [21], which is why we prepared it in nanotube formulations. Therefore, in this study, the modification of titanium in the form of Na TNT is an in vitro and in vivo study on both bacterial and fungal infections that need to be investigated.

The purpose of this work was to examine the antibacterial and antifungal activities of a sodium titanate biomaterial generated by the hydrothermal process against a variety of infections that affect bone in humans and animals.

2. Materials and Methods

2.1. Materials

Strains: All fungal isolates used in this investigation were obtained from the reference collection of the Fungal Research Institute (Doki, Giza, Cairo, Egypt), while the bacterial strains were obtained from the American Type Culture Collection (ATCC) at the Cairo Microbiology Research Center. Strains used for phylogenetic reconstruction represented all relevant Mucorales taxa, including the clinically significant species, CNRMA 03894 *Mucor rhizopus*, which was used in this study. This study examined the effects of NaTNT as a preventive agent against wound infection for osteomyelitis and bone infection prevention. The reference standard for doxorubicin was supplied by Pharma Swede Pharmaceutical Company, while cyclohexamide served as the standard antifungal medication. Gram-positive strains including *St. pneumonia* (ATCC 49619), *S. aureus* (ATCC 25913), *Listeria monocytogenes* (ATCC 19115), and Gram-negative strains including *E. coli* (ATCC 25922), *Haemophilus influenza* (ATCC 49766), and *Bacillus subtilis* were utilized for antibacterial research (ATCC 35021). Regional Center for Mycology and Biotechnology (RCMB) isolates for Aspergillosis included *Aspergillus flavus* RCMB 02783, *Aspergillus fumigatus* RCMB 02564, and *Aspergillus niger* RCMB 02588, *Candida albicans* RCMB 05035 for Candidacies, *Mucor rhizopus* CNRMA 03.894 for Mucormycosis, and *Pencillieum notatum* (NCPF 2881). The bacterial isolates were incubated at 37 °C for 24 h using Muller Hinton broth and Muller Hinton Agar for bacterial growth. For fungal growth, Sabaroud Dextrose Agar and broth were employed with the conventional antifungal medication (cyclohexamide) at 25 °C for five days. Before the experiments, each tube was sanitized using an autoclave.

2.2. Synthesis of Sodium Titanate Nanotubes

All chemicals involved in the preparation step were of analytical grade and obtained from Sigma Aldrich Co. They were used without further purification. Na-TNT was synthesized using the hydrothermal method [22]. Firstly, 10 g of anatase TiO_2 powder was stirred for 30 min with 500 mL of 10.0 M NaOH until a milky suspension appeared. This milky suspension was allowed to react hydrothermally in a Teflon-lined stainless-steel autoclave with a 500 mL volume for 23 h at 160 °C to produce Na-TNT. The autoclave was then cooled to ambient temperature. Afterward, the prepared Na-TNT was filtered, washed several times with distilled water, and finally dried at 80 °C overnight.

Characterization of Na-TNT was performed using several techniques. PANalytical (Empyrean) XRD using Cu Ka radiation (wavelength = 0.154 cm^{-1}) was used to obtain the X-ray diffraction pattern at an accelerating voltage of 40 kV, a current of 35 mA, scan angle ranging from 5 to 80°, and scan step of 0.04°. The FT-IR spectrum was measured in the range of 400–4000 cm^{-1} on a VERTEX 70 FT-IR spectrometer (Bruker Optics, Ettlingen, Germany) via the KBr pellet technique. Zeta potential was detected using Zetasizer Nano-ZS90 (Malvern, UK). Quanta FEG 250 (Thermo Fisher Scientific, Basel, Switzerland) electron microscope was used for FESEM imaging. High-resolution transmission electron microscope (HRTEM) imaging was performed using a JEOL-JEM 2100 (Tokyo, Japan) electron microscope operating at 200 kV. Brunauer-Emmett-Teller (BET) surface area was detected by the N_2 sorption technique using Micromeritics TriStar II.

2.3. Anti-Microbial Measurements

2.3.1. Fungal Isolates and Bacterial Inoculum Preparations

Recent cultures of *Aspergillus flavus* RCMB 02782, *Aspergillus fumigatus* RCMB 02564, *Aspergillus niger* RCMB 02568, *Candida albicans* RCMB 05035, *Mucor rhizopus* CNRMA 03.894, and *Pencillieum notatum* (NCPF 2881) were used to create suspensions, which were plated on Sabouraud's Dextrose Agar (SDA). After incubation, about 4–5 yeast colonies were transferred (using a sterile loop) to test tubes containing 5 mL of 0.9% saline solution. The final inoculum's turbidity was standardized using a suspension of barium sulphate 1.175% and sulphuric acid 1% (tube 0.5 on the McFarland scale, turbidity or standard tube). The final concentration was approximately 1.5×10^8 colony-forming units per milliliter (CFU/mL) [23].

To prepare the bacterial inoculum, *St. pneumonia* (ATCC 49619), *S. aureus* (ATCC 25913), *Listeria monocytogenes* (ATCC 19115), Gram-negative *E. coli* (ATCC 25922), *Haemophilus influenza* (ATCC 49766), and *Bacillus subtilis* (ATCC 35021) cultures were plated on Muller Hinton agar media and incubated at 37 °C for 24 h. About six colonies were then transferred to saline to obtain 10^8 CFU/mL, using conventional tube matching, as described in fungal inoculum preparation.

To determine antibacterial activity, the microdilution susceptibility test in Muller–Hinton Broth (Oxoid) was employed to estimate the minimal inhibitory concentration (MIC) for bacteria. Sabouraud's Liquid Medium (Oxoid) was used to estimate the MIC for fungus. Stock-tested chemical solutions were prepared in saline. The stock solution was subsequently diluted with standard method broth (Difco) to manufacture twofold serial dilutions of the broth containing approximately 10^8 CFU/mL of test microorganisms. The solution was then applied to each well of the 96-well Microtiter plate. The microplates were sealed and incubated for 24 h at 37 °C in a humid room. Prior to the conclusion of the incubation period, the MIC values were determined to be the lowest concentrations of the chemical that did not produce visible turbidity. Uninoculated medium served as the control in studies conducted under the same conditions as the test chemicals. To confirm their reproducibility, each experiment was conducted three times. Means and standard deviation (SD) values were calculated using SPSS version 21, and *p*-values less than 0.05 were considered statistically significant.

2.3.2. Minimal Bactericidal Concentration (MBC)

On Muller Hinton Agar Plates, the MIC dilution and at least two of the more concentrated tested NaTNT dilutions are plated and viable CFU/mL are determined. MBC is the lowest concentration of NaTNT at which no viable bacterial colonies are seen following a 24 h incubation at 37 °C (bactericidal activity).

2.3.3. Minimum Inhibitory Concentration for Fungal Isolates (MIC-$_f$)

Using the broth microdilution method to determine the MIC of fungi [23]. 100 µL of Sabouraud's Dextrose broth medium (SDB) was dispensed into each well of a 96-well microdilution plate with a "U" shaped bottom. Then, 100 µl of the tested nanomaterials emulsion was added to the first horizontal row of plate wells. A 100 µL aliquot extracted from the most concentrated well and transferred to the next well resulted in concentrations ranging from 1000 to 1.9 µg/mL. In the end, 10 µL of an inoculum suspension containing different tested strains was put into each well of the plate, where each column represented a fungal strain. In the presence of the conventional antifungal Cyclohexamide standard antifungal treatment for rapid-growing fungi were a positive control (medium without fungal strains) and a negative control (fungal strains without Na TNT). On SDB plates, each well contained 100 µL of SDB with various concentrations of tested nanomaterials in 2-fold serial dilutions (1000, 500, 250, 125, 62.5, 31.25, 15.62, 7.81, 3.95, and 1.95 µg/mL). A total of 10 µL solutions containing 1.5×10^8 fungal strains/mL were injected after dilution.

The U-shaped plates were incubated at 25 °C for 72 h. After the required period of incubation, the presence (or lack) of growth was visually evaluated. Consideration was given to the creation of cell clusters or "buttons" in the plate wells. The MIC was determined as the lowest concentration that inhibited fungal growth visibly. According to the criteria established by Morales et al., the antibacterial activity of the nanomaterials tested was evaluated (considered active or inactive) [24]: Strong/excellent activity (MIC < 1000 µg/mL).

2.4. Sorbitol Assay-Effect of NaTNT on the Cell Wall of Different Tested Fungal Strains

The assay was conducted using sorbitol-containing and sorbitol-free (control) media to examine potential antifungal processes involved in the nanomaterials' effect on the cell walls of various fungi. The culture medium (peptone water medium) was supplemented with sorbitol at a concentration of 0.8 M sorbitol (5 g/L added to peptone water media 15 g/L). The test was conducted using the microdilution technique in "U"-shaped 96-well plates. The plates were aseptically sealed and incubated at 35 °C, and readings were obtained on the fifth day of incubation. Based on the ability of sorbitol to act as an osmotic protective agent for the fungal cell wall, the higher MIC values reported in the medium with added sorbitol compared to the standard medium suggested that the cell wall is one of the potential cell targets for the NaTNT. Cyclohexamide was utilized as the placebo. The assay was run in triplicate and the findings were represented as the arithmetic mean [25].

2.4.1. Minimum Fungicidal Concentration Assay (MFC)

To evaluate the MFC, we inoculated SDA-coated Petri dishes with 100 µL aliquots of MIC, MIC 2, and MIC 4 of the investigated nanomaterials, cyclohexamide, and the negative control for fungal growth. After 72 h of incubation at 25 °C, the MFC was evaluated based on the development of the control organisms. The minimal fungicidal concentration (MFC) was defined as the lowest product concentration that prevented the growth of the tested microorganisms, resulting in either 50 or 99.9% fungicidal activity [26]. Assays of biological activity were conducted in triplicate, and the results were represented as the arithmetic mean of the MIC and MFC concentrations. Using both dilution procedures, it was feasible to identify whether the chemical is active; however, it is not possible to determine whether the substance will kill the fungus or simply slow its growth. The minimum fungicidal concentration (MFC) test is performed for this purpose. Small aliquots from each broth dilution test are subcultured on a rich solid medium and incubated for a predetermined amount of time and temperature, depending on the tested fungus species. According to papers standardized by the Chemical and Laboratory Standard Institute (CLSI), MFC is regarded as the lowest concentration of the drug in which no observed subculture growth occurs. MFC could also provide information regarding fungicide or fungiostatic activity. If the MFC and MIC are the same, the substance is a compound fungicide; if the MFC is higher than the MIC, it is fungiostatic [27].

2.4.2. Disc Diffusion Assay

For the standard size (50 mm diameter) disc diffusion analysis of all tested microorganisms, Whatman filter paper discs were made and then stored in 10 screw-capped wide-mouthed containers to assure sterilization. The bottles were then placed in a 150 °C hot air oven. Following this, the standard discs of the sterilized filter paper were impregnated with a 1000 µg/mL solution of the test substance (NaTNT) in saline. Then, they were placed in duplicate on nutrient agar plates seeded with the appropriate test organism. For the antibacterial assay, the usual conditions of 10^8 CFU/mL (Colony Forming Units per milliliter) were applied. Utilizing Petri dishes with a diameter of 12 cm, two discs of filter paper were inoculated in each dish. Gram-positive *St. pneumonia* (ATCC 49619), *S. aureus* (ATCC 25913), *Listeria monocytogenes* (ATCC 19115), and Gram-negative *E. coli* (ATCC 25922), *Haemophillus influenza* (ATCC 49766), and *Bacillus subtilis* were utilized as test organisms (ATCC 35021). Doxycycline was used as a reference antibiotic against Gram-negative bacteria, Gram-positive bacteria, and fungi, in that order. For bacteria and fungi, the plates were incubated at 37 °C for 24 h and at 25 °C for 5 days, respectively.

The twofold serial dilution approach revealed a considerable growth inhibition zone for the derivative.

2.4.3. Agar Diffusion Method for Fungal Isolates

The Agar diffusion technique is a semi-quantitative assay that involves applying a sample with a known concentration to a Sabaroud Agar Surface that has been inoculated with a standard number of fungal cells (*Aspergillus flavus* RCMB 02782, *Aspergillus fumigatus* RCMB 02564, and *Aspergillus niger* RCMB 02782), Candidacies (*Candida albicans* RCMB 05). Various procedures can be used to apply the sample, including disc diffusion, in which discs made of sterile filter paper (6 mm) are soaked with the sample and then applied to the agar surface in the presence of cyclohexamide, the standard antifungal. Following inoculation, the samples disperse into the agar medium, forming a circular concentration gradient. If the sample exhibits antifungal action, a zone of growth inhibition will emerge around the disc as the fungus multiplies. This inhibitory zone is measured in millimeters, and it is categorized by some writers as entire inhibition, partial inhibition, or no inhibition [28,29].

2.4.4. Antifungal Assay

Agar dilution method for detecting antifungal activity of various tested nanomaterials. According to the method of eff-Agboola et al. [30], the antifungal efficacy of NaTNT against randomly selected fungus isolates was examined after 72 h of growth on SDA at 25 degrees Celsius, the examined fungi were suspended in physiological saline (0.9% NaCl), and adjusted to 1.5×10^8 CFU. After preparing and autoclaving SDA at 121 °C for 15 min and storing it at 55 °C, the tested nanomaterials were created and mixed with SDA based on the concentration tested. NaTNT was prepared at 1, 2, and 3% concentrations. The 20 mL of solidified Sabaroud-agar medium was then put into sterilized Petri dishes. On the agar plates, equal volumes of the fungal suspensions were inoculated and speared. The plates were then incubated for 72 h at 25 °C before being evaluated on the fifth day of incubation.

2.5. *In Vivo Study with Wound Healing, Antimicrobial Evaluation, and Histopathological Investigations*

Antibacterial efficacy is determined by the best in vitro (*S. aureus* and *M. indices*) and in vivo (wound healing) results from this study (*S. aureus* and *M. indices*). The Institutional Animal Care and Use Committee (IACUC) of Beni-Suef University approved all animal experiments for research and testing. All animal handling, care, infliction of wounds, and treatment were conducted in accordance with the IACUC's requirements for approval. A total of 24 six-week-old adult male rats weighing between 150 and 200 gm were purchased from the faculty of pharmacy lab animals at Beni-Suef University. Each group consisted of three rats and was divided into eight groups (4 groups for *S. aureus* and 4 groups for *M. indices*). The rats were separated into four different groups as follows; Group 1 (G1) were control negative non-infected normal rats, group 2 (G2) were treated with Na TNT ointment with 10% Vaseline, group 3 (G3) rats were treated with commercial standard ointment as woundplast (fucidin) for *S. aureus* infection or with cyclohexamide ointment for *M. Rhizopus* infection, and finally G4 were control positive infected non-treated rats in both tested microorganisms. After anaesthesia with ketamine (90 mg/kg b.wt.) and xylazine (5 mg/kg b.wt.), we used a 1:1 mL ratio and injected 0.1 mg/100 gm b.wt., intraperiotineally; subsequently, after induction of an 1×1 cm wound area (at the back in *S. aureus* and in the top leg surface in *M. indices*), 100 μL of *S. aureus* and *M. indices* (1×10^8 CFU/mL) were administered to the wounds. At the wound site of the treated groups, the final concentration of NaTNT ointment was 10 gm:90 gm Vaseline. Rates of wound contraction were measured daily and every three days until the 12th day. All animals are maintained in sanitary and regulated circumstances. All rats were examined on a daily basis for wound fluid, signs of infection, and other abnormalities. In order to evaluate wound-healing activity, wound contraction % and wound closure time were utilized. On days Zero, 3, 6, 9, and 12 following surgery, the size of the wound was measured [31] (Equation (1)).

$$\text{Percentage of woundsize} = \frac{\text{Wound area on day X}}{\text{Wound area on day zero}} \times 100 \quad (1)$$

At 2, 6, and 12 days of therapy, samples of infected and treated wounds were collected in Muller Hinton broth media and incubated at 37 °C for 24 h. Then, the spread-plate method was used to determine the quantity of bacteria in solution, whereas for fungi, the plate count method was applied (*Mucor rhizopus*). The shape of the fungal isolate cultivated from debrided tissue was evaluated on potato dextrose agar (PDA) at 30 °C in the dark, and temperature tolerance was evaluated on Sabouraud's dextrose agar (SAB). There was no growth at 40 degrees Celsius, which was the optimal temperature. After 72 h at 30 °C, the diameter of the colonies was roughly 6.3 cm. The colonies on PDA were a light brown color with elevated mycelia. A microscopic inspection revealed yellowish-brown sporangia with walls that were finely roughened, ranging in diameter from 35 to 75 μm. The rats were photographed at 3, 6, and 12 days and slaughtered so that the wound tissues could be extracted for H&E staining and histological examinations using 10% formalin. The processed samples and acquired sections (5 mm) were stained with hematoxylin and eosin (H&E) and analyzed microscopically for cellular or immunological infiltration or macrophages in the wound region, collagen or fibroblast percentage, and vascularization rate [32].

2.6. Statistical Analysis

The data were presented as the mean standard deviation of the mean (S.E.M.). According to Snedecor, statistical significance was assessed using a one-way analysis of variance (ANOVA) [33]. Tukey's post-hoc test for multiple comparisons was then performed using SPSS (version 20.0) software (IBM SPSS Statistic 20.0, Armonk, NY, USA). *p*-values below 0.05 were deemed statistically significant.

3. Results and Discussion

3.1. Nano Material Characterization

Figure 1 presents the HRTEM and FESEM images of Na-TNT. The images reveal that the synthesized nanotubes are partially agglomerated to a low extent and are relatively thick and smooth. The HRTEM images show multiwall open-ended nanotubes with an average length between 100 and 200 nm. The inner diameter of the prepared nanotubes is about 4 nm with an outer diameter of about 10 nm. These findings support that alkaline hydrothermal treatment is an efficient method for converting nano-particulate morphology into a nanotubular structure. Additionally, EDX analysis confirmed the presence of Ti, O, and Na elements in the prepared nanotubes, as shown in Figure 1.

Figure 2a represents the FT-IR spectra of TiO_2 and Na-TNT. The FT-IR spectrum of Na-TNT shows the same main peaks of TiO_2 with increased intensity for peaks corresponding to the hydroxyl groups of Na-TNT. The broad peak appears at around 3370.0 cm^{-1} and corresponds to the O-H stretching vibration, indicating the presence of a high number of O-H functional groups in Na-TNT. The strong adsorption band at 1630 cm^{-1} is attributed to the bending vibration of hydroxyl groups [34]. Another characteristic peak that appears at 910 cm^{-1} is assigned to the Ti-O-Na bond [35]. The peak appears around the wave number of 730 cm^{-1} and reflects the anatase phase of titanate. Furthermore, the peak around 466 cm^{-1} could be attributed to the Ti-O-Ti crystal phonons due to the tubular structure of Na-TNT [36].

Figure 2b illustrates the XRD pattern of Na-TNT, which shows peaks centered at 2θ values of 9.9°, 24.4°, 28.4°, 48.2°, and 61.9°, corresponding to the crystal planes (200), (110), (600), (020), and (002), respectively. These results confirm the formation of Na-TNT with an orthorhombic unit cell, according to ICDD card no 00-057-0123 [22]. The prepared sample shows a crystallite size of 14.7 nm, according to the XRD results.

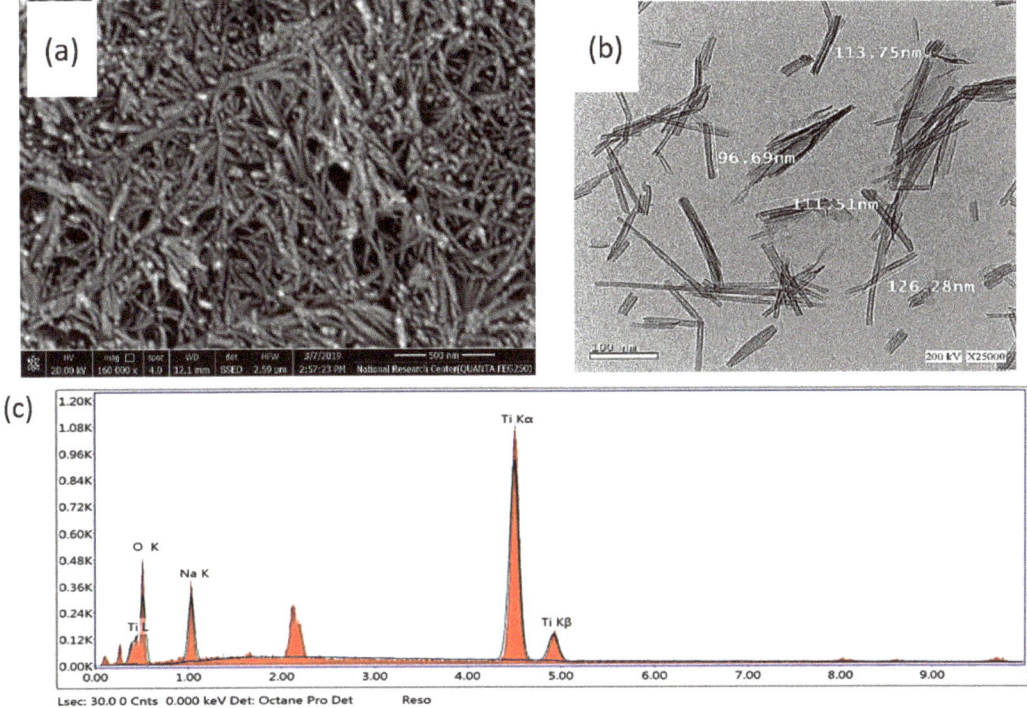

Figure 1. FESEM (**a**), HRTEM (**b**) and EDX elemental composition of Na-TNT (**c**).

Further investigation of Na-TNT was performed using N2 sorption analysis to identify the porous nature of the material and its specific surface area. Figure 2c presents the nitrogen adsorption/desorption isotherms of Na-TNT with a pore size distribution curve as an inset figure. The adsorption isotherm of Na-TNT shows a type IV isotherm pattern with a noticeable hysteresis loop, reflecting the mesoporous nature of Na-TNT. According to the IUPAC classification, the hysteresis loop of Na-TNT can be classified as a combination of H1 and H3 types. The H1 type hysteresis loop is characteristic of mesoporous materials that have a narrow range of uniform cylindrical-like pores, reflecting the tubular structure of Na-TNT. On the other hand, the H3 type refers to a wide range of slit-shaped pores with non-uniform size; such pores arise from solids consisting of non-rigid agglomerates or aggregates of plate-like particles [37]. The pore size distribution curve shows two types of pores: the first type is a narrow range of pores around 4 nm, which refers to the pores inside the nanotubes and is in good agreement with the inner diameter obtained from the HRTEM images, while the second type is a broad distribution of larger pores that may be attributed to the pores between the nanotubes. The shape of the isotherm of Na-TNT, as well as its hysteresis loop, are in agreement with those previously published for titanate nanotubes [38]. Furthermore, the textural properties are summarized in Table 1.

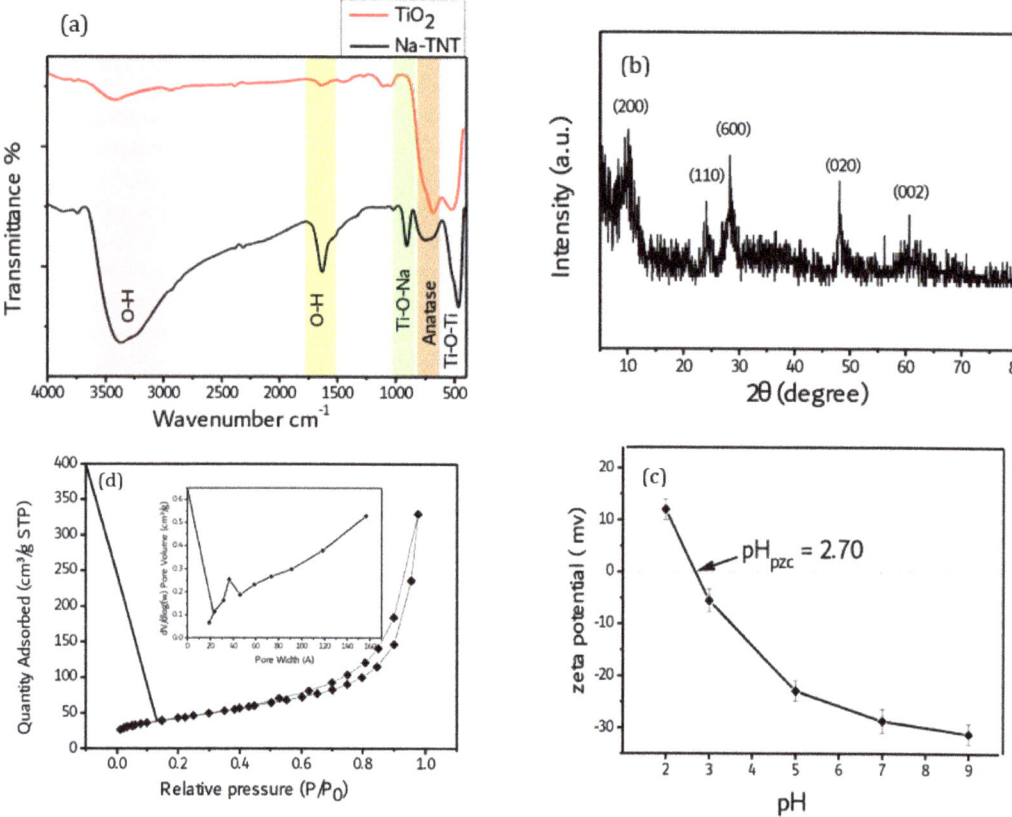

Figure 2. FT-IR Spectra (**a**), XRD pattern (**b**), nitrogen adsorption/desorption isotherm with inset pore size distribution curve (**c**) and Zeta potential (**d**) all for Na-TNT.

Table 1. Textural parameters of Na-TNT.

S_{BET} (m$^2 \cdot$g^{-1})	Average Pore Size (nm)	Total Pore Volume (cm^3/g)
154.85	5.791	0.21732

According to the zeta potential results of several previous studies, the TiO$_2$ surface is positively charged in the acidic medium and negatively charged in and near an alkaline medium with an isoelectric pH (pH$_{PZC}$). The zeta potential of Na-TNT as a function of pH was measured at room temperature and the results are indicated in Figure 2d. The results indicate that the synthesized material is positively charged in the low pH medium (pH = 2) [39]. At a low pH solution (pH = 2), a high concentration of H$^+$ leads to a protonation reaction of hydroxyl groups on the surface of the material, giving rise to positively charged particles at this pH, while at pH 3–9, Na-TNT is negatively charged as a result of a deprotonation reaction at this pH. Chemical reactions that occur on the surface of the particles are described in Equations (2) and (3).

The isoelectric pH (pH$_{PZC}$) value of Na-TNT is 2.7, implying particles of a neutral surface at this pH. Overall, the zeta potential results revealed the formation of a dominant-negative charge on the surface of Na-TNT particles at the pH range from 3 to 9.

$$-Ti–OH + H^+ \rightarrow -Ti–OH_2^+ \quad \text{(protonation reaction)} \qquad (2)$$

$$-Ti-OH + OH^- \rightarrow -Ti-O^- + H_2O \quad \text{(deprotonation reaction)} \tag{3}$$

3.2. Antimicrobial Investigations

Anti-Bacterial Assay

In terms of comparative efficacy and bone penetration, investigations on animals have shed light on the management of bone infections. The absence of debridement in the animals, the large initial inoculum, and the lack of experience with recurring or persistent infection are limitations of these studies. Similarly, experimental models do not permit long-term follow-up. Invariably, *S. aureus* is chosen as the infecting organism to research anti-Gram-positive drugs, which is representative of many but not all patient infections; hence, the results cannot be immediately applicable to streptococcal infections. The relevance of peak bone concentrations in relation to the MIC for the isolate is not well understood, and this does not necessarily match with the clinical outcome in animal investigations. In spite of these restrictions, useful data about antibiotic bone and serum concentrations, time to sterilization, and percentage cure have been published. There will be a discussion of studies on the most frequently used antibiotics for bone and joint infections.

The MIC and MBC of the examined NaTNT against different bacterial isolates are depicted in Figure 3. The figure reveals that the MIC value of the tested NaTNT varied significantly from one species to the next. Additionally, the recorded values of MBC and MIC are comparable for *L. monocytogenes*, indicating its bactericidal activity; however, they were significantly different for *S. aureus*, *St. Pyogens*, and the tested Gram-negative species. The maximum MIC value was slightly above 250 µg/mL and was recorded for *E. coli*, followed by *B. subtilis* and *H. influenza*, while the minimum MIC value was approximately 15 µg/mL for *Staphylococcus aureus* and *St. pneumoniae*. Therefore, *Staphylococcus aureus*, *Streptococcus pneumoniae*, and *Listeria monocytogenes* had better values for MIC than *E. coli*, *B. subtilis*, and *H. influenza*. Similarly, for MBC, *E. coli* also had the highest MBC value, followed by *B. subtilis* and *H. influenza*, while *Staphylococcus aureus* and *Streptococcus pneumoniae* had the lowest MBC values followed by *L. monocytogenes*, which shows the bactericidal action of NaTNT, as shown in Figure 3.

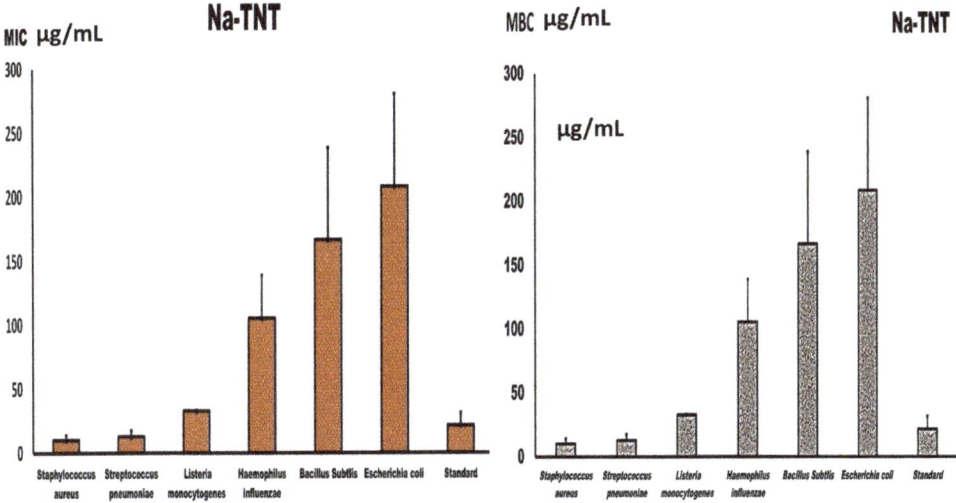

Figure 3. Presents the MIC and MBC values of NaTNT against both Gram-positive bacteria and Gram-negative bacteria (Mean ± SE). The best obtained results as shown by the MIC and MBC was achieved by Na TNT against *S. aureus*, *St. pyogens*, and *L. monocytogenes*.

Plates containing several strains of bacteria, including Gram-positive *St. pneumonia* (ATCC 49619), *S. aureus* (ATCC 25913), *Listeria monocytogenes* (ATCC 19115), and Gram-negative *E. coli* (ATCC 25922), *Haemophillus influenza* (ATCC 49766), and Bacillus subtilis (ATCC 35021). In addition, the figure illustrates the inhibition zone of each strain at different NaTNT doses. The inhibition zone was determined by the Agar diffusion technique in millimeters. Overall, the measured diameters of different species were distinct. As such, Figure 4 is a bar graph depicting the computed mean of the inhibition zone (mm) at various concentrations of NaTNT (1000, 500, 250, and 125 µg/mL) vs. the distinct types of bacteria stated before on the X-axis. Overall, the effect of NaTNT on the examined strains was inconsistent. Regarding Gram-positive bacteria, *S. aureus*, *Bacillus subtilis*, and Staphylococcus had the highest response rates, while *L. monocytogenes* had the lowest. Second, the reaction of Gram-negative H. influenza was greater than that of *E. coil*. In addition, the picture illustrates that the inhibition zone was precisely proportional to the NaTNT concentration in all tested species. *S. aureus* had the largest inhibitory zone, measuring roughly 28.5 mm, while *L. monocytogenes* exhibited the smallest, measuring around 26 mm. Notably, the tested NaTNT was compared to doxycycline for both Gram-negative and Gram-positive organisms (24 mm), and the results revealed that the effect of NaTNT and the compared standard drug was hardly the same in both Gram-negative and positive organisms, with NaTNT being more effective against *Bacillus subtilis*. From this perspective, the researched NaTNT could serve as an effective alternative to traditional antibiotics in combating bacterial resistance.

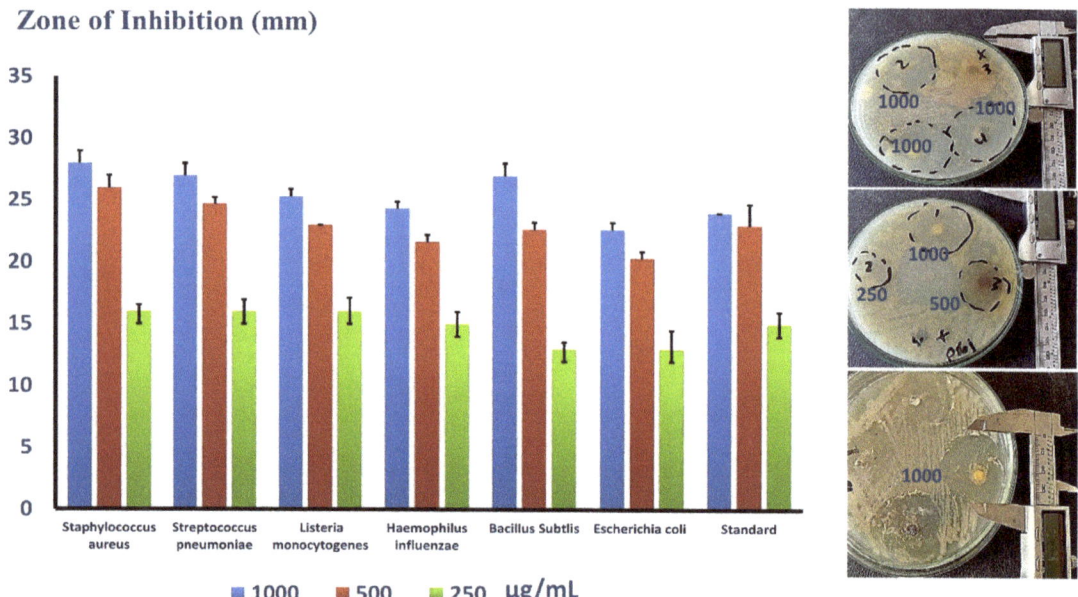

Figure 4. Illustrates the calculated mean of the inhibition zone (mm) at different concentrations of NaTNT versus diverse species of bacteria, and the mean of the inhibition zone against standard antibiotics (Doxycycline for both Gram-negative and Gram-positive) (Mean ± SE). Representative clear zone of inhibition appeared in the agar plates. "1–4": the tested different concentrations used for NaTNT as a key on the plates which meet (1000, 500 & 250 µg/mL).

Regarding the fungal broth micro dilution assay for NaTNT, a number of studies have explored the interaction of nanomaterials with bacteria, but few have examined their impact on fungi. This may be related to the comparative simplicity of bacterial and fungal systems [40].

The Mucor strain is one of the most severely affected fungi by NaTNT, according to this study's antifungal examination of NaTNT. Comparable to other invasive fungal illnesses, Mucor contagious species cause immunosuppression (especially delayed and excessive neutropenia, a serious hematological disease with or without stem cell transplantation, and the delayed use of corticosteroids) that predisposes to Mucormycosis [41]. Inadequately treated diabetes mellitus with or without diabetic ketoacidosis, iron overload, and medication with the iron chelator deferoxamine are additional risk factors [42]. Mucormycosis' most prevalent mode of transmission is the inhalation of fungal spores, manifesting as aspiratory or rhino-orbito-cerebral forms. Diseases caused by Mucorales spp. have been monitored for expansion following significant injuries, including burns [43], induced by direct spore inoculation into the tissue. In certain instances, infections can arise without other risk factors. In rare instances, spores infiltrated the tissue through tiny injuries like insect bites or animal scratches [44]. Mucormycosis of the gastrointestinal tract has also been described, particularly from swallowed spores [45]. A significant characteristic shared by all varieties of mucormycosis is the invasion of blood vessels and consequent thrombosis and necrosis of tissue. Angio-invasion also explains the often seen spread of infection in Mucormycosis [46]. Mucormycosis is distinguished from other forms of illnesses, such as conspicuous aspergillosis, by its unique histological alterations, its rapidly dynamic character, and the widespread tissue rot that often accompanies it. In addition, diabetes, press overload, and deferoxamine medication are unique risk factors for Mucormycosis. Due to the threat posed by this fungus, it is essential to seek innovative antifungal substances that may cure or prevent this sort of severe fungal infection.

The MICs for *A. niger* and *Fumigates*, other than *C. albicans*, were identical to the MFCs, confirming the fungicidal action of NaTNT, as shown in Figure 5, but were somewhat higher for the other examined isolates. The nanomaterial NaTNT proved efficient against all fungal species, particularly Mucor and Penicillium strains (20 and 15 µg/mL, respectively). In higher doses, they exhibited antifungal action against additional species, such as Candida (66 µg/mL) and *A. niger* (125 µg/mL). As shown in Figure 5, MFC for NaTNT had a good antifungal efficacy against Penicillium and Mucor (27 and 31 µg/mL, respectively). Other examined isolates were likewise impacted by NaTNT, but at greater doses.

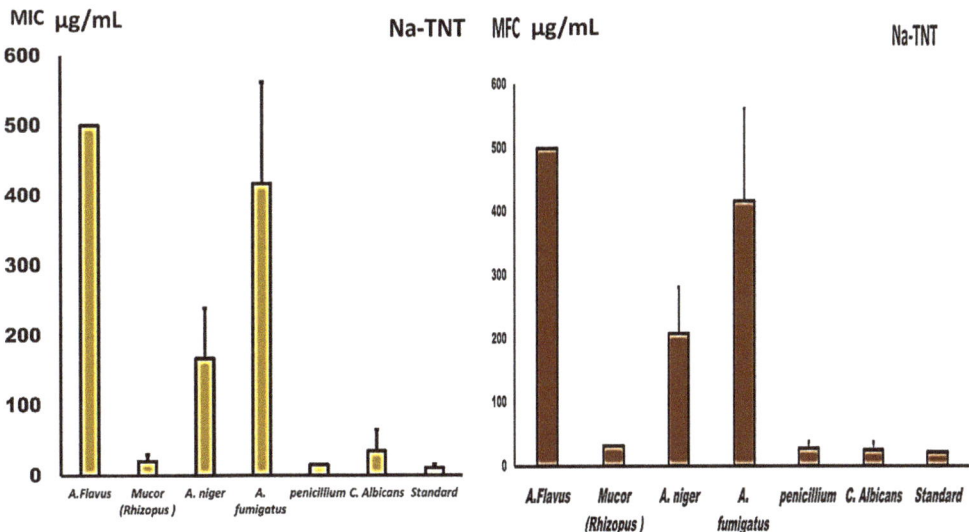

Figure 5. Presents the MIC and MFC values (µg/mL) of NaTNT against both different fungal isolates (Mean ± SE). The best obtained results for NA TNT were obtained against Mucor and pencillium species while fumigatus and flavus needed higher concentrations.

To investigate the antifungal activity of the tested nanomaterial (mechanism of action of NaTNT as an antifungal agent), the experiment was conducted, repeated, and quantified using sorbitol. The MIC data were repeated on a different sorbitol medium to clarify the specific mechanism of action of the tested substances against various fungal strains, the lower values of effective MIC are an indication of the impact on the fungal cell wall. After evaluating the MIC in various mediums with more added sorbitol, the findings indicated that NaTNT was more active against Penicillium, Mucor, and Candida at concentrations of 10, 10, and 17 μg/mL, as opposed to the previously reported higher values in the current normal MIC (15.20 & 66 μg/mL, respectively). Figure 6. Sorbitol is an osmotic stabilizer used to stabilize the protoplasts of fungi. Specific fungal cell wall inhibitors have the property that their antifungal activities are nullified in sorbitol-containing media [47]. In the presence of fungal cell wall inhibitors, cells protected by sorbitol may proliferate, but growth would be impeded in the absence of sorbitol. This impact is recognized by the decrease in MIC values reported in media containing sorbitol compared to media without sorbitol (standard medium) [48]. Osmotic destabilizing agents and disruption of the cell wall result in the reorganization of the cell wall, allowing for the survival of fungal cells [49]. The studied substances seemed to operate on the cell wall, altering its structure, limiting its manufacture, and inducing cell death, as well as impeding spore germination, proliferation, and cellular respiration.

In addition to lower effective fungicidal concentrations against Mucor and Penicillium, the investigated MFC findings utilizing various mediums with additional sorbitol concentrations revealed lower fungicidal concentrations against Mucor and Penicillium. As also shown in Figure 6, for Penicillium and Mucor, the MFC concentrations decreased to 16 and 16 μg/mL from 27 and 31 μg/mL for the other fungal strains.

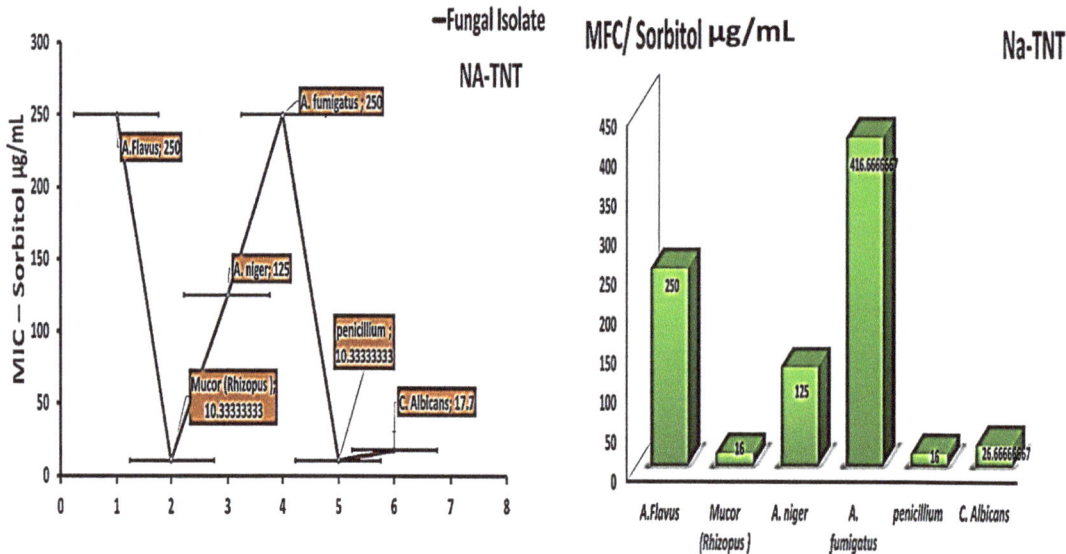

Figure 6. Presents the MIC and MFC values (μg/mL) of NaTNT on Sorbitol media against both different fungal isolates (Mean ± SE). The best obtained results for NA TNT were obtained on the Mucor and pencillieum species while fumigatus and flavus needed higher concentrations, MIC results with sorbitol decreased, indicating its action on the fungal cell wall.

The disc diffusion method is regarded as one of the most precise techniques for measuring antifungal or antibacterial activity. On SDA plates, inhibition zones against several fungal strains were tested, and numerous concentrations are shown in Figure 7.

They were evaluated at doses of 1000, 500, and 250 µg/mL; NaTNT demonstrated a good zone of inhibition against Mucor, Candida, and *A. niger* in comparison to the conventional antifungal for rapidly growing fungus (cyclohexamide). As shown in Figure 7, NaTNT showed promising antifungal effectiveness against the other fungal strains.

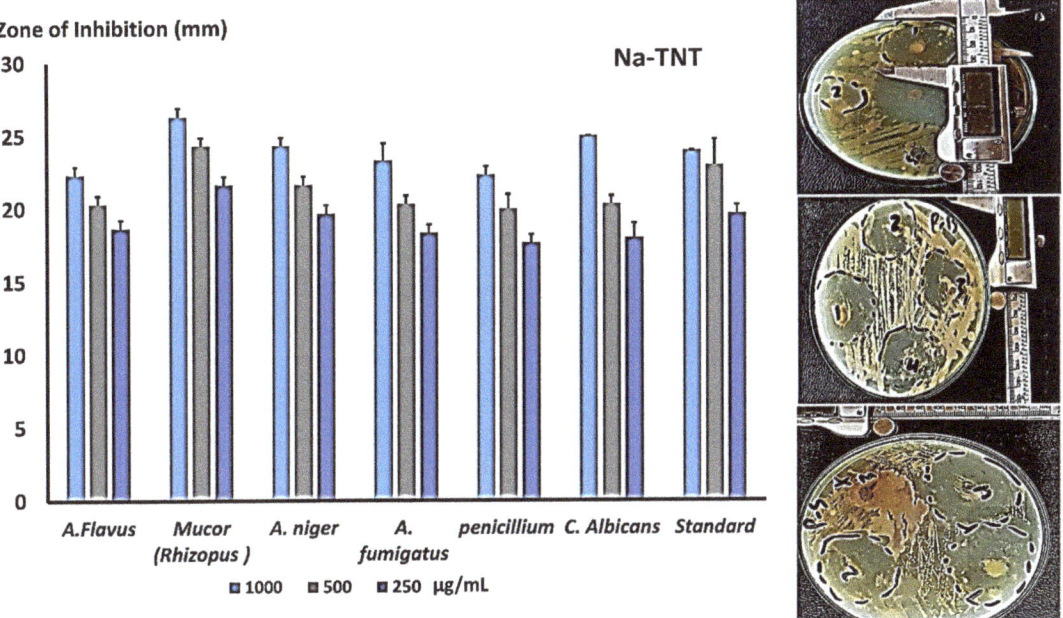

Figure 7. Illustrates the calculated mean of the inhibition zone (mm) at different concentrations of NaTNT versus diverse species of fungi, and the mean of the inhibition zone against standard antibiotics (cyclohexamide) (Mean ± SE). Representative clear zone of inhibition appeared in the agar plates. "1–4": different testes concentration 1 = 1000; 2 = 500 & 3–4 = 250.

Concerning antifungal activity (inhibition percentage), on the basis of the measurement of antifungal activity following the addition of materials to media, the percentage of fungal inhibition was calculated and shown in Figure 8. Mucor was inhibited at a rate of 98% by NaTNT, whereas candida was inhibited at a rate of 83%. The antifungal action of NaTNT is a result of its unique features, including its tiny size, wide surface area, and uniform dispersion.

After investigating the distinctive structure of NaTNT, we assessed it's in vitro and in vivo antibacterial activities. The in vitro antibacterial activity of NaTNT was evaluated using the conventional colony counting technique on two different microorganism strains, one bacterial (*S. aureus*) and the other a severe fungus isolate (*M. Rhizopus*). In this study, the (in vitro) antimicrobial activity of NaTNT displayed outstanding inhibitory activity against both *S. aureus* and *Mucor rhizopus* (in vitro study). Using rats with *S. aureus* and *Mucor rhizopus*-infected skin lesions as a model, we next examined the in vivo antibacterial effectiveness of NaTNT. Photographs of the wounds of rats in the control group and the NaTNT group at 3, 6, and 12 days were shown in Figure 9. Compared to the control groups, the NaTNT group demonstrated a significant decrease in wound area after 3 days. Comparably; after 12 days, wound area reduced to 5% in the NaTNT group, suggesting the high antibacterial action of NaTNT. In addition, the number of CFU in the NaTNT group after 12 days was significantly lower than in the control group with 0% inhibition percentages (Figure 9), further proving their antibacterial activity against multidrug-resistant bacteria in vivo. These findings indicated that NaTNT, a new antimicrobial agent, had excellent antibacterial and antifungal properties.

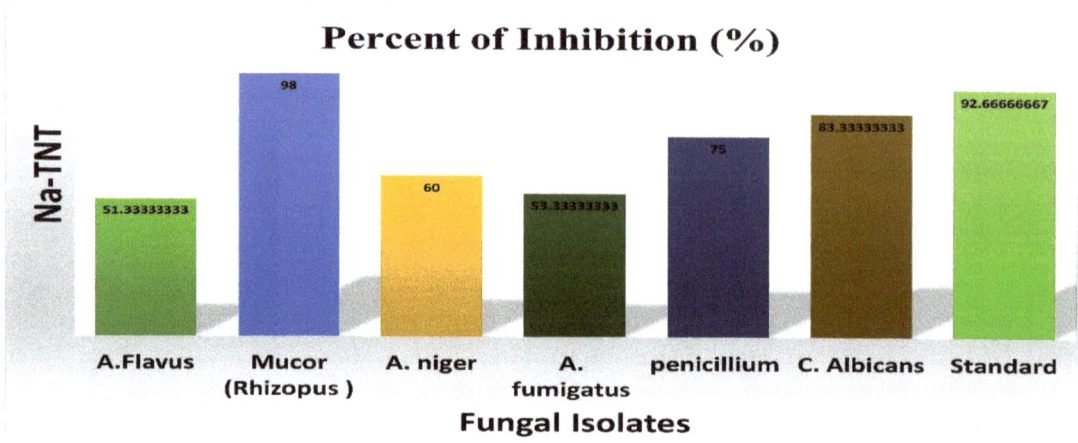

Figure 8. Percent of inhibition (%) of NaTNT in SDA media against multiple fungal strains. The best inhibitory percentage was against the Mucor type.

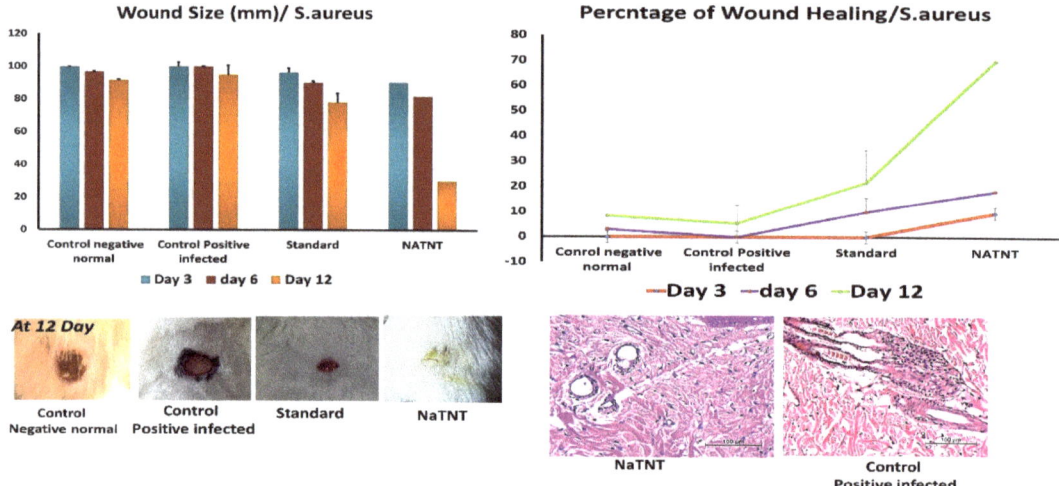

Figure 9. Size of the infected wound with *S. aureus* (10^8 CFU/mL), percentages of wound healing, and histopathological investigations (Mean ± SE). Percentages of wound healing were the best obtained for Na TNT at day 12 of the experiment when compared to the standard and control positive groups.

The wound pictures of rats in each group at 3, 6, and 12 days for NaTNT antifungal activity were shown in Figure 10. Compared to the normal control and infected untreated groups, the NaTNT group showed a significant decrease in wound area after 3 days. After 6 days, the wound area in the NaTNT group reduced below 20% (Figure 10), indicating more rapid healing. In addition, wound tissues from each group were collected at 0 and 12 days. At 12 days, the number of colony-forming units (CFU) in the NaTNT group was much lower than in the control and standard groups (Figure 11), revealing the remarkable antibacterial activity of NaTNT against in vivo multidrug-resistant bacteria. Additionally, we evaluated the antibacterial therapeutic effects of NaTNT by histological examination. After 12 days of therapy, rats in each group had their wounds extracted for H&E staining. On H&E staining, there are fewer infected tissues in the NaTNT group than in the control infected group (Figures 9 and 10). Moreover, throughout the wound's healing phase, these findings indicated that NaTNT exhibited remarkable antibacterial activity in vivo, indicating its considerable potential for treating illnesses caused by bacteria that are resistant to many drugs. NaTNT resulted in full wound healing with normal epithelial formation and vasculature, as determined by histopathological examinations of skin samples from the various treatments. In addition, the same healing activity was seen in a conventional group, albeit at a lesser efficiency than in the two experimental groups. Other untreated groups of rats had inadequate wound healing, including congestion and epithelial rupture (Figures 9 and 10).

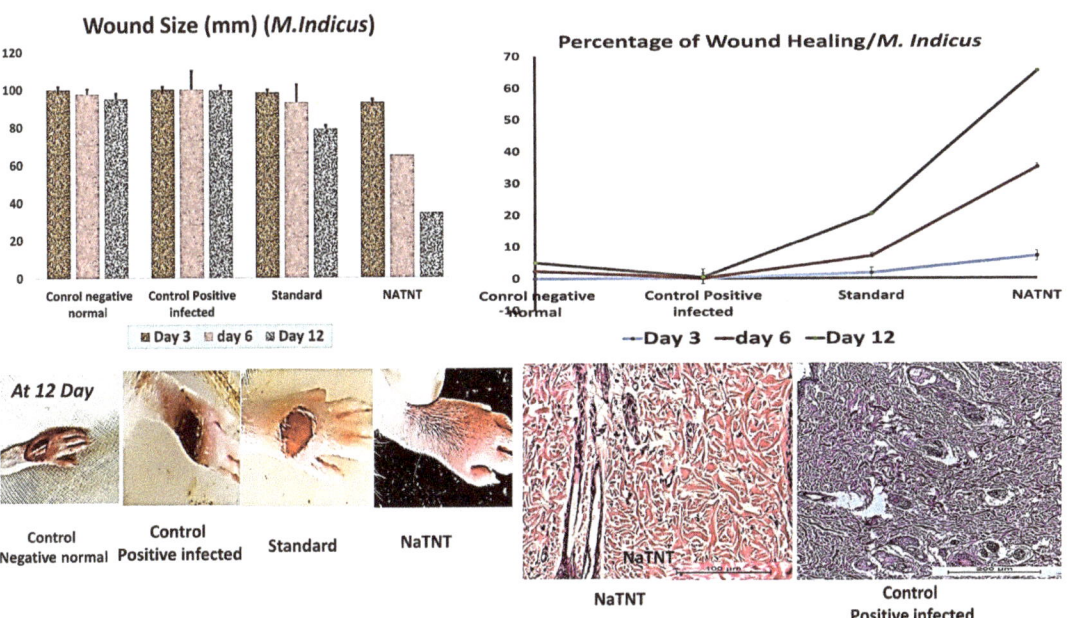

Figure 10. Size of the infected wound with *M. Rhizopus* (10^8 CFU/mL), percentages of wound healing, and histopathological investigations. (Mean ± SE). Higher healing percentages for the infected wound was achieved by Na TNT at the 12th day of treatment when compared to other groups.

During daily life, microorganisms such as bacteria, fungi, and viruses often infect humans. The use of antimicrobial drugs is essential for imparting sterility (e.g., hospital trays) and avoiding infection (e.g., wound dressing) along one path to bone infection. Antibacterial compounds, including a variety of natural and inorganic substrates, have been extensively researched [19]. TiO_2 has gained more attention than other antimicrobial chemicals due to its superior stability, environmental friendliness, safety, and extensive antibiosis [20]. The use of tiny TiO_2 particles in antibacterial compositions has been the topic of much investigation. Nonetheless, the powder TiO_2 catalyst has the problem of slurry separation post-application following photoreaction [20]. Consequently, surface-immobilized TiO_2 with a high specific surface area is more advantageous for antibacterial applications [21].

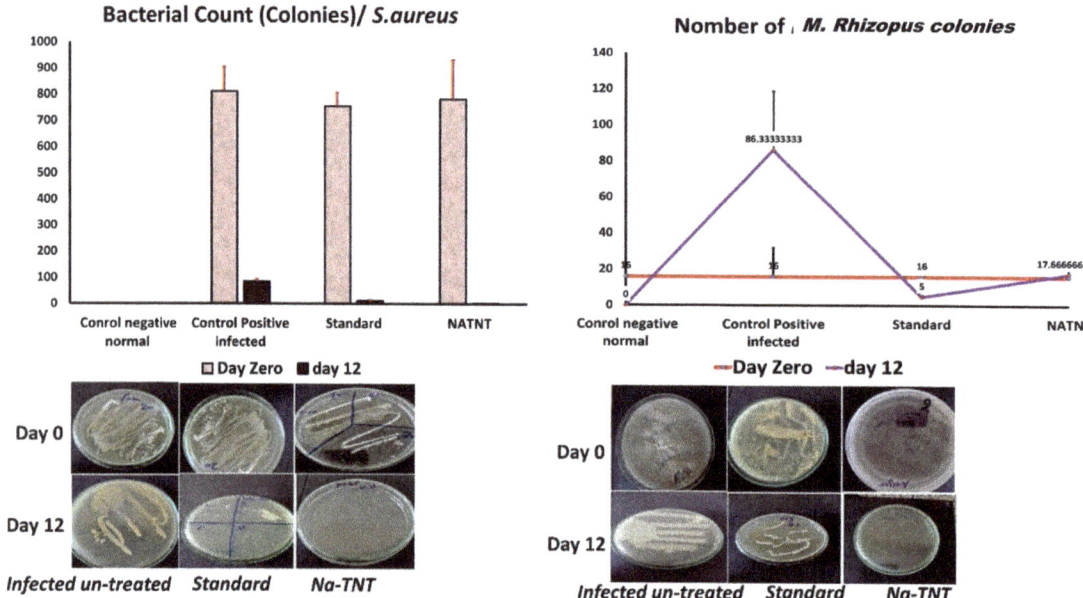

Figure 11. Bacterial and fungal colonies from the infected wound at Day Zero and on the last day of treatment (Day 12). (Mean ± SE). No colony growth appeared on the 12th day in the Na TNT groups. The highest bacterial colonies were obtained in the control positive infected non-treated group.

Wound healing and bone affections continue to be demanding clinical issues for which effective wound management and care are required. Moreover, successful wound and tissue regeneration remains a significant healthcare and biological problem in the twenty-first century. In addition to being a burden on the healthcare system's resources, infected or chronic wounds often result in death due to the inability to fulfil the targeted function and the rise in pain intensity [50]. Therefore, the discovery of procedures or medications that may aid in expediting the wound healing process and decreasing the time required for full wound recovery would reveal a treatment of major value. In addition to histopathological results, the percentage of healing activity and the size of wound closure over the course of 12 days were employed as a marker for wound healing activity. NaTNT demonstrated a quick and complete wound healing process in a shorter period of time than the standard alone and the untreated group after topical application. The effective healing properties of NaTNT may be linked to the nanomaterial's high wound-penetrating ability, which is a result of its enhanced surface area. Infections with bacteria are the primary cause of unhealed wounds [51]. Thus, the hunt for new materials that are effective against Gram-positive and Gram-negative bacteria is crucial. Staphylococcus is one of the most prevalent bacterial pathogens responsible for the vast majority of wound infections and is one of the leading causes of hospital-acquired infections. Bacteremia, sepsis, and/or toxic shock syndrome may result from the ineffectiveness of antimicrobial drugs or their low invading capability [52]. Histopathological studies revealed that the NaTNT exhibited rapid contraction, which is crucial for the quick healing of wounds, particularly in animals with loose skin (mice, rats). Re-epithelialization was a common step in the wound healing process and contact epithelial surface for all species. To the best of our knowledge, no prior trials on the effectiveness of NaTNT for wound infections have been published [53].

The benefits of topical treatment include the capacity to give a high local concentration with minimal dosages of the drug, especially in patients with limb ischemia, so as to avoid the first-pass action in the gastrointestinal tract and minimize the risk of systemic adverse effects. Very high local concentrations are achieved using topical preparations [54]. No clinical evidence supports the use of topical treatments for the prevention of infection recurrence in bone or wound or bone pathologies. All open wounds are colonized by bacteria, which impact the healing process in general. However, if the colonization progresses into a local infection, which then becomes systemic, the outcome might be fatal. Therefore, wound care includes not only cleaning, debridement, and therapy of the underlying etiology, but also steps to reduce the likelihood of colonized wounds becoming locally or even systemically infected in order to avoid osteomyelitis or arthritis [55]. Local antibiotic therapies have been shown to promote healing, however, treatment of the underlying etiology remains essential [56]. The number of bacteria present on a wound's surface is a local factor that might impede healing.

Despite the fact that the actual mechanism or interaction between metal inorganic framework structures and various infections has never been described, several demonstrations might be proposed. Consistent with earlier research, the inhibitory antibacterial activity of NaTNT may be attributed to the generation of reactive oxygen species. *M. Rhisopus* and *S. aureus* have their adhesion inhibited in nanotube films due to the high wettability and roughness of the nanoscale of the films. The antibacterial activity of NaTNT may have been due to the spontaneous release of free radicals such as ROS, inducing oxidative stress-mediated cell damage. Consider the possibility that cell membrane damage was generated by the electrochemical manner of interaction between the Na+ ions and the phosphate group in the lipid layers, hence weakening cell membrane integrity and generating membrane leakage. Similar to the suggested process, Gram-positive bacteria with numerous pores (Porins) may have let NaTNT enter into the cell, leading to membrane disruption, cell content release, and eventually cell death [57].

Similar to that of bacteria, the antifungal activity of NaTNT may be the result of the electrostatic interaction between the phosphate group in the cell membrane and Na+, the penetration of NaTNT into the cell, and the subsequent binding of Na+ with the thiol group of proteins, which results in their denaturation. In addition, NaTNT may have triggered cell death through ROS-mediated oxidative stress. These assumptions need close examination. On the other hand, NaTNT may play a substantial role, in particular, its antibacterial efficacy has been proven. In addition, it was shown that NaTNT caused permanent alterations in membrane characteristics (charge, intra and extracellular permeability, and physicochemical properties). Changes in cell surface hydrophobicity, charge, increased PI uptake, and K+ leakage with local rupture or hole formation in the cell membranes of Gram-negative and -positive bacteria were established as the mechanism for the antibacterial action of NaTNT [58].

These findings are consistent with earlier research about the precise mechanism of action for the antibacterial activity of NaTNT. The production of reactive oxygen species (ROS) such as the hydroxyl radical explains the antibacterial action of nanomaterials based on titanium. The antibacterial action of -OH radicals is linked to their capacity to destroy the cell wall. Thus, it stimulates its perforation, destruction of the cytoplasmic membrane, and cell lysis, resulting in the organism's total mineralization. Additionally, H_2O_2 may permeate the cell membrane, react with biological macromolecules, and serve as a precursor to -OH. Therefore, the production of ROS may account for the enhanced antibacterial action of the tested nanomaterials. Kuhn et al. [59] demonstrated that the superior antibacterial activity was due to the direct action of the ROS generated by the photocatalytic process, which caused peroxidation of the lipid components of the cell wall, including lipopolysaccharides, phospholipids, and lipoproteins of the outer membrane, as well as plasma membrane phospholipids [60].

Hydrophobicity plays a crucial role in the attachment of several bacterial species to their substrates, which is another factor for the antibacterial action of NaTNT [11,47]. According to studies, there is significant interaction between bacteria and hydrophobic surfaces, resulting in high cell attachment rates [61]. In a hospital setting, bacterial adherence to biotic and abiotic surfaces may be a cause of dangerous infections [61]. Therefore, it is desirable to produce super hydrophilic surfaces that reduce the contact between bacteria and substrates. In a physiological environment, super hydrophilic surfaces create a thin layer of water that may prevent the development of bacterial biofilms by inhibiting bacterial adhesion [62]. Ji et al. [18] found that increasing the hydrophilicity of titanium surfaces decreased *E. coli* adherence. Additionally, surface roughness might affect bacterial adhesion. According to studies, nanoscale roughness has anti-adhesive properties. This was found in research on both Gram-negative and Gram-positive bacteria. Thus, the roughness of the nanotube films may have also contributed to their ability to impede bacterial attachment [63].

In this research, sodium titanate nanotubes (NaTNT) had the highest antibacterial activity; few studies have indicated antimicrobial activity for titanate nanostructures. Titanate nanotubes show substantial antibacterial activity against Gram-positive bacteria and also Gram-negative bacteria, but at a lesser level based on the observed zone of inhibition as compared to Gram-positive bacteria, as reported by Kundu et al. in prior research [64]. Titanate nanotubes have a considerable antibacterial impact against *Bacillus subtilis*, which may be due to their interaction with the microorganism's cell wall composition. In contrast to the findings of Kundu et al., this investigation demonstrates that the activity of titanate nanostructures against Gram-positive bacteria is not necessarily superior to that against Gram-negative bacteria [64]. The interaction between nanostructures and the bacterial cell wall is mostly driven by the zeta potential. Regardless of the surface area and crystallite size, the surface charge will influence the electrostatic attraction or repulsion between the nanostructures' surface and the bacterial cell wall. This will determine the kind of interaction (bacteria/fungi—nanoparticles) and, therefore, the MIC for each strain of bacteria. Finally, NaTNT is the most effective agent for treating both Gram-positive and Gram-negative bacteria.

In conclusion, NaTNT structures enhance several research applications; the current work focused on one of these structures, namely NaTNT in terms of synthesis, characterization, and application. The study attempted to evaluate the antibacterial efficacy of NaTNT against types of serious disease-causing microorganisms such as Mucor and staph that damage bone and joints by entering infected wounds. In light of this, the research implies that NaTNT has the potential for wound protection against both bacterial and fungal infections.

Gram-positive and mucormycosis infections are responsible for the majority of bone and joint infections, particularly in immunocompromised individuals. Antibiotics penetrate effectively into the synovial fluid of infected joints, and after drainage, septic arthritis may be treated with two to three weeks of intravenous and oral medication. Nanomaterial penetration into bone is more varied and reliant on a number of variables. In addition to the removal of all contaminated tissue, osteomyelitis treatment needs weeks to months of antibiotic treatment. Traditionally, the whole course of parenteral antibiotics has been recommended to attain adequate bone concentrations. The ultimate choice of antibiotic, usage of oral treatment, and course length are determined by microbiological, surgical, and patient considerations, and should be reviewed with the physician and medical microbiology for each individual patient. The prevalence of more resistant infecting organisms is worrisome, both in terms of patient care and broader implications for cross-infection. Although the first studies are promising, the effectiveness of the 'new' antibiotics in treating orthopaedic infections has yet to be shown.

4. Future Study

In the future, the most effective and commonly used coating material for immunecompromised patients with COVID-19 or other immunosuppressive diseases, as well as diabetic patients, will be nano-synthesized NaTNT. This material has been proven to have antifungal and antibacterial properties against life-threatening mucormycoses and other bacterial or fungal infections that can cause bone damage.

Author Contributions: Conceptualization, A.H.A., W.H.H., A.B., A.F. and F.I.A.E.-E.; methodology, R.M.S., A.E.A., A.A., R.M. and F.I.A.E.-E.; software, O.A., S.L., A.H.E.H. and W.H.H.; validation, S.L., M.M.G., A.H.E.H. and R.M.; formal analysis, R.M., A.F., A.H.A. and S.L.; investigation, O.A., S.L., A.H.E.H., A.B., A.F. and M.M.G.; resources, R.M., A.F. and A.H.A.; data curation, O.A., S.L., A.H.E.H. and M.M.G.; writing—original draft preparation, R.M.S., A.E.A. and A.A.; writing—review and editing, all authors; visualization, all authors; supervision, A.B., A.F. and A.H.E.H.; project administration, A.H.A. and A.B. funding acquisition, A.H.A., A.B., M.M.G., A.H.E.H. and S.L. All authors have read and agreed to the published version of the manuscript.

Funding: The King Salman Center for Disability Research has supported this work through the KSRG-2022-067 Research Group.

Institutional Review Board Statement: All animal handling and treatment at this study was approved via the IACUC; Institutional of Animal Care and Use Committee of Beni-Suef University, faculty of Veterinary Medicine ((022-387)-03-2023).

Data Availability Statement: All data are provided in the manuscript.

Acknowledgments: The authors express their appreciation to the King Salman Center for Disability Research for funding this work through the KSRG-2022-067 Research Group.

Conflicts of Interest: The authors declare no conflict of interest.

References

1. Calhoun, J.H.; Manring, M.; Shirtliff, M. Osteomyelitis of the long bones. In *Seminars in Plastic Surgery*; Thieme Medical Publishers: New York, NY, USA, 2009; Volume 23, pp. 59–72.
2. Sax, H.; Lew, D. Osteomyelitis. *Curr. Infect. Dis. Rep.* **1999**, *1*, 261–266. [CrossRef] [PubMed]
3. Waldvogel, F.; Vasey, H. Osteomyelitis: The past decade. *N. Engl. J. Med.* **1980**, *303*, 360–370. [CrossRef] [PubMed]
4. Goldenberg, D.L. Septic arthritis. *Lancet* **1998**, *351*, 197–202. [CrossRef] [PubMed]
5. Homed, K.A.; Tam, J.Y.; Prober, C.G. Pharmacokinetic optimisation of the treatment of septic arthritis. *Clin. Pharmacokinet.* **1996**, *31*, 156–163. [CrossRef]
6. Oliker, R.; Cunha, B.A. Streptococcus pneumoniae septic arthritis and osteomyelitis in an HIV-seropositive patient. *Heart Lung* **1999**, *28*, 74–76. [CrossRef]
7. Darley, E.S.; MacGowan, A.P. Antibiotic treatment of gram-positive bone and joint infections. *J. Antimicrob. Chemother.* **2004**, *53*, 928–935. [CrossRef]
8. Massarotti, E.; Dinerman, H. Septic arthritis due to Listeria monocytogenes: Report and review of the literature. *J. Rheumatol.* **1990**, *17*, 111–113.
9. Raff, M.J.; Melo, J.C. Anaerobic osteomyelitis. *Medicine* **1978**, *57*, 83. [CrossRef]
10. Goldstein, E.J. Bite wounds and infection. *Clin. Infect. Dis.* **1992**, *14*, 633–640. [CrossRef]
11. Taj-Aldeen, S.J.; Gamaletsou, M.N.; Rammaert, B.; Sipsas, N.V.; Zeller, V.; Roilides, E.; Kontoyiannis, D.P.; Henry, M.; Petraitis, V.; Moriyama, B.; et al. Bone and joint infections caused by mucormycetes: A challenging osteoarticular mycosis of the twenty-first century. *Med. Mycol.* **2017**, *55*, 691–704. [CrossRef]
12. Koehler, P.; Tacke, D.; Cornely, O.A. Aspergillosis of bones and joints–a review from 2002 until today. *Mycoses* **2014**, *57*, 323–335. [CrossRef] [PubMed]
13. Horsburgh, C.R., Jr.; Cannady, P.B., Jr.; Kirkpatrick, C.H. Treatment of fungal infections in the bones and joints with ketoconazole. *J. Infect. Dis.* **1983**, *147*, 1064–1069. [CrossRef] [PubMed]
14. Joshi, B.; Regmi, C.; Dhakal, D.; Gyawali, G.; Lee, S.W. Efficient inactivation of Staphylococcus aureus by silver and copper loaded photocatalytic titanate nanotubes. *Prog. Nat. Sci. Mater. Int.* **2018**, *28*, 15–23. [CrossRef]
15. Franco, B.M.R.; Souza, A.P.O.; Molento, C.F.M. Welfare-friendly Products: Availability, labeling and opinion of retailers in Curitiba, Southern Brazil. *Rev. Econ. Sociol. Rural* **2018**, *56*, 9–18. [CrossRef]
16. Xin, W.; Zhu, D.; Liu, G.; Hua, Y.; Zhou, W. Synthesis and characterization of Mn-C-codoped TiO_2 nanoparticles and photocatalytic degradation of methyl orange dye under sunlight irradiation. *Int. J. Photoenergy* **2012**, *2012*, 767905. [CrossRef]
17. Park, S.; Park, J.; Heo, J.; Lee, S.-E.; Shin, J.-W.; Chang, M.; Hong, J. Polysaccharide-based superhydrophilic coatings with antibacterial and anti-inflammatory agent-delivering capabilities for ophthalmic applications. *J. Ind. Eng. Chem.* **2018**, *68*, 229–237. [CrossRef]
18. Ji, X.-W.; Liu, P.-T.; Tang, J.-C.; Wan, C.-J.; Yang, Y.; Zhao, Z.-L.; Zhao, D.-P. Different antibacterial mechanisms of titania nanotube arrays at various growth phases of E. coli. *Trans. Nonferrous Met. Soc. China* **2021**, *31*, 3821–3830. [CrossRef]
19. Yoshinari, M.; Oda, Y.; Kato, T.; Okuda, K. Influence of surface modifications to titanium on antibacterial activity in vitro. *Biomaterials* **2001**, *22*, 2043–2048. [CrossRef]
20. Liu, H.; Chen, Q.; Song, L.; Ye, R.; Lu, J.; Li, H. Ag-doped antibacterial porous materials with slow release of silver ions. *J. Non-Cryst. Solids* **2008**, *354*, 1314–1317. [CrossRef]

21. Murakami, Y.; Matsumoto, T.; Takasu, Y. Salt Catalysts Containing Basic Anions and Acidic Cations for the Sol–Gel Process of Titanium Alkoxide: Controlling the Kinetics and Dimensionality of the Resultant Titanium Oxide. *J. Phys. Chem.* **1999**, *103*, 1836–1840. [CrossRef]
22. Saleh, R.; Zaki, A.H.; El-Ela, F.I.A.; Farghali, A.A.; Taha, M.; Mahmoud, R. Consecutive removal of heavy metals and dyes by a fascinating method using titanate nanotubes. *J. Environ. Chem. Eng.* **2021**, *9*, 104726. [CrossRef]
23. Hadacek, F.; Greger, H. Testing of antifungal natural products: Methodologies, comparability of results and assay choice. *Phytochem. Anal. Int. J. Plant Chem. Biochem. Tech.* **2000**, *11*, 137–147. [CrossRef]
24. Morales, G.; Paredes, A.; Sierra, P.; Loyola, L.A. Antimicrobial activity of three Baccharis species used in the traditional medicine of Northern Chile. *Molecules* **2008**, *13*, 790–794. [CrossRef]
25. Leite, M.C.A.; Bezerra, A.P.d.B.; Sousa, J.P.; Guerra, F.Q.S.; Lima, E.O. Evaluation of antifungal activity and mechanism of action of citral against *Candida albicans*. *Evid.-Based Complement. Altern. Med.* **2014**, *2014*, 378280. [CrossRef]
26. Espinel-Ingroff, A.; Chaturvedi, V.; Fothergill, A.; Rinaldi, M. Optimal testing conditions for determining MICs and minimum fungicidal concentrations of new and established antifungal agents for uncommon molds: NCCLS collaborative study. *J. Clin. Microbiol.* **2002**, *40*, 3776–3781. [CrossRef] [PubMed]
27. Alexander, B.D. *Reference Method for Broth Dilution Antifungal Susceptibility Testing of Filamentous Fungi*; Clinical and Laboratory Standards Institute: Wayne, PA, USA, 2017.
28. De Souza, G.C.; Haas, A.; Von Poser, G.; Schapoval, E.; Elisabetsky, E. Ethnopharmacological studies of antimicrobial remedies in the south of Brazil. *J. Ethnopharmacol.* **2004**, *90*, 135–143. [CrossRef] [PubMed]
29. Kalemba, D.; Kunicka, A. Antibacterial and antifungal properties of essential oils. *Curr. Med. Chem.* **2003**, *10*, 813–829. [CrossRef] [PubMed]
30. Jeff-Agboola, Y.; Onifade, A.; Akinyele, B.; Osho, I. In vitro antifungal activities of essential oil from Nigerian medicinal plants against toxigenic *Aspergillus flavus*. *J. Med. Plants Res.* **2012**, *6*, 4048–4056. [CrossRef]
31. Walker, H.L.; Mason, A.D., Jr. A standard animal burn. *J. Trauma Acute Care Surg.* **1968**, *8*, 1049–1051. [CrossRef]
32. Sasidharan, S.; Nilawatyi, R.; Xavier, R.; Latha, L.Y.; Amala, R. Wound Healing Potential of Elaeis guineensis JacqLeaves in an Infected Albino Rat Model. *Molecules* **2010**, *15*, 3186–3199. [CrossRef]
33. Snedecor, G.; Cochran, W. *Statistical Methods*, 7th ed.; The IOWA State Univ Press: Ames, IA, USA, 1982; Volume 507, pp. 53–57.
34. Hua, S.; Yu, X.; Li, F.; Duan, J.; Ji, H.; Liu, W. Hydrogen titanate nanosheets with both adsorptive and photocatalytic properties used for organic dyes removal. *Colloids Surf. Physicochem. Eng. Asp.* **2017**, *516*, 211–218. [CrossRef]
35. Wu, C.; Cai, Y.; Xu, L.; Xie, J.; Liu, Z.; Yang, S.; Wang, S. Macroscopic and spectral exploration on the removal performance of pristine and phytic acid-decorated titanate nanotubes towards Eu (III). *J. Mol. Liq.* **2018**, *258*, 66–73. [CrossRef]
36. Subramaniam, M.; Goh, P.; Abdullah, N.; Lau, W.; Ng, B.; Ismail, A. Adsorption and photocatalytic degradation of methylene blue using high surface area titanate nanotubes (TNT) synthesized via hydrothermal method. *J. Nanopart. Res.* **2017**, *19*, 220. [CrossRef]
37. Martínez-Klimov, M.E.; Hernández-Hipólito, P.; Martínez-García, M.; Klimova, T.E. Pd catalysts supported on hydrogen titanate nanotubes for Suzuki-Miyaura cross-coupling reactions. *Catal. Today* **2018**, *305*, 58–64. [CrossRef]
38. Hernández-Hipólito, P.; Juárez-Flores, N.; Martínez-Klimova, E.; Gómez-Cortés, A.; Bokhimi, X.; Escobar-Alarcón, L.; Klimova, T.E. Novel heterogeneous basic catalysts for biodiesel production: Sodium titanate nanotubes doped with potassium. *Catal. Today* **2015**, *250*, 187–196. [CrossRef]
39. Sheng, G.; Ye, L.; Li, Y.; Dong, H.; Li, H.; Gao, X.; Huang, Y. EXAFS study of the interfacial interaction of nickel (II) on titanate nanotubes: Role of contact time, pH and humic substances. *Chem. Eng. J.* **2014**, *248*, 71–78. [CrossRef]
40. Aguilar-Méndez, M.A.; Martín-Martínez, S.; Ortega-Arroyo, L.; Cobián-Portillo, G.; Sánchez-Espíndola, E. Synthesis and characterization of silver nanoparticles: Effect on phytopathogen Colletotrichum gloesporioides. *J. Nanopart. Res.* **2011**, *13*, 2525–2532. [CrossRef]
41. Petrikkos, G.; Skiada, A.; Lortholary, O.; Roilides, E.; Walsh, T.J.; Kontoyiannis, D.P. Epidemiology and clinical manifestations of mucormycosis. *Clin. Infect. Dis.* **2012**, *54*, S23–S34. [CrossRef] [PubMed]
42. Binder, U.; Maurer, E.; Lass-Flörl, C. Mucormycosis–from the pathogens to the disease. *Clin. Microbiol. Infect.* **2014**, *20*, 60–66. [CrossRef]
43. Kronen, R.; Liang, S.Y.; Bochicchio, G.; Bochicchio, K.; Powderly, W.G.; Spec, A. Invasive fungal infections secondary to traumatic injury. *Int. J. Infect. Dis.* **2017**, *62*, 102–111. [CrossRef]
44. Arnáiz-García, M.; Alonso-Peña, D.; del Carmen González-Vela, M.; García-Palomo, J.; Sanz-Giménez-Rico, J.; Arnáiz-García, A. Cutaneous mucormycosis: Report of five cases and review of the literature. *J. Plast. Reconstr. Aesthet. Surg.* **2009**, *62*, e434–e441. [CrossRef]
45. Kaur, H.; Ghosh, A.; Rudramurthy, S.M.; Chakrabarti, A. Gastrointestinal mucormycosis in apparently immunocompetent hosts—A review. *Mycoses* **2018**, *61*, 898–908. [CrossRef]
46. Revisión Bibliográfica Narrativa: Mortalidad y Complicaciones de Mucormicosis en Zonas Rino-Orbital y Rinocerebral en Pacientes Inmunocomprometidos Con Leucemia. 2021. Available online: http://repositorio.puce.edu.ec:80/handle/22000/18876 (accessed on 1 February 2023).
47. Frost, D.J.; Brandt, K.D.; Cugier, D.; Goldman, R. A whole-cell *Candida albicans* assay for the detection of inhibitors towards fungal cell wall synthesis and assembly. *J. Antibiot.* **1995**, *48*, 306–310. [CrossRef] [PubMed]

48. Svetaz, L.; Agüero, M.B.; Alvarez, S.; Luna, L.; Feresin, G.; Derita, M.; Zacchino, S. Antifungal activity of Zuccagnia punctata Cav.: Evidence for the mechanism of action. *Planta Med.* **2007**, *73*, 1074–1080. [CrossRef] [PubMed]
49. Reference Method for Broth Dilution Antifungal Susceptibility Testing of Yeasts, Approved Standard. CLSI Document M27-A2. 2002. Available online: https://cir.nii.ac.jp/crid/1570854176048718848 (accessed on 1 February 2023).
50. Cortivo, R.; Vindigni, V.; Iacobellis, L.; Abatangelo, G.; Pinton, P.; Zavan, B. Nanoscale particle therapies for wounds and ulcers. *Nanomedicine* **2010**, *5*, 641–656. [CrossRef]
51. Xu, R.; Luo, G.; Xia, H.; He, W.; Zhao, J.; Liu, B.; Tan, J.; Zhou, J.; Liu, D.; Wang, Y.; et al. Novel bilayer wound dressing composed of silicone rubber with particular micropores enhanced wound re-epithelialization and contraction. *Biomaterials* **2015**, *40*, 1–11. [CrossRef] [PubMed]
52. Deepachitra, R.; Lakshmi, R.P.; Sivaranjani, K.; Chandra, J.H.; Sastry, T.P. Nanoparticles embedded biomaterials in wound treatment: A review. *J. Chem. Pharm. Sci.* **2015**, *8*, 324–329.
53. Parham, S.; Wicaksono, D.H.; Bagherbaigi, S.; Lee, S.L.; Nur, H. Antimicrobial treatment of different metal oxide nanoparticles: A critical review. *J. Chin. Chem. Soc.* **2016**, *63*, 385–393. [CrossRef]
54. Abbas, M.; Uçkay, I.; Lipsky, B.A. In diabetic foot infections antibiotics are to treat infection, not to heal wounds. *Expert Opin. Pharmacother.* **2015**, *16*, 821–832. [CrossRef] [PubMed]
55. Robson, M.C. Wound infection: A failure of wound healing caused by an imbalance of bacteria. *Surg. Clin. N. Am.* **1997**, *77*, 637–650. [CrossRef] [PubMed]
56. Singh, A.; Halder, S.; Chumber, S.; Misra, M.C.; Sharma, L.K.; Srivastava, A.; Menon, G.R. Meta-analysis of randomized controlled trials on hydrocolloid occlusive dressing versus conventional gauze dressing in the healing of chronic wounds. *Asian J. Surg.* **2004**, *27*, 326–332. [CrossRef] [PubMed]
57. Madeira MD, P.; Gusmão, S.B.; de Lima, I.S.; Lemos, G.M.; Barreto, H.M.; Abi-chacra, É.D.A.; Osajima, J.A. Deposition of sodium titanate nanotubes: Superhydrophilic surface and antibacterial approach. *J. Mater. Res. Technol.* **2022**, *19*, 2104–2114. [CrossRef]
58. Mohamed, H.; Zaki, A.; El-Ela, F.I.A.; El-dek, S. Effect of hydrothermal time and acid-washing on the antibacterial activity of Sodium titanate nanotubes. In *IOP Conference Series: Materials Science and Engineering*; IOP Publishing: Bristol, UK, 2021; Volume 1046, p. 012025.
59. dos Reis, C.M.; da Rosa, B.V.; da Rosa, G.P.; Carmo, G.D.; Morandini, L.M.B.; Ugalde, G.A.; Kuhn, K.R.; Morel, A.F.; Jahn, S.L.; Kuhn, R.C. Antifungal and antibacterial activity of extracts produced from Diaporthe schini. *J. Biotechnol.* **2019**, *294*, 30–37. [CrossRef]
60. Hafshejani, T.M.; Zamanian, A.; Venugopal, J.R.; Rezvani, Z.; Sefat, F.; Saeb, M.R.; Vahabi, H.; Zarintaj, P.; Mozafari, M. Antibacterial glass-ionomer cement restorative materials: A critical review on the current status of extended release formulations. *J. Control. Release* **2017**, *262*, 317–328. [CrossRef] [PubMed]
61. Maikranz, E.; Spengler, C.; Thewes, N.; Thewes, A.; Nolle, F.; Jung, P.; Bischoff, M.; Santen, L.; Jacobs, K. Different binding mechanisms of Staphylococcus aureus to hydrophobic and hydrophilic surfaces. *Nanoscale* **2020**, *12*, 19267–19275. [CrossRef]
62. Hwangbo, S.; Jeong, H.; Heo, J.; Lin, X.; Kim, Y.; Chang, M.; Hong, J. Antibacterial nanofilm coatings based on organosilicate and nanoparticles. *React. Funct. Polym.* **2016**, *102*, 27–32. [CrossRef]
63. Yang, K.; Shi, J.; Wang, L.; Chen, Y.; Liang, C.; Yang, L.; Wang, L.-N. Bacterial anti-adhesion surface design: Surface patterning, roughness and wettability: A review. *J. Mater. Sci. Technol.* **2022**, *99*, 82–100. [CrossRef]
64. Kundu, S.; Sain, S.; Choudhury, P.; Sarkar, S.; Das, P.K.; Pradhan, S.K. Microstructure characterization of biocompatible heterojunction hydrogen titanate-Ag_2O nanocomposites for superior visible light photocatalysis and antibacterial activity. *Mater. Sci. Eng.* **2019**, *99*, 374–386. [CrossRef]

Disclaimer/Publisher's Note: The statements, opinions and data contained in all publications are solely those of the individual author(s) and contributor(s) and not of MDPI and/or the editor(s). MDPI and/or the editor(s) disclaim responsibility for any injury to people or property resulting from any ideas, methods, instructions or products referred to in the content.

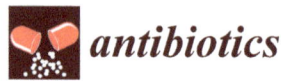

Article

New Ionic Liquid Microemulsion-Mediated Synthesis of Silver Nanoparticles for Skin Bacterial Infection Treatments

Fayez Althobaiti [1], Ola A. Abu Ali [2], Islam Kamal [3], Mohammad Y. Alfaifi [4], Ali A. Shati [4], Eman Fayad [1], Serag Eldin I. Elbehairi [3,5], Reda F. M. Elshaarawy [6,7,*] and W. Abd El-Fattah [8,9,*]

1. Department of Biotechnology, Faculty of Sciences, Taif University, P.O. Box 11099, Taif 21944, Saudi Arabia
2. Department of Chemistry, College of Science, Taif University, P.O. Box 11099, Taif 21944, Saudi Arabia
3. Department of Pharmaceutics, Faculty of Pharmacy, Port Said University, Port Said 42526, Egypt
4. Biology Department, Faculty of Science, King Khalid University, Abha 62529, Saudi Arabia
5. Cell Culture Lab, Egyptian Organization for Biological Products and Vaccines (VACSERA Holding Company), 51 Wezaret El-Zeraa St., Agouza, Giza 12654, Egypt
6. Department of Chemistry, Faculty of Science, Suez University, Suez 43533, Egypt
7. Institut für Anorganische Chemie und Strukturchemie, Heinrich-Heine Universität Düsseldorf, 40204 Düsseldorf, Germany
8. Chemistry Department, College of Science, IMSIU (Imam Mohammad Ibn Saud Islamic University), P.O. Box 5701, Riyadh 11432, Saudi Arabia
9. Department of Chemistry, Faculty of Science, Port Said University, Port Said 42526, Egypt
* Correspondence: reda.elshaarawy@suezuniv.edu.eg (R.F.M.E.); wabdulfatah@imamu.edu.sa (W.A.E.-F.); Tel.: +20-101-7377216 (R.F.M.E.)

Abstract: This work reports a new approach for the synthesis of extremely small monodispersed silver nanoparticles (AgNPs) (2.9–1.5) by reduction of silver nitrate in a new series of benzyl alkyl imidazolium ionic liquids (BAIILs)-based microemulsions (3a–f) as media and stabilizing agents. Interestingly, AgNPs isolated from the IILMEs bearing the bulkiest substituents (*tert*-butyl and *n*-butyl) (3f) displayed almost no nanoparticle agglomeration. In an in vitro antibacterial test against ESKAPE pathogens, all AgNPs-BAIILs had potent antibiotic activity, as reflected by antibacterial efficiency indices. Furthermore, when compared to other nanoparticles, these were the most effective in preventing biofilm formation by the tested bacterial strains. Moreover, the MTT assay was used to determine the cytotoxicity of novel AgNPs-BAIILs on healthy human skin fibroblast (HSF) cell lines. The MTT assay revealed that novel AgNPs-BAIILs showed no significant toxic effects on the healthy cells. Thus, the novel AgNPs-BAIILs microemulsions could be used as safe antibiotics for skin bacterial infection treatments. AgNPs isolated from BAIIL (3c) was found to be the most effective antibiotic of the nanoparticles examined.

Keywords: benzyl alkyl imidazolium ionic liquids; microemulsions; silver nanoparticles; antibacterial; skin bacterial infection treatments

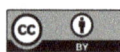

1. Introduction

The exponential increase in bacterial-induced pathogenic infection has created a serious threat to global human health. The ESKAPE pathogens (*Staphylococcus aureus* (SA), *Klebsiella pneumoniae* (KP), *Pseudomonas aeruginosa* (PA), *Enterococcus faecium* (EF), Acinetobacter baumannii (AB), and Enterobacter species) have been assigned as the most deadly bacteria by the Infectious Diseases Society of America (IDSA). Antimicrobial agents (AMAs) effectively protect humans from these potentially fatal pathogenic micro-organisms [1,2]. However, many bacterial strains acquired tolerance to antibiotics long before humans began mass-producing them to prevent and cure infectious illnesses [3]. Further, the emergence of antimicrobial-resistant microbes has sparked a worldwide crisis due to antibiotic overuse and the limited effectiveness of conventional antibiotic therapy. Consequently, research for novel antimicrobial agents is urgently required to address this issue.

Recently, nanomaterials (NMs) have attracted a lot of attention from scientists and found widespread usage in many biological applications [4–7]. Among the different nanomaterials, noble metal nanoparticles (NMNPs) have gained great attention in the development of a diversity of smart multifunctional NMs for biomedical applications, owing to their non-toxicity and excellent intrinsic properties [8]. Aside from being surface active, NMNPs can release bioactive metal ions into biological systems, resulting in the induction of multiple modes of bioactivity.

There has been extensive research into nanosystems for drug delivery because of its attractive biodegradability, biocompatibility, specificity/selectivity, and low toxicity. In addition to its useful properties including biocompatibility and durability, non-immunogenicity, a large surface area, a high drug loading capacity, and a minimal leakage of medications, they can also be employed to the targeted administration of pharmaceuticals [9]. Over the past two decades, the use of metal nanoparticles (MNPs) as nanocarriers has drastically evolved due to their numerous advantages and benefits. Their unique physical, chemical, and biological properties are in the forefront of these advantages. Additionally, their small size allows them to traverse through biological barriers and release drugs at a desired target site [10]. Moreover, MNPs possess high loading capacity, surface-area-to-volume ratio, and can be easily functionalized with a variety of ligands to modulate the drug release profile. Therefore, MNPs have been successfully used in a range of drug delivery systems, including transdermal, oral, and injectable delivery [11]. Despite the advantages, the use of MNPs as nanocarriers is still in its infancy due to several current challenges. For example, the toxicity of MNPs, the difficulty in controlling their size and shape, and poor biocompatibility are several factors that need to be addressed [10].

Despite several studies reporting on the biological and therapeutic applications of NMNPs, particularly AgNPs [12–14], there have been very few reports on the use of ionic liquid-supported AgNPs (PdNPs-ILs) in these disciplines. For instance, Dorjnamjin et al. reported the synthesis of uniform monodisperse crystalline Ag nanoparticles mediated by two different series of hydroxyl functionalized ionic liquids (HFILs) and hydroxyl functionalized cationic surfactants (HFCSs). AgNPs isolated from various ionic liquids exhibited promising in vitro antimicrobial activities against a range of Gram-positive and Gram-negative bacteria and fungi [15]. In addition, a room temperature ionic liquid (2-amino-1-dodecylpyridinium bromide) was used to prepare AgNPs (2–20 nm) with excellent antibacterial activity against *S. aureus, E. coli,* and *P. aeruginosa* [16]. AgNPs anchored in poly(ionic liquid) mesoporous nanocomposite (Ag-PIL) were recently synthesized by in situ reduction of AgNO$_3$ in PIL and used for controlled anticancer drug delivery with an antimicrobial effect. The Ag-PIL nanocomposite demonstrated outstanding bacteriostatic and bactericidal activity against both *E. coli* and *S. aureus* [17].

Notably, one of the drawbacks of using MNPs is their proclivity to agglomerate and aggregate as a result of the Ostwald ripening process [18]. This significantly reduces their stability and limits their utility in pharmaceutical applications [19]. Therefore, the MNPs should be stabilized either sterically or electrostatically to prevent agglomeration [19]. Benzyl alkyl ionic liquids (BAILs) could offer a promising solution for steric and electrostatic stabilizing of MNPs [20]. Electrostatic and steric interactions between MNPs and ILs contribute to their stabilization without affecting surface characteristics [21,22]. Furthermore, the ILs' strong ionic strength, polarity, and dielectric constant make them suitable mediums for the preparation and stabilization of MNPs [22]. On the other hand, among the various reported methods for synthesizing NMNPs [23], the microemulsion approach has attracted the attention of many researchers worldwide due to its simplicity, cost-effectiveness, and efficiency to produce stable NPs [24,25].

Motivated by these astounding facts and as a new step in our ongoing journey to explore and develop novel pharmacological agents [26–28], the present study reports the synthesis of new BAIILs for application in the preparation and stabilization of AgNPs. In this study, several BAIIL aggregation effects will be investigated as a function of the phenyl and imidazyl substituents. Furthermore, the effects of various produced AgNPs on ESKAPE pathogens as well as healthy human skin fibroblast (HSF) cell lines will be examined.

2. Results and Discussion

2.1. Synthesis

Using substituted alkylbenzenes and alkyl imidazoles as building blocks, a three-step methodology is developed to produce the desired benzyl alkyl ionic liquids (BAIILs) (See Figure 1). First, alkylbenzenes (cumene and tert-butylbenzene) were chloromethylated with a chloromethylating agent mixture of dimethoxymethane-chlorosulfonic acid-ZnI to produce the appropriate chlorobenzyl derivatives (**1a–c**). Following that, N-benzyl imidazolium chlorides (**2a–f**) were synthesised by quaternizing 1-alkylimidazoles with chlorobenzyl derivatives under refluxing conditions in an inert atmosphere. Eventually, the counterparts imidazolium bis-((trifluoromethyl)sulfonyl) imide ionic liquids (**3a–f**) were obtained by subjecting these ILs to anion (chloride) metathesis with LiTf$_2$N at room temperature. On the other hand, the AgNPs were successfully produced using hydrazine hydrate-catalyzed AgNO$_3$ reduction in BAIILs/TX-100/H$_2$O microemulsions. The colour change of water-BAIIL microemulsion containing Ag+ ions from a light yellow to a brownish yellow is indicative of the AgNPs formation. In this reduction process, BAIIL acts as a green solvent and stabilizing agent (Figure 1).

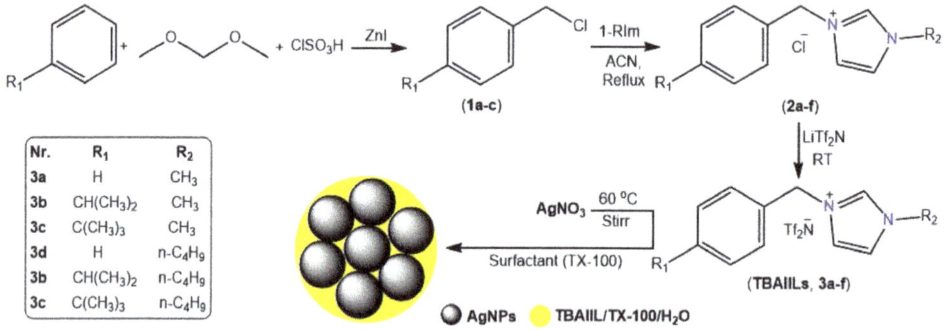

Nr.	R$_1$	R$_2$
3a	H	CH$_3$
3b	CH(CH$_3$)$_2$	CH$_3$
3c	C(CH$_3$)$_3$	CH$_3$
3d	H	n-C$_4$H$_9$
3b	CH(CH$_3$)$_2$	n-C$_4$H$_9$
3c	C(CH$_3$)$_3$	n-C$_4$H$_9$

Figure 1. Stepwise synthesis of BAIILs (**3a–f**) their applications in the synthesis of AgNPs.

2.2. Physical Characterization

BAIILs were produced in excellent yields (85–95%) overall and they were physically characterized based on their appearance, solubility, lipophilicity, viscosity, and thermal stability measurements.

2.2.1. Physical Appearance, Solubility, and Lipophilicity

It is well established that the aqueous solubility and lipophilic properties of a new pharmacological agent are directly related to its pharmacokinetics and pharmacodynamics. It was for this reason that the room-temperature aqueous solubility of the novel BAIILs was studied. All BAIILs were found to be soluble in water, though each BAIIL dissolved in different degree depending on its structure. The degree to which they are soluble in water is controlled by the type of alkyl substituent present on the benzene and imidazole rings (see Table 1). For example, the tert-butylbenzylimidazolium cation (**3f**), which bears the most hydrophobic side chain (n-butyl), is the least soluble of the group (LogS = −8.163), while the benzylmethylimidazolium cation (**3a**) has the highest solubility (LogS = −5.719).

Table 1. Physicochemical characteristics of new BAIILs.

TAAI.	MW (g/mol)	Appearance	LogS [a]	CLogP [b]	D (g/cm^3) [c]	η (cP) [d]	T$_{dec}$ (°C) [e]
3a	453.37	Yellow oil	−5.719	−0.352	1.468	421.15	407
3b	495.46	Orange oil	−6.820	−0.262	1.397	426.85	402
3c	509.48	Yellow oil	−7.150	0.137	1.551.	439.25	412
3d	495.46	Orange oil	−6.735	−0.102	1.298	512.67	397
3e	537.54	Brown oil	−7.834	1.325	1.213	521.83	394
3f	551.56	Orange oil	−8.163	1.724	1.311	543.25	401

[a,b] calculated using ChemDraw 16; [c] density measured using COSMOtherm at 50 °C; [d] viscosity measured at 25 °C using a capillary viscometer; [e] decomposition temperature from DTG curves.

CLogP measurements demonstrate that the benzyl-alkylimidazolium cation is the least lipophilic cation, with a range from (−0.352) to (−0.102) depending on the nature of the alkyl substituent used (see Table 1). In contrast, replacing the hydrogen atom on the benzene ring with more hydrophobic groups such as *iso*-propyl and *tert*-butyl has significantly increased the CLogP values to be in the range of (−0.262)–(1.325) and (0.137)–(1.724), respectively, confirming their great lipophilic character. Interestingly, ionic liquids interact strongly with the outer lipophilic layer of microbial cell surfaces when they have a high CLogP value, and consequently their lipophilicity is increased [29].

2.2.2. Viscosity and Thermal Stability

Notably, IL-viscosity exhibits a great influence on the formation, molecular diffusion, and stability of nanoparticles. The stability of nanoparticles is greatly enhanced by the fact that their diffusion is greatly reduced in extremely viscous media like ionic liquids, which results in a lifetime increase of a factor of 10–1000 compared to that in traditional low viscosity solvents [30]. Ionic liquids also have the added benefit of reducing the likelihood of agglomeration of colloidal nanoparticles by suppressing their thermal motion due to the high viscosity. Therefore, the viscosities of new BAIILs were measured at 25 °C, and the results are shown in Table 1. High viscosity values (421.15–543.25 cP) were observed for all imidazolium ILs; however, these values varied according to the cation's intrinsic structural characteristics. For example, out of all of the examined ionic liquids, the one with the lowest viscosity (428.75 cP) was BAIIL 3a, which was made up of the simplest cation (benzyl-methylimidazolium). In contrast, tert-butylbenzyl group-containing BAIIL 3f showed the greatest viscosity (543.25 cP). The very hydrophobic Tf$_2$N anion exerts stronger ion–ion interactions with the hydrophobic tert-butylbenzyl-methylimidazolium cation, which leads to the observed behavior of an increase in viscosity [29].

On the other hand, the thermal stabilities of BAIILs (3a–f) were verified using their thermogravimetric (TG) curves (Figure S1, Supplementary Materials). All BAIILs are clearly thermally stable up to about 400 °C before undergoing a sudden decline in their masses between 400 and 450 °C. Table 1 and Figure S1 (Supplementary Materials) show that BAIILs with long side chains (n-butyl) linked to the imidazolium ring (3e–f) had more complex thermal degradation patterns and lower decomposition temperatures than BAIILs containing methylimidazolium cation (3a–c).

2.3. Structural Characterization

Spectral investigations (FTIR, NMR (^{1}H, ^{13}C, ^{19}F), and ESI-MS) were used to deduce the structural formulae of all the synthesized BAIILs.

2.3.1. Mass Spectrometry

To acquire a first perception of the characteristics of their cation and anion' structures, the electrospray ionization mass spectra (ESI-MS) of BAIILs can be a helpful tool. In light of this, the ESI-MS of BAIIL (3f) (Figure 2A) was extensively studied as a representative of new BAIILs. The major peak was found at an *m/z* value of 271.3, which corresponds to the molar mass of a single-charged cation, [M − Tf$_2$N$^-$]$^+$, generated by the elimination of the bonded anion. In addition, the fragmentation peaks that can be seen at m/z 214.4, 157.5, and 57.3 (base peak) could be assigned to consecutive removal of butyl side chains and benzyl-butylimidazolium radicals from the parent molecule, respectively, $[M - Tf_2N^- - C_4H_9{}^\cdot]^+$, $[M - Tf_2N^- - 2\,(C_4H_9{}^\cdot)]^+$, and $[M - Tf_2N^- - BnBIm^\cdot]^+$.

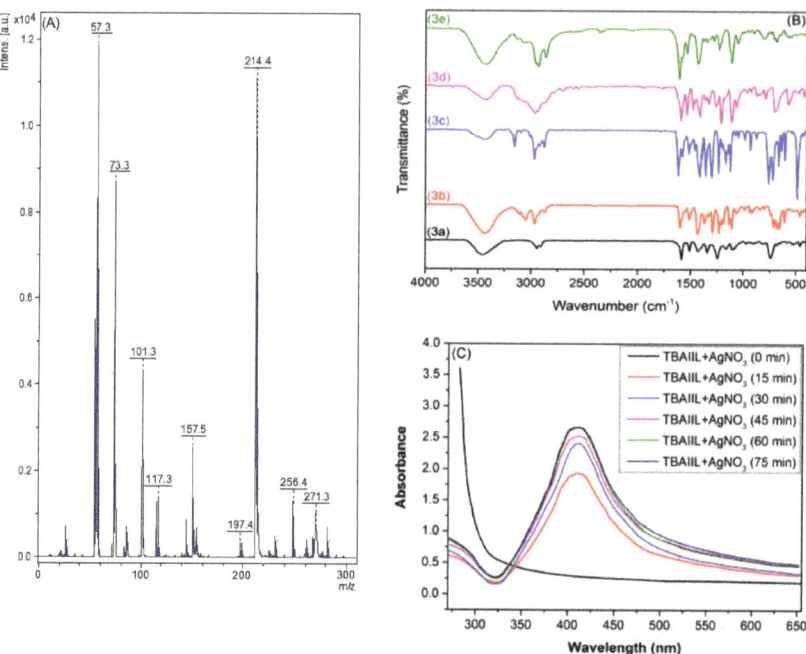

Figure 2. (A) A positive mode electrospray ionization mass spectra (ESI-MS (+ve)) of BAIIL (3f); (B) FTIR spectra of the native BAIILs (3a–f); and (C) UV-Vis spectrum AgNPs produced by BAIIL (3f).

2.3.2. FTIR Spectroscopy

The FTIR spectra of the new BAIILs (Figure 2B) were studied in an effort to learn more about the structural features of the cations and anions that make them up. The spectra of the TAILs exhibit absorption bands that are analogous to those of previously reported imidazolium-based ILs [31–33]. The common absorption peaks that can be seen in the FTIR spectra of BAIILs at 3110, 2970, 1591, 1245, 875, and 707 cm^{-1} could be attributed to the vibrational modes of the benzylimidazolium cation fragments, including imidazolium C2-H, alkyl C-H, imidazolium C=N, and the benzyl moiety, respectively [31]. In addition, the distinctive vibration bands of (TN$_2$f) anion may be observed in the regions of 1271 ± 3 cm^{-1} ascribed to $\nu_{as}(CF_3 + SO_2)$; 1224 ± 2 cm^{-1} due to $\nu_s(CF_3 + SO_2)$; 1139 ± 4 cm^{-1} typical for $\nu_{as}(CF_3 + CS)$; 1024 ± 3 and 911 ± 3 cm^{-1} for $\nu(N-S)$; 710 ± 5 cm^{-1} for $\delta(CF_3)$; and 747 ± 3 cm^{-1} assigned to $\nu(C-S)$ [34].

2.3.3. UV-Vis Spectroscopy

Figure 2C shows UV-Visible spectra of the BAIIL (3f)-based microemulsion containing AgNO$_3$ at time intervals as well as the progress in the formation of BAIIL-stabilized AgNPs with time. The appearance of a new peak at 430 nm in the microemulsion spectrum, which is characteristic of the surface plasmon resonance (SPR) of AgNPs [35], verifies the synthesis of AgNPs. Further, the SPR peak intensity rises with time, reflecting an increase in AgNPs yield, until it reaches a maximum value at 60 min. Thereafter, the peak intensity almost stops rising, denoting the end of the reaction.

2.3.4. NMR Spectroscopy

NMR spectra of new BAIILs were utilized to verify their successful production and provide a striking visual representation of the structure of their ions. However, due to the fact that all new BAIILs have nearly identical NMR spectra, with the exception of the peak of alkyl side chains, the ^{1}H/^{13}C NMR spectra of BAIIL (**3e**) (Figure 3) were analyzed in more detail as a representative of new BAIILs. As shown in the ^{1}H NMR spectrum of **3e**, the proton resonance of imidazolium (C2-H) can be seen as a singlet at 9.91 ppm. Furthermore, a group of signals was detected in the chemical shift region of 7.93–7.12 ppm, assignable to the resonances of the imidazolium and phenyl protons. In addition, the benzylic protons can be seen as a singlet peak at 5.64. As for the protons of alkyl side chains (isopropyl and n-butyl groups), the methine and methyl protons of the isopropyl group emerged as septet (3.28 ppm) and doublet (1.21 ppm), respectively. While the methylene and methyl protons of the n-butyl group can be observed as a set of multiplets in the high-field region (4.26–0.91 ppm). The ^{13}C NMR spectrum of **3e**, on the other hand, shows the carbon map in detail for both the central benzylimidazolium cation and the alkyl substituents. The carbon signals characteristic of the benzylimidazolium cation can be detected in the low-field region (146.03–122.54 ppm) for the resonances of the imidazolium and phenyl carbon atoms, while it is 55.75 for benzylic carbon. In contrast, the peaks distinctive of C-atom of alkyl substituents can be seen in the high-field region, 32.38 and 23.23 ppm for methine and methyl carbons of the isopropyl group; and 47.45, 31.82, 19.84, and 13.76 ppm for carbon atoms of n-butyl group. It is worth noting that the low-field carbon signal observed at 149.65 could be assigned to CF$_3$ of Tf$_2$N anion [29].

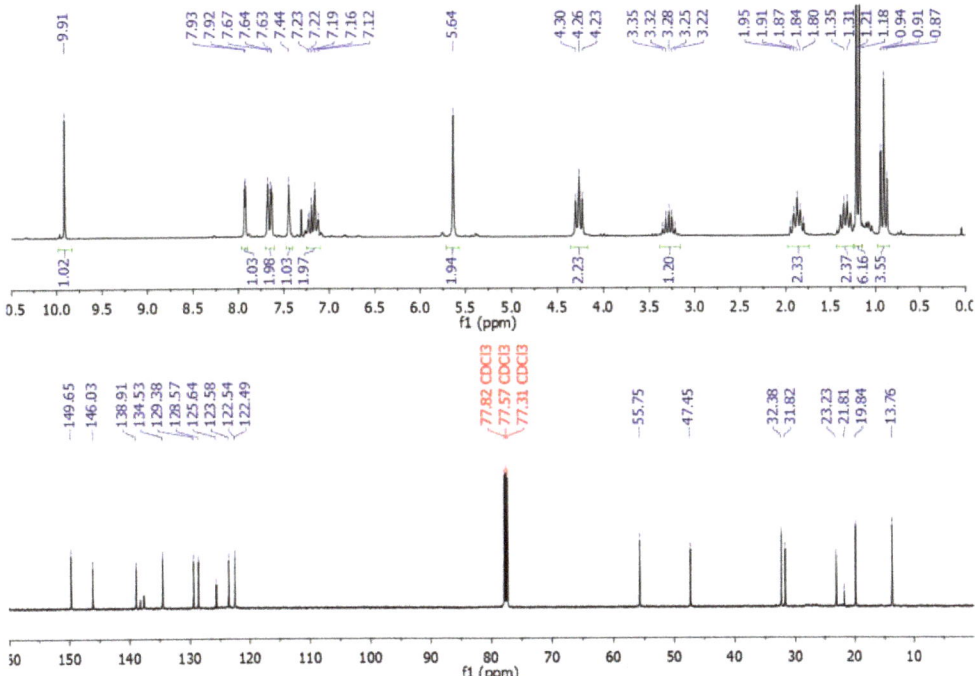

Figure 3. ^{1}HNMR (200 MHz) and ^{13}CNMR (125 MHz) of BAIIL (**3e**) in CDCl$_3$.

2.4. Morphological Characterization

2.4.1. Transmission Electron Microscopy (TEM) Analysis

Representative TEM images of AgNPs obtained from hydrazine reduction of $AgNO_3$ in various BAIILs are shown in Figure 4. When $AgNO_3$ is reduced in the presence of new BAIILs, discrete AgNPs with diameters in the range of 2.9–1.5 nm are formed (from TEM). More agglomeration can be seen in the AgNPs made from the methylimidazolium-supported BAIILs (**3a–c**) (Figure 4A–C) than in those made from the butylimidazolium-supported BAIILs (**3d–f**) (Figure 4D–F). Meanwhile, the primary AgNPs produced by 4-iso-propylbenzyl- or 4-tert-butylbenzyl-substituted BAIILs (**3b**, **3c**, **3e**, and **3f**) were more separated than those produced by unsubstituted benzyl-based BAIILs (**3a,d**). This could be due to the electrostatic and steric interactions between AgNPs and BAIILs, which contribute to their stabilization without affecting surface characteristics by forming a protecting layer that prevents AgNPs coalescence [21,22]. Unlike more traditional approaches, this synthetic process permits the synthesis of AgNPs networks with narrower particle size dispersion. Interestingly, AgNPs isolated from the BAIIL bearing the bulkiest substituents (*tert*-butyl and *n*-butyl) (**3f**) displayed almost no NPs agglomeration (see Figure 4E).

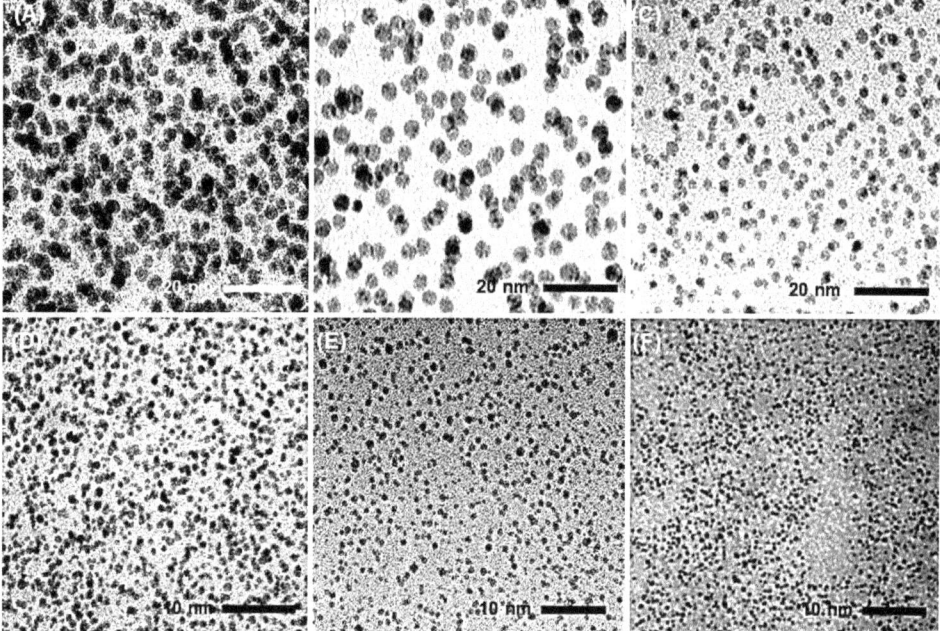

Figure 4. TEM images of AgNPs generated by the hydrazine-reduction of $AgNO_3$ in different BAIILs-based microemulsions: (**A**) 3a, (**B**) 3b, (**C**) 3c, (**D**) 3d, (**E**) 3e, and (**F**) 3f.

2.4.2. Particle Size Distribution (PSD)

The size histograms of the AgNPs obtained by BAIILs (Figure 5) show that the nanoparticles have a very narrow PSD and are either not agglomerated or exhibit very little agglomeration. Uniformly dispersed AgNPs with a mean diameter of 1.5 ± 0.5 nm were produced by using the BAIIL **3f** with the highest surface steric energy (69.772 kcal/mol) as a stabilizing agent. In contrast, when using BAIIL **3a** of lowest surface steric energy (50.029 kcal/mol) as a medium for AgNPs production, the AgNPs with a mean diameter of 2.9 ± 0.6 nm were obtained coupled with few agglomerated big AgNPs cluster of 4–5 nm.

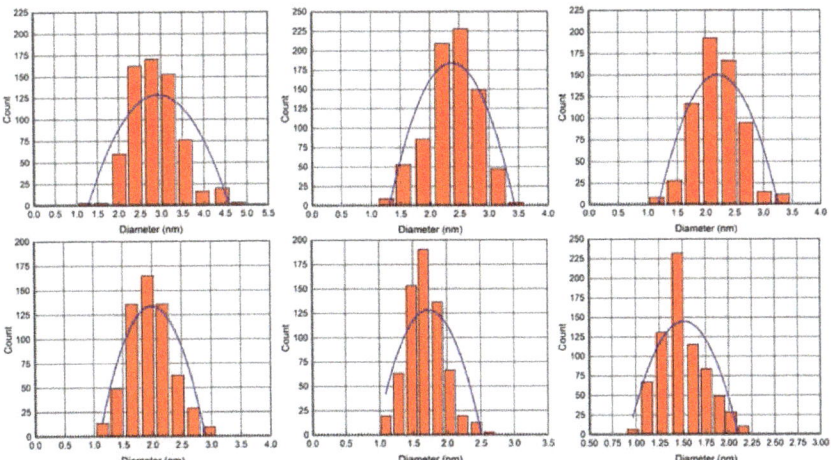

Figure 5. PSD histograms of AgNPs obtained using different BAIILs-based microemulsions.

2.5. Antibacterial Assay

The in vitro antibacterial activity of BAIILs-coated AgNPs was evaluated in comparison to that of Ciprofloxacin (Cipro) (a clinical antibiotic used for treating skin bacterial infections) using three of the most common ESKAPE infections found in contaminated food. Initially, the antibacterial efficacy of each sample was measured using the inhibition zone diameter (IZD, mm). As can be seen in Figure 6, all AgNPs have the capacity to limit the growth of all tested bacterial cells; however, their efficacy varies depending on the kind of bacterium, BAIIL structural characteristics, and AgNPs' mean size. Noteworthy, the gram-positive (G$^+$) bacterial strain (*SA*) was generally more susceptible to all treatments than gram-negative (G$^-$) ones (*PA* and *KP*). The structural differences between the outer bacterial walls of the two types may be to blame for the different inclination of bacterial membrane permeability and, as a result, bactericidal effects. Particularly, unlike the G$^+$—bacterial wall that contains only a thin peptidoglycan layer, G$^-$ - bacteria have a more sophisticated outer membrane that may operate as a barrier to the invasion of antibiotics into bacterial cells due to the presence of phospholipids (PLs), lipopolysaccharides (LPS), and lipoproteins (LPs) [36]. Interestingly, the IZD data indicate that the antibacterial activity of AgNPs improves as their mean size falls. For example, the AgNPs of the smallest size (1.5 nm), obtained using BAIIL **3f**, exhibit the highest activity against *SA* (43.59 ± 1.48 mm). In contrast, the antistaphylococcal activity (24.31 ± 0.79 mm) is lowest for the biggest AgNPs (2.9 nm), which were made using BAIIL **3a**. The findings of CFU method and CFU/mL values are in good consistency with the results obtained by AWD method. As shown in Figure 6A–C and S2 (SM†), a remarkable bacterial reduction was observed in all bacterial cells after treatment with BAIIL-coated AgNPs; however, the performance depends on the bacterial strain type, the ionic liquid coating, and the AgNPs' sizes. Overall, the G$^+$ strain (*SA*) was more sensitive to AgNPs, and its bacterial colony count was reduced by a value of 72–92% after treatment. In contrast, G$^-$ bacteria (*PA* and *KP*) were less responsive to AgNPs treatments and showed bacterial colony reductions (BCR) of 58–81% and 54–75%, respectively, in AgNPs-treated PA and KP samples in comparison to growth controls.

It is worth noting that the butylimidazolium-coated AgNPs (AgNPs-3d, AgNPs-3e, and AgNPs-3f) (BCR 68–92%) are more potent antibiotics than methylimidazolium-coated AgNPs (AgNPs-3a, AgNPs-3b, and AgNPs-3c) (BCR 54–77%). Antibiotic activity (BCR 71–92%) is greatest for AgNPs with a mean particle size of 1.5 nm.

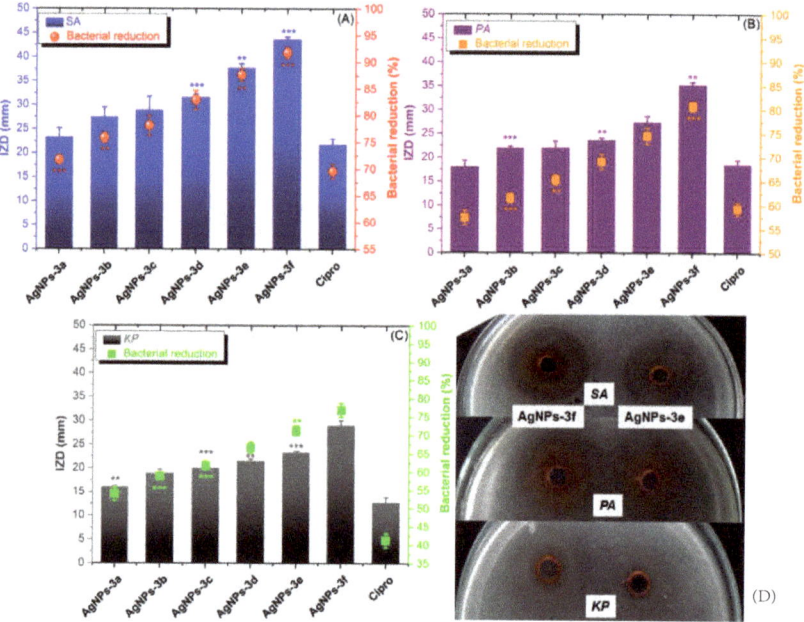

Figure 6. Graph for the inhibition zone diameter (IZD, mm) and the percentage of bacterial colonies reduction (%) for the examined AgNPs against (**A**) G⁺ bacteria (*SA*), (**B**) G⁻ bacteria (*PA*), and (**C**) G⁻ bacteria (*KP*) (** $p < 0.005$, *** $p < 0.001$). (**D**) Photographs of inhibition zones for the most active antibiotics (**AgNPs-3e** and **AgNPs-3f**).

Once more, Table 2 MIC and MBC values demonstrate that G⁺-bacterium was more sensitive to AgNPs than G⁻ species. The presence of negatively charged phosphate groups on its surface may also play a role in this [37]. The positively charged nanoparticles can interact strongly with these groups. The extent to which AgNPs exhibited bactericidal or bacteriostatic actions was also significantly influenced by the type of tested bacteria and the NPs size. For example, the AgNPs coated by 4-tert-butylbenzyl-substituted BAIIL (**3f**) were the most potent antibiotic for *SA* (MIC/MCB = 0.25 ± 0.12/0.35 ± 0.16 µg/mL).

Table 2. MIC and MBC values (µg/mL) of new BAIILs-supported AgNPs against ESKAPE pathogens, as compared to clinical antibiotics (GM and TC).

Sample	Size (nm)	SA		PA		KB	
		MIC ± SD	MBC ± SD	MIC ± SD	MBC ± SD	MIC ± SD	MBC ± SD
AgNPs-3a	2.9	3.25 ± 0.25	3.75 ± 0.31	8.76 ± 0.32	8.85 ± 0.35	9.32 ± 0.34	9.50 ± 0.37
AgNPs-3b	2.4	2.25 ± 0.12	2.25 ± 0.15	7.07 ± 0.19	7.15 ± 0.45	8.87 ± 0.11	8.05 ± 0.25
AgNPs-3c	2.2	1.95 ± 0.15	2.07 ± 0.19	5.85 ± 0.25	5.95 ± 0.33	7.35 ± 0.37	7.48 ± 0.33
AgNPs-3d	2.0	1.76 ± 0.15	1.95 ± 0.11	5.55 ± 0.29	5.65 ± 0.37	7.15 ± 0.21	7.23 ± 0.25
AgNPs-3e	1.7	0.85 ± 0.11	0.95 ± 0.23	2.75 ± 0.36	2.85 ± 0.45	4.45 ± 0.29	4.55 ± 0.41
AgNPs-3f	1.5	0.25 ± 0.12	0.35 ± 0.18	1.36 ± 0.27	1.39 ± 0.28	2.22 ± 0.15	2.25 ± 0.19
Cipro	-	5.20 ± 0.16	5.75 ± 0.25	7.75 ± 0.23	8.05 ± 0.31	10.13 ± 0.56	10.55 ± 0.48

NA = not assigned.

On the other hand, AgNPs obtained by nascent benzyl-imidazolium BAIIL (**3a**) were the least active anti-staphylococcal agent (MIC/MCB = 3.25 ± 0.25/3.75 ± 0.31 µg/mL). It is worth noting that with MIC/MCB values between 2.22 ± 0.15/2.25 ± 0.19 µg/mL and 9.32 ± 0.34/9.50 ± 0.37 µg/mL, *KP* is the most drug-resistant strain of bacteria.

2.6. Anti-Biofilm Activity

The ability of the most potent antibiotics (**AgNPs-3d**, **AgNPs-3e**, and **AgNPs-3f**) to prevent the development of bacterial biofilm on polystyrene surfaces was evaluated in vitro as compared to a positive control (Cipro) and a growth control (deionized water, DIW). As can be seen in Figure 7, all of the materials studied strongly limit the formation of bacterial biofilms, albeit this capacity varies depending on material structure and bacterial type. Specifically, the G$^+$ bacterial biofilm (*staphylococcal* biofilm) formation is inhibited by AgNPs more so than by G$^-$ bacterial (*PA* and *KP*) biofilms. Furthermore, it is evident that AgNPs impeded *PA* biofilm formation more so than *KP* biofilm production ($p < 0.005$). Among the tested AgNPs, (tert-butyl)benzyl)-butylimidazolium-coated AgNPs (**AgNPs-3f**) was the most effective anti-biofilm agent, inhibiting bacterial biofilm formation by approximately 96%, 89%, and 78% for *SA*, *PA*, and *KP*, respectively, which was 1.5- to 2-fold higher than the effects induced by the positive control (Cipro). These findings suggest that the increased activity of AgNPs in preventing bacterial biofilm formation is due to its strong antimicrobial impact on the bacterial cells submerged in cultures or biofilms, and their ability to restrict adhesion of bacterial cells onto the NPs-coated polystyrene surfaces.

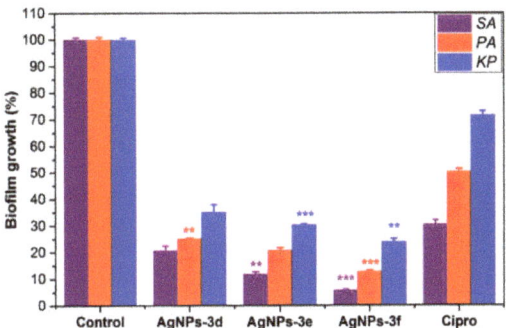

Figure 7. Inhibition of bacterial biofilm formation by the most potent antibiotics (AgNPs-3d, AgNPs-3e, and AgNPs-3f) as compared to a positive control (Cipro) and negative control (DI water), (** $p < 0.005$, *** $p < 0.001$).

2.7. In Vitro Cytotoxicity

New BAIILs-coated AgNPs were tested for cytotoxicity against normal (HSF) cells using the MTT assay in comparison to the positive control, cisplatin (CDDP). It is common practice to conduct initial single-dose studies of novel drugs for cytotoxic effects in human cell lines. Therefore, we looked at how BAIILs-coated AgNPs affected HSF cell proliferation when used in a single dose (10 μg/mL) (Figure 8A). The cytotoxicity data showed that all BAIILs-coated AgNPs are significantly ($p < 0.0001$) less toxic than CDDP toward HSF cells. In addition, the AgNPs derived from the butylimidazolium-supported BAIILs (**3d–f**) (AgNPs-3d, AgNPs-3e, and AgNPs-3f) are more toxic for HSF cells than the AgNPs obtained from the methylimidazolium-supported BAIILs (**3a–c**). Meanwhile, according to IC$_{50}$ values (Figure 8B), the clinical drug (CDDP) is more toxic to healthy cells than all new TBAIILs-AgNPs. BAIIL coatings are proving to be an effective tool in reducing the toxic effects of silver nanoparticles on normal cells. This new innovative solution is based on using BAIILs covalently bound to the silver nanoparticles. These ILs act to reduce the release of silver ions, which are typically the most toxic components. According to our findings, this study provides hope for the future development of safe and promising BAIILs-AgNPs-based microemulsions as bacterial infection medications, particularly for skin bacterial infections.

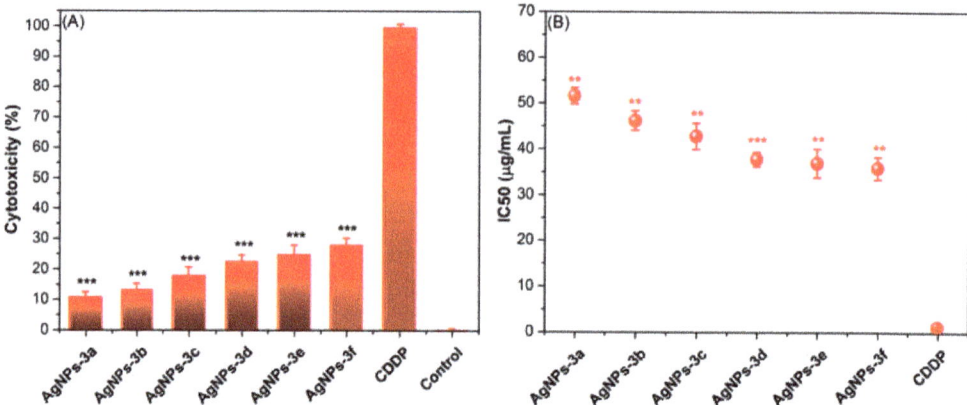

Figure 8. (**A**) A single dose (10 μg/mL) inhibitory impacts of BAIILs-AgNPs on the proliferation of HSF cell lines. (**B**) Values of IC_{50} (μg/mL) for BAIILs-AgNPs against HSF in comparison to CDDP (** p < 0.005, *** p < 0.001).

2.8. Proposed Mechanism for Pharmacological Activity of New BAIILs-AgNPs

There is still much uncertainty about how NMNPs exert their beneficial effects on bacteria or cancer. However, the high biocompatibility and excellent photothermal effects of AgNPs may greatly contribute to their superior bioactivity [38]. In addition, the ability of BAIIL-coated AgNPs to adhere to the bacterial membrane by electrostatic binding between the negatively charged bacterial cell and the positively charged NPs and BAIIL is critical for their bactericidal activity. This breaks the integrity of the bacterial membrane, leading to cell death [39]. Moreover, the extremely small sizes (2.9–1.5 nm) and unique hydrophobic coatings (**BAIILs**) enable these NPs to enter bacterial cells without being ingested by endocytosis and to subsequently aggregate within the cells, where they can exert a wide range of antimicrobial effects [39,40]. According to Jiang et al., silver nanoparticles release silver ions that interact with the thiol groups of many enzymes, rendering most of the respiratory chain enzymes inactive and thereby triggering the formation of reactive oxygen species (ROS), which in turn triggers the bacterial cell's own self-destruction and that of the cancer cell as well [41]. Additionally, silver works as a soft acid that interacts readily with the nitrogen, sulphur, and phosphorus bases of DNA to inactivate its replication, so rendering the nuclear machinery of the cell inoperable [42]. Eventually, it could be speculated that the surface area to volume ratio of AgNPs has a significant impact in providing pharmacological activity. The presence of BAIILs capping nanoparticles confers a unique surface functionality, causing them to interact with various cell types in a predetermined fashion (see Figure 9). The effectiveness of pharmacological activity increases as particle size decreases. Additionally, the BAIIL coating plays an important role in the enhancing the antibacterial action of AgNPs in multiple possible ways: (i) the effects on bacterial cell walls due to interactions between cationic imidazolium group and their negative charge; (ii) the capabilities of hydrophobic alkyl substituents to aid AgNPs in penetrating lipophilic cell membranes [43]; and (iii) changes in membrane structure and dynamics as a result of exposure to imidazolium-based ionic liquids. Specifically, the imidazolium-based ionic liquids caused changes in the lipid bilayer of the cell membrane, leading to an increase in membrane permeability and cellular damage [44].

Comparing the antibacterial activity of newly developed BAIILs-capped AgNPs with that of previously reported counterparts (see Table S1, Supplementary Materials), [45,46] revealed that the BAIILs-AgNPs had significantly higher antibacterial efficacies (with MIC/MBC values in the range of 0.25/0.35–2.22/2.25 μg/mL) than the previously reported AgNPs (with MIC/MBC values in the range of 16/16–256/256 μg/mL). These results demonstrate that the new AgNPs have both higher MIC values as well as higher MBC values in comparison to previously reported ionic liquid-coated AgNPs. This indicates that the new AgNPs are more effective in controlling bacteria growth than their previously studied counterparts. Thus, the new AgNPs could potentially be an effective and safe alternative to treat bacterial infections more effectively.

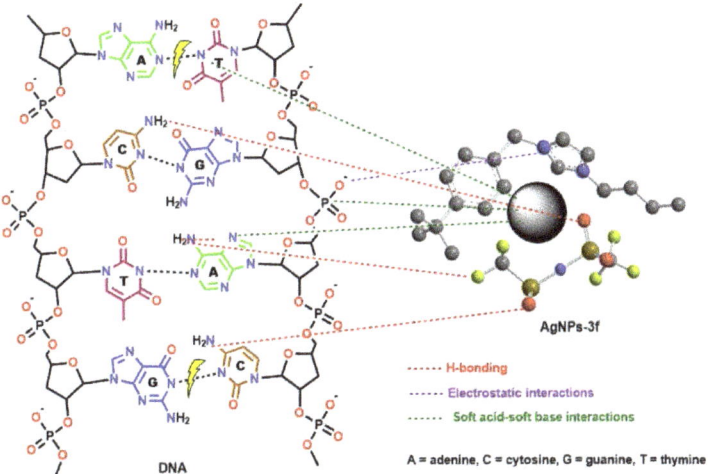

Figure 9. The proposed mechanism for DNA-cleavage activity of new thiazolium AgNPs-3f.

Notably, the alkyl chain length of BAIILs plays vital roles both in the steric stabilization of AgNPs as well as their antibacterial capabilities. The findings of the previous studies indicate that increasing the chain length of the ionic liquid can enhance the steric stabilization of AgNPs, which can be attributed to the increased number of hydrophobic interactions between the ionic liquid molecules and the AgNPs [45,46]. In addition, increasing the alkyl chain length of an imidazolium ionic liquid can lead to an increase in its antimicrobial effectiveness. The findings are in agreement with a study conducted by Docherty and Kulpa [47] which revealed that chain length has a significant impact on the antimicrobial potency of the ionic liquids. The researchers found that increasing the chain length from C1 to C4 resulted in a significant increase in antibacterial activity against Gram-positive and Gram-negative bacteria. In particular, the C4 derivative was observed to be the most effective with a minimum inhibitory concentration (MIC) of 8.25 mM against G$^+$-bacteria and 4.03 mM against G$^-$-bacteria. The increased antibacterial activity was due to an increased partition coefficient of the ionic liquid, which allowed it to be more effectively absorbed by the cellular membrane of the bacteria.

3. Materials and Methods

Chemical and solvent suppliers and their details were provided in the Supplementary Materials (Supplementary Materials). In addition, the preparation and characterization of benzyl chloride (R^1BnCl) derivatives (**1a–c**) and benzyl alkyl imidazolium chloride [R^1BnImR^2]$^+$Cl$^-$ ionic liquids (**2a–f**) were described in the Supplementary Materials.

The new BAIILs were structuraly chracterized based upon the spectral analyses (FTIR, UV-Vis, NMR (^{1}HNMR, ^{13}CNMR, ^{19}FNMR), and ESI-MS) and physical measurements. The detail for these instruments were also provided in the Supplementary Materials.

3.1. Synthesis of Tunable Benzyl Alkyl Imidazolium Ionic Liquids (BAIILs, 3a–f)

While vigorously stirring, a solution of lithium bis(trifluoromethanesulfonimide) (LiTf$_2$N) (6.66 g, 0.03 mol) in a combination of ACN (10 mL) and deionized water (DIW) (10 mL) was added dropwise to a solution of [R^1BzR^{2}Im]Cl (**2a–f**) (0.03 mol) in DIW. The resulting mixture was then magnetically stirred overnight at room temperature. After the reaction time was completed and the aqueous layer was discarded, the oily residues were dissolved in dichloromethane (DCM) and repeatedly washed with DIW until there was no precipitation of the AgNO$_3$ solution with the washing water. The resulting oily products were subsequently vacuum-dried for 48 hours at 343 K to remove any leftover water. Samples of the produced BAIILs (**3a–f**) were chracterized as follow:

3-benzyl-1-methylimidazolium bis((trifluoromethyl)sulfonyl)amide [BnMIm][Tf$_2$N] (**3a**): Obtained in a 95% yield. ^{1}H NMR (500 MHz, CDCl$_3$) δ (ppm); 9.41 (1H, s, Im-H), 7.90 (1H, d, J = 1.8 Hz, Im-H), 7.72 (1H, d, J = 1.8 Hz, Im-H), 7.70–7.49 (5H, m, Ar-H), 5.38 (2H, 2, Ph-C$\underline{H_2}$), 3.87 (3H, s, N-C$\underline{H_3}$). ^{13}C NMR (75 MHz, CDCl$_3$) δ (ppm): 149.87, 139.96, 137.38, 131.42, 129.56, 126.21, 124.51, 122.98, 56.39, and 37.63. ^{19}F NMR (565 MHz, CDCl$_3$): singlet at δ −81.67 ppm (Tf$_2$N-C$\underline{F_3}$). ESI-MS (positive mode): 173.2 m/z [M − Tf$_2$N$^-$, C$_{11}$H$_{13}$N$_2$]$^+$.

3-(4-isopropylbenzyl)-1-methylimidazolium bis((trifluoromethyl)sulfonyl)amide [^{iso}PBnMIm][Tf$_2$N] (**3b**): Obtained in a 87% yield. ^{1}H NMR (500 MHz, CDCl$_3$) δ (ppm); 9.35 (1H, s, Im-H), 7.96 (1H, d, J = 1.9 Hz, Im-H), 7.74 (1H, d, J = 1.9 Hz, Im-H), 7.38–7.16 (4H, m, Ar-H), 5.39 (2H, 2, Ar-C$\underline{H_2}$), 3.98 (3H, s, N-C$\underline{H_3}$), 3.78 (1H, p, J = 1.9 Hz, C$\underline{H}$(CH$_3$)$_2$), 1.24 (6H, d, J = 6.9 Hz, CH(C$\underline{H_3}$)$_2$). ^{13}C NMR (75 MHz, CDCl$_3$) δ (ppm): 148.92, 146.07, 137.61, 133.88, 130.64, 126.33, 123.06, 122.31, 56.31, 37.17, 33.31, and 23.21. ^{19}F NMR (565 MHz, CDCl$_3$): singlet at δ −81.69 ppm (Tf$_2$N-C$\underline{F_3}$). ESI-MS (positive mode): 215.2 m/z [M − Tf$_2$N$^-$, C$_{14}$H$_{19}$N$_2$]$^+$.

3-(4-(^{tert}butyl)benzyl)-1-methylimidazolium bis((trifluoromethyl)sulfonyl)amide [^{tert}BBnMIm][Tf$_2$N] (**3c**): Obtained in a 91% yield. ^{1}H NMR (500 MHz, CDCl$_3$) δ (ppm); 9.88 (1H, s, Im-H), 7.93 (1H, d, J = 2.0 Hz, Im-H), 7.74 (1H, d, J = 2.0 Hz, Im-H), 7.49–7.23 (4H, m, Ar-H), 5.39 (2H, 2, Ar-C$\underline{H_2}$), 3.89 (3H, s, N-C$\underline{H_3}$), 1.38 (9H, s, C(C$\underline{H_3}$)$_3$). ^{13}C NMR (126 MHz, CDCl$_3$) δ (ppm): 149.76, 148.57, 138.64, 131.95, 129.13, 125.15, 123.88, 122.96, 55.63, 37.74, 34.34, and 31.91. ^{19}F NMR (565 MHz, CDCl$_3$): singlet at δ −81.65 ppm (Tf$_2$N-C$\underline{F_3}$). ESI-MS (positive mode): 229.2 m/z [M − Tf$_2$N$^-$, C$_{15}$H$_{21}$N$_2$]$^+$.

3-benzyl-1-butylimidazolium bis((trifluoromethyl)sulfonyl)amide [BnBIm][Tf$_2$N] (**3d**): Obtained in a 91% yield. ^{1}H NMR (500 MHz, CDCl$_3$) δ (ppm); 9.26 (1H, s, Im-H), 7.84 (1H, d, J = 1.8 Hz, Im-H), 7.78 (1H, d, J = 1.7 Hz, Im-H), 7.61–7.36 (5H, m, Ar-H), 5.35 (2H, 2, Ph-C$\underline{H_2}$), 4.19 (2H, t, J = 7.2 Hz, N-C$\underline{H_2}$CH$_2$CH$_2$CH$_3$), 1.79 (2H, p, J = 7.2 Hz, N-CH$_2$C$\underline{H_2}$CH$_2$CH$_3$), 1.27 (2H, m$_{(6)}$, N-CH$_2$CH$_2$C$\underline{H_2}$CH$_3$), 0.91 (3H, t, J = 7.3 Hz, N-CH$_2$CH$_2$CH$_2$C$\underline{H_3}$). ^{13}C NMR (126 MHz, CDCl$_3$) δ (ppm): 149.68, 137.93, 134.63, 129.24, 128.74, 126.02, 123.14, 122.89, 55.24, 47.44, 31.60, 19.16, and 13.60. ^{19}F NMR (565 MHz, CDCl$_3$): singlet at δ −81.66 ppm (Tf$_2$N-C$\underline{F_3}$). ESI-MS (positive mode): 215.2 m/z [M − Tf$_2$N$^-$, C$_{14}$H$_{19}$N$_2$]$^+$.

3-(4-isopropylbenzyl)-1-butylimidazolium bis((trifluoromethyl)sulfonyl)amide [^{iso}PBnBIm][Tf$_2$N] (**3e**): Obtained in a 85% yield. ^{1}H NMR (500 MHz, CDCl$_3$) δ (ppm); 9.91 (1H, s, Im-H), 7.92 (1H, d, J = 2.2 Hz, Im-H), 7.72 (1H, d, J = 2.1 Hz, Im-H), 7.44–7.19 (4H, m, Ar-H), 5.64 (2H, 2, Ar-C$\underline{H_2}$), 4.26 (2H, t, J = 7.4 Hz, N-C$\underline{H_2}$CH$_2$CH$_2$CH$_3$), 3.28 (1H, p, J = 6.9 Hz, C$\underline{H}$(CH$_3$)$_2$), 1.85 (2H, p, J = 7.2 Hz, N-CH$_2$C$\underline{H_2}$CH$_2$CH$_3$), 1.33 (2H, m$_{(6)}$, N-CH$_2$CH$_2$C$\underline{H_2}$CH$_3$), 1.19 (6H, d, J = 7.1 Hz, CH(C$\underline{H_3}$)$_2$) 0.91 (3H, t, J = 7.3 Hz, N-CH$_2$CH$_2$CH$_2$C$\underline{H_3}$). ^{13}C NMR (126 MHz, CDCl$_3$) δ (ppm): 149.65, 146.03, 138.91, 134.53, 129.38, 128.57, 125.64, 123.58, 122.54, 55.75, 47.45, 32.38, 31.82, 23.23, 21.81, and 13.85. ^{19}F NMR (565 MHz, CDCl$_3$): singlet at δ −81.67 ppm (Tf$_2$N-C$\underline{F_3}$). ESI-MS (positive mode): 257.3 m/z [M − Tf$_2$N$^-$, C$_{17}$H$_{25}$N$_2$]$^+$

3-(4-(^{tert}butyl)benzyl)-1-butylimidazolium bis((trifluoromethyl)sulfonyl)amide [^{tert}BBnBIm][Tf$_2$N] (**3f**): Obtained in a 89% yield. ^{1}H NMR (500 MHz, CDCl$_3$) δ (ppm); 9.84 (1H, s, Im-H), 7.91 (1H, d, J = 2.1 Hz, Im-H), 7.74 (1H, d, J = 2.1 Hz, Im-H), 7.49–7.27 (4H, m, Ar-H), 5.61 (2H, 2, Ar-C$\underline{H_2}$), 4.28 (2H, t, J = 7.3 Hz, N-C$\underline{H_2}$CH$_2$CH$_2$CH$_3$), 1.83 (2H, p, J = 7.1 Hz, N-CH$_2$C$\underline{H_2}$CH$_2$CH$_3$), 1.40 (9H, s, C(C$\underline{H_3}$)$_3$), 1.31 (2H, m$_{(6)}$, N-CH$_2$CH$_2$C$\underline{H_2}$CH$_3$), 1.19 (6H, d, J = 6.9 Hz, CH(C$\underline{H_3}$)$_2$) 0.90 (3H, t, J = 7.2 Hz, N-CH$_2$CH$_2$CH$_2$C$\underline{H_3}$). ^{13}C NMR (126 MHz, CDCl$_3$) δ (ppm): 149.72, 148.51, 137.92, 131.65, 129.42, 125.64, 123.63, 122.91,

55.68, 47.52, 34.41, 33.34, 31.43, 21.21, and 13.87. ^{19}F NMR (565 MHz, CDCl$_3$): singlet at δ −81.69 ppm (Tf$_2$N-C$\underline{F}_3$). ESI-MS (positive mode): 271.3 m/z [M − Tf$_2$N$^-$, C$_{18}$H$_{27}$N$_2$]$^+$

3.2. Preparation of IILMEs-Mediated AgNPs

With a minor tweak, we used the optimum conditions adopted from previously reported investigations [48–50] to fabricate the AgNPs in situ in the microemulsions containing the BAIILs (**3a–f**). In brief, the BAIIL/TX-100/H$_2$O microemulsions (IILMEs) were first prepared by mixing 0.1 g of BAIIL and 1.4 g of TX-100 in deionized water (8.5 g) for 20 min at room temperature to ensure proper blending and formation of homogeneous solutions. Afterward, a 0.1 mmol aqueous AgNO$_3$ solution was added to this microemulsion and the mixture was agitated for 10 min. A diluted hydrazine hydrate solution (1 mL) was added and the reaction mixture was then stirred at 60 °C for 1 h. The solution color changes from a light yellow to a brownish yellow, which is evidence of the creation of silver nanoparticles. To ensure full reduction, a small amount of hydrazine hydrate was added. Moreover, UV-Visible spectroscopy scanning verified the production of AgNO$_3$. Silver nanoparticles were recovered after being stabilized in a microemulsion system composed of AgNO$_3$/BAIILs/TX-100/H$_2$O by centrifuging.

3.3. Antimicrobial Study

Three representative ESKAPE pathogens *PA* (ATCC-27853), *KP* (ATCC-13883), and *SA* (ATCC-29737) were utlized to test the antimicrobial power of the new BAIIL-supported AgNPs. Ciprofloxacin (Cipro), the most common antibiotic used for skin bacterial treatments, was served as the "positive" control. The NODCAR in Cairo, Egypt, kindly supplied all of the bacterial species used in this study, and these bacteria were routinely cultured in nutrient broth agar (NBA). First, we inoculated Mueller–Hinton Broth (MHB) with a bacterial solution containing ~10^6 CFU/mL and incubated the mixture at 37 °C in a 5% CO$_2$ environment to establish the initial bacterial culture. We then used the Well diffusion assay (WDA) and colony forming unit (CFU) methods outlined in our previous work [51] to determine which bacterial strains were most sensitive to the novel AgNPs. The sizes of the inhibition zones (IZD, mm) were the most important factors in determining the NPs' antibacterial effectiveness. For the CFU method, we used the following formula (Equation (1)) to determine the relative decline in bacterial colony numbers (R%):

$$R\% = \frac{BC_{CT} - BC_{TT}}{BC_{CT}} \qquad (1)$$

where BC_{CT} and BC_{TT} are the number of bacterial colonies in growth control and treatment test tubes, respectively. The obtained results were determined using mean SEM from triplicates of each trial.

Minimal Inhibitory/Bactericidal Concentrations (MIC/MBC)

The antibacterial efficacy indicators, MIC and MBC, of new compounds against tested bacterial strains were determined using the microtitre broth dilution technique as described in our prior study [52]. In brief, the bacterial suspension was treated with AgNPs and antibiotics, separately, that had been pre-dispersed in DMSO and prediluted Mueller–Hinton Broth (MHB). After transferring 190 µL bacterial suspensions (10^6 CFU/mL) to 96-well microtiter plates, AgNPs with concentrations in the range of 0.25–50.0 g/mL were added, then the plates were left to incubate at 37 °C for 24 h; controls consisted of wells that had not been treated. The Well turbidity measurements were used to calculate MIC and MBC concentrations. In order to calculate the MIC and MBC, multiple independent replicates of each sample were evaluated. The results are shown as the mean ± SEM.

3.4. Anti-Biofilm Study

According to our previously published work [52], the ability of the most effective antibiotics (**AgNPs-3d**, **AgNPs-3e**, and **AgNPs-3f**) to inhibit bacterial biofilm formation and eradicate the biofilms created by the tested bacterial strains (SA, PA, and KP) was studied.

3.5. In Vitro Cytotoxicity Study

3.5.1. Cell Cultures

Healthy human skin fibroblast (HSF) cell lines were obtained from the American Type Cell Culture Collection (ATCC, Manassas, USA). Dulbecco's Modified Eagle's Medium (DMEM, Invitrogen/Life Technologies) was used to cultivate these cell lines, supplemented with 10% fetal bovine serum, 100 U/mL of penicillin, and 100 g/mL of streptomycin (HyClone, Thermo Scientific). The cells were maintained in a Thermo Scientific Heracell VIOS CO_2 incubator maintained at 37 °C with 5% CO_2 humidity.

3.5.2. In Vitro Anti-Proliferative Activity

The new BAIIL-supported AgNPs were tested for their anti-breast cancer action in vitro using the MTT assay. Briefly, a 96-well plate (Falcon, NJ, USA) was used to treat cell lines (10^5 cells/well) with a range of doses (1.56 – 50 μg/mL) of the tested substance, a positive control cisplatin (CDDP), and a negative control (DMSO). Sets of wells (consisting of three wells each) were assigned for each sample. Cells were incubated for 48 h at 37 °C in a 5% CO_2 atmosphere, after which they were fixed, washed, and stained with MTT reagent, and then re-incubated for an additional 4 h. The staining media was carefully removed from the plate after incubation, and 180 μL of acidified isopropanol/well was added. The plate was then agitated at ambient temperature with a MaxQ 2000 plate shaker (Thermo Fisher Scientific Inc., MI, USA) to dissolve the formazan crystals that had formed. In order to determine the vitality of the cells, the plate was next subjected to a spectrophotometric analysis using a Stat FaxR 4200 plate reader (Awareness Technology, Inc., FL, USA).

4. Conclusions

This work presents the synthesis and characterization of a new class of imidazolium-supported BAIILs. (**3a–f**) by employing spectral (FTIR, NMR, and ESI-MS), thermal, and viscosity techniques. BAIILs were used as media and stabilizing agents for hydrazine-hydrate-catalyzed $AgNO_3$ reduction in BAIILs/TX-100/H_2O microemulsions into extremely small AgNPs. Unlike more traditional approaches, this synthetic process permits the synthesis of AgNPs networks with narrower PSD. Interestingly, AgNPs isolated from the BAIIL bearing the bulkiest substituents (*tert*-butyl and *n*-butyl) (**3f**) displayed almost no NPs agglomeration. This study demonstrates that a simple step can be taken to achieve well-separated AgNPs—the addition of an electron-donating bulky para-substituent on the phenyl ring of the benzylimidazolium cation. All of the AgNPs-BAIILs tested in the in vitro antibacterial assay against ESKAPE pathogens showed very strong antibiotic properties, as evidenced by their DIZ and MIC/MBC values. Additionally, Gram-negative bacterial strains were more treatment-resistant than Gram-positive ones. Human skin fibroblast (HSF) cell lines were employed in an MTT experiment to measure the growth inhibitory effects of new drugs. The MTT cytotoxicity assay showed that the novel AgNPs had no great effect on the HSF cells. Consequently, the BAIIL-coated AgNPs could offer safe and promising antibiotic candidates for skin bacterial infection treatments.

Supplementary Materials: The following supporting information can be downloaded at: https://www.mdpi.com/article/10.3390/antibiotics12020247/s1, Figure S1: TG curves of TBAIILs. Figure S2: Photographs of inhibition zones for the most active antibiotics (**AgNPs-3e** and **AgNPs-3f**). Table S1: MIC and MBC values (μg/mL) of new BAIILs-supported AgNPs against different pathogens, in comparison to previously reported ones.

Author Contributions: F.A., funding acquisition, supervision, visualization, analyzing the data, and writing the original draft paper; O.A.A.A., funding acquisition, supervision, visualization, analyzing the data, and writing the original draft paper; I.K., methodology, analyzing the data, visualization, and writing the original draft paper; M.Y.A., funding acquisition, coordinating the biological studies work, and analyzed the data; E.F., visualization, analyzing the data, software, and writing the original draft paper; A.A.S. and S.E.I.E., biological studies, visualization, analyzing the data, and writing the original draft paper; R.F.M.E., coordinating the work, performed the synthesis and characterization, and writing the original draft paper, review & editing; W.A.E.-F., synthesis and the preliminary characterization, analyzing the data, visualization, analyzing the data, and writing the original draft paper. All authors have read and agreed to the published version of the manuscript.

Funding: This study was supported by Taif University Researchers Supporting Project number (TURSP-2020/222), Taif University, Taif, Saudi Arabia, and King Khalid University funding under grant number (R.G.P. 2/59/44).

Institutional Review Board Statement: Not applicable.

Informed Consent Statement: Not applicable.

Data Availability Statement: Not applicable.

Acknowledgments: The authors extend their appreciation to the Deanship of Scientific Research at Taif University for funding this work through Taif University Researchers Supporting Project number (TURSP-2020/222), Taif University, Taif, Saudi Arabia. In addition, the authors thank the Deanship of Scientific Research at King Khalid University for funding this work through large Groups (Project under grant number R.G.P. 2/59/44).

Conflicts of Interest: The authors declare no conflict of interest.

References

1. Ribeiro, A.I.; Dias, A.M.; Zille, A. Synergistic effects between metal nanoparticles and commercial antimicrobial agents: A Review. *ACS Appl. Nano Mater.* **2022**, *5*, 3030–3064. [CrossRef] [PubMed]
2. Ju, J.; Xie, Y.; Yu, H.; Guo, Y.; Cheng, Y.; Qian, H.; Yao, W. Synergistic interactions of plant essential oils with antimicrobial agents: A new antimicrobial therapy. *Crit. Rev. Food Sci. Nutr.* **2022**, *62*, 1740–1751. [CrossRef] [PubMed]
3. Larsson, D.; Flach, C.-F. Antibiotic resistance in the environment. *Nat. Rev. Microbiol.* **2022**, *20*, 257–269. [CrossRef] [PubMed]
4. Kailasa, S.K.; Joshi, D.J.; Kateshiya, M.R.; Koduru, J.R.; Malek, N.I. Review on the biomedical and sensing applications of nanomaterial-incorporated hydrogels. *Mater. Today Chem.* **2022**, *23*, 100746. [CrossRef]
5. Mohammadzadeh, V.; Barani, M.; Amiri, M.S.; Taghvizadeh Yazdi, M.E.; Hassanisaadi, M.; Rahdar, A.; Varma, R.S. Applications of plant-based nanoparticles in nanomedicine: A review. *Sustain. Chem. Pharm.* **2022**, *25*, 100606. [CrossRef]
6. Hassan, Y.A.; Khedr, A.I.M.; Alkabli, J.; Elshaarawy, R.F.M.; Nasr, A.M. Co-delivery of imidazolium Zn(II)salen and Origanum Syriacum essential oil by shrimp chitosan nanoparticles for antimicrobial applications. *Carbohydr. Polym.* **2021**, *260*, 117834. [CrossRef]
7. Azharuddin, M.; Zhu, G.H.; Das, D.; Ozgur, E.; Uzun, L.; Turner, A.P.F.; Patra, H.K. A repertoire of biomedical applications of noble metal nanoparticles. *Chem. Commun.* **2019**, *55*, 6964–6996. [CrossRef]
8. Iravani, S.; Varma, R.S. Advanced Drug Delivery Micro- and Nanosystems for Cardiovascular Diseases. *Molecules* **2022**, *27*, 5843. [CrossRef]
9. Chandrakala, V.; Aruna, V.; Angajala, G. Review on metal nanoparticles as nanocarriers: Current challenges and perspectives in drug delivery systems. *Emergent Mater.* **2022**, *5*, 1593–1615. [CrossRef]
10. Carvalho, S.G.; Araujo, V.H.S.; Dos Santos, A.M.; Duarte, J.L.; Silvestre, A.L.P.; Fonseca-Santos, B.; Villanova, J.C.O.; Gremião, M.P.D.; Chorilli, M. Advances and challenges in nanocarriers and nanomedicines for veterinary application. *Int. J. Pharm.* **2020**, *580*, 119214. [CrossRef]
11. Ye, L.; Cao, Z.; Liu, X.; Cui, Z.; Li, Z.; Liang, Y.; Zhu, S.; Wu, S. Noble metal-based nanomaterials as antibacterial agents. *J. Alloys Compd.* **2022**, *904*, 164091. [CrossRef]
12. Huq, M.A.; Ashrafudoulla, M.; Rahman, M.M.; Balusamy, S.R.; Akter, S. Green Synthesis and Potential Antibacterial Applications of Bioactive Silver Nanoparticles: A Review. *Polymers* **2022**, *14*, 742. [CrossRef] [PubMed]
13. Naganthran, A.; Verasoundarapandian, G.; Khalid, F.E.; Masarudin, M.J.; Zulkharnain, A.; Nawawi, N.M.; Karim, M.; Che Abdullah, C.A.; Ahmad, S.A. Synthesis, Characterization and Biomedical Application of Silver Nanoparticles. *Materials* **2022**, *15*, 427. [CrossRef] [PubMed]
14. Dorjnamjin, D.; Ariunaa, M.; Shim, Y.K. Synthesis of Silver Nanoparticles Using Hydroxyl Functionalized Ionic Liquids and Their Antimicrobial Activity. *Int. J. Mol. Sci.* **2008**, *9*, 807–820. [CrossRef] [PubMed]

15. Patil, R.S.; Kokate, M.R.; Salvi, P.P.; Kolekar, S.S. A novel one step synthesis of silver nanoparticles using room temperature ionic liquid and their biocidal activity. *Comptes Rendus Chim.* **2011**, *14*, 1122–1127. [CrossRef]
16. Aliakbari, E.; Nural, Y.; Zamiri, R.E.; Yabalak, E.; Mahdavi, M.; Yousefi, V. Design and synthesis of silver nanoparticle anchored poly(ionic liquid)s mesoporous for controlled anticancer drug delivery with antimicrobial effect. *Int. J. Environ. Health Res.* **2022**, *32*, 1–13. [CrossRef]
17. Ostwald, W. Blocking of Ostwald ripening allowing long-term stabilization. *Phys. Chem.* **1901**, *37*, 385.
18. Długosz, O.; Szostak, K.; Staroń, A.; Pulit-Prociak, J.; Banach, M. Methods for Reducing the Toxicity of Metal and Metal Oxide NPs as Biomedicine. *Materials* **2020**, *13*, 279. [CrossRef]
19. Ahrens, S.; Peritz, A.; Strassner, T. Tunable aryl alkyl ionic liquids (TAAILs): The next generation of ionic liquids. *Angew. Chem. Int. Ed.* **2009**, *48*, 7908–7910. [CrossRef]
20. Verma, C.; Ebenso, E.E.; Quraishi, M. Transition metal nanoparticles in ionic liquids: Synthesis and stabilization. *J. Mol. Liq.* **2019**, *276*, 826–849. [CrossRef]
21. Hassanpour, M.; Shahavi, M.H.; Heidari, G.; Kumar, A.; Nodehi, M.; Moghaddam, F.D.; Mohammadi, M.; Nikfarjam, N.; Sharifi, E.; Makvandi, P.; et al. Ionic liquid-mediated synthesis of metal nanostructures: Potential application in cancer diagnosis and therapy. *J. Ion. Liq.* **2022**, *2*, 100033. [CrossRef]
22. de Oliveira, P.F.M.; Torresi, R.M.; Emmerling, F.; Camargo, P.H.C. Challenges and opportunities in the bottom-up mechanochemical synthesis of noble metal nanoparticles. *J. Mater. Chem. A* **2020**, *8*, 16114–16141. [CrossRef]
23. Mangaiyarkarasi, R.; Priyanga, M.; Santhiya, N.; Umadevi, S. In situ preparation of palladium nanoparticles in ionic liquid crystal microemulsion and their application in Heck reaction. *J. Mol. Liq.* **2020**, *310*, 113241. [CrossRef]
24. Capek, I. Preparation of metal nanoparticles in water-in-oil (w/o) microemulsions. *Adv. Colloid Interface Sci.* **2004**, *110*, 49–74. [CrossRef]
25. Elshaarawy, R.F.M.; Eldeen, I.M.; Hassan, E.M. Efficient synthesis and evaluation of bis-pyridinium/bis-quinolinium metallosalophens as antibiotic and antitumor candidates. *J. Mol. Struct.* **2017**, *1128*, 162–173. [CrossRef]
26. Elshaarawy, R.F.M.; El-Azim, H.A.; Hegazy, W.H.; Mustafa, F.H.A.; Talkhan, T.A. Poly(ammonium/pyridinium)-chitosan Schiff base as a smart biosorbent for scavenging of Cu2+ ions from aqueous effluents. *Polym. Test.* **2020**, *83*, 106244. [CrossRef]
27. Refaee, A.A.; El-Naggar, M.E.; Mostafa, T.B.; Elshaarawy, R.F.M.; Nasr, A.M. Nano-bio finishing of cotton fabric with quaternized chitosan Schiff base-TiO2-ZnO nanocomposites for antimicrobial and UV protection applications. *Eur. Polym. J.* **2022**, *166*, 111040. [CrossRef]
28. Alfaifi, M.Y.; Shati, A.A.; Elbehairi, S.E.I.; Elshaarawy, R.F.M.; Gad, E.M. Fine-tuning of the pharmacological potential of novel thiazolium ionic liquids by anion alteration. *RSC Adv.* **2022**, *12*, 458–469. [CrossRef]
29. Kraynov, A.; Müller, T.E. Concepts for the stabilization of metal nanoparticles in ionic liquids. *Appl. Ionic Liquids Sci. Technol.* **2011**, *9*, 235–260.
30. Sidek, N.; Manan, N.S.A.; Mohamad, S. Efficient removal of phenolic compounds from model oil using benzyl Imidazolium-based ionic liquids. *J. Mol. Liq.* **2017**, *240*, 794–802. [CrossRef]
31. El-Sayed, W.N.; Alkabli, J.; Althumayri, K.; Elshaarawy, R.F.M.; Ismail, L.A. Azomethine-functionalized task-specific ionic liquid for diversion of toxic metal ions in the aqueous environment into pharmacological nominates. *J. Mol. Liq.* **2021**, *322*, 114525. [CrossRef]
32. Ibrahim, H.K.; El-Tamany, S.H.; El-Shaarawy, R.F.; El-Deen, I.M. Synthesis and investigation of mass spectra of some novel benzimidazole derivatives. *Maced. J. Chem. Chem. Eng.* **2008**, *27*, 65–79. [CrossRef]
33. Vitucci, F.M.; Trequattrini, F.; Palumbo, O.; Brubach, J.B.; Roy, P.; Paolone, A. Infrared spectra of bis(trifluoromethanesulfonyl)imide based ionic liquids: Experiments and DFT simulations. *Vib. Spectrosc.* **2014**, *74*, 81–87. [CrossRef]
34. Amendola, V.; Bakr, O.M.; Stellacci, F. A Study of the Surface Plasmon Resonance of Silver Nanoparticles by the Discrete Dipole Approximation Method: Effect of Shape, Size, Structure, and Assembly. *Plasmonics* **2010**, *5*, 85–97. [CrossRef]
35. Galbraith, H.; Miller, T.B. Physicochemical effects of long chain fatty acids on bacterial cells and their protoplasts. *J. Appl. Bacteriol.* **1973**, *36*, 647–658. [CrossRef]
36. Clements, A.; Gaboriaud, F.; Duval, J.F.; Farn, J.L.; Jenney, A.W.; Lithgow, T.; Wijburg, O.L.; Hartland, E.L.; Strugnell, R.A. The major surface-associated saccharides of Klebsiella pneumoniae contribute to host cell association. *PLoS ONE* **2008**, *3*, e3817. [CrossRef]
37. Szewczyk, O.K.; Roszczenko, P.; Czarnomysy, R.; Bielawska, A.; Bielawski, K. An overview of the importance of transition-metal nanoparticles in cancer research. *Int. J. Mol. Sci.* **2022**, *23*, 6688. [CrossRef]
38. Gopinath, K.; Karthika, V.; Gowri, S.; Senthilkumar, V.; Kumaresan, S.; Arumugam, A. Antibacterial activity of ruthenium nanoparticles synthesized using Gloriosa superba L. leaf extract. *J. Nanostructure Chem.* **2014**, *4*, 83. [CrossRef]
39. Lewinski, N.; Colvin, V.; Drezek, R. Cytotoxicity of Nanoparticles. *Small* **2008**, *4*, 26–49. [CrossRef]
40. Jiang, H.S.; Zhang, Y.; Lu, Z.W.; Lebrun, R.; Gontero, B.; Li, W. Interaction between Silver Nanoparticles and Two Dehydrogenases: Role of Thiol Groups. *Small* **2019**, *15*, 1900860. [CrossRef]
41. Prabhu, S.; Poulose, E.K. Silver nanoparticles: Mechanism of antimicrobial action, synthesis, medical applications, and toxicity effects. *Int. Nano Lett.* **2012**, *2*, 32. [CrossRef]
42. Riduan, S.N.; Zhang, Y. Imidazolium salts and their polymeric materials for biological applications. *Chem. Soc. Rev.* **2013**, *42*, 9055–9070. [CrossRef] [PubMed]

43. Bakshi, K.; Mitra, S.; Sharma, V.K.; Jayadev, M.S.K.; Sakai, V.G.; Mukhopadhyay, R.; Gupta, A.; Ghosh, S.K. Imidazolium-based ionic liquids cause mammalian cell death due to modulated structures and dynamics of cellular membrane. *Biochim. Et. Biophys. Acta (BBA)-Biomembr.* **2020**, *1862*, 183103. [CrossRef] [PubMed]
44. Gholami, A.; Shams, M.S.; Abbaszadegan, A.; Nabavizadeh, M. Ionic liquids as capping agents of silver nanoparticles. Part II: Antimicrobial and cytotoxic study. *Green Process. Synth.* **2021**, *10*, 585–593. [CrossRef]
45. Avirdi, E.; Paumo, H.K.; Kamdem, B.P.; Singh, M.B.; Kumari, K.; Katata-Seru, L.M.; Bahadur, I. Influence of cation (imidazolium based ionic liquids) as "smart" stabilizers for silver nanoparticles and their evaluation as antibacterial activity on Escherichia coli, Staphylococcus aureus and Enterobacter cloacae. *J. Mol. Liq.* **2023**, *369*, 120695. [CrossRef]
46. Docherty, K.M.; Kulpa, J.C.F. Toxicity and antimicrobial activity of imidazolium and pyridinium ionic liquids. *Green Chem.* **2005**, *7*, 185–189. [CrossRef]
47. Corrêa, C.M.; Bizeto, M.A.; Camilo, F.F. Direct synthesis of silver nanoparticles in ionic liquid. *J. Nanopart. Res.* **2016**, *18*, 132. [CrossRef]
48. Setua, P.; Pramanik, R.; Sarkar, S.; Ghatak, C.; Rao, V.G.; Sarkar, N.; Das, S.K. Synthesis of silver nanoparticle in imidazolium and pyrolidium based ionic liquid reverse micelles: A step forward in nanostructure inorganic material in room temperature ionic liquid field. *J. Mol. Liq.* **2011**, *162*, 33–37. [CrossRef]
49. Sun, X.; Qiang, Q.; Yin, Z.; Wang, Z.; Ma, Y.; Zhao, C. Monodispersed silver-palladium nanoparticles for ethanol oxidation reaction achieved by controllable electrochemical synthesis from ionic liquid microemulsions. *J. Colloid Interface Sci.* **2019**, *557*, 450–457. [CrossRef]
50. Elshaarawy, R.F.; Tadros, H.R.; Abd El-Aal, R.M.; Mustafa, F.H.; Soliman, Y.A.; Hamed, M.A. Hybrid molecules comprising 1,2,4-triazole or diaminothiadiazole Schiff-bases and ionic liquid moieties as potent antibacterial and marine antibiofouling nominees. *J. Environ. Chem. Eng.* **2016**, *4*, 2754–2764. [CrossRef]
51. Elshaarawy, R.F.; Lan, Y.; Janiak, C. Oligonuclear homo-and mixed-valence manganese complexes based on thiophene-or aryl-carboxylate ligation: Synthesis, characterization and magnetic studies. *Inorg. Chim. Acta* **2013**, *401*, 85–94. [CrossRef]
52. Elshaarawy, R.F.M.; Ismail, L.A.; Alfaifi, M.Y.; Rizk, M.A.; Eltamany, E.E.; Janiak, C. Inhibitory activity of biofunctionalized silver-capped N-methylated water-soluble chitosan thiomer for microbial and biofilm infections. *Int. J. Biol. Macromol.* **2020**, *152*, 709–717. [CrossRef] [PubMed]

Disclaimer/Publisher's Note: The statements, opinions and data contained in all publications are solely those of the individual author(s) and contributor(s) and not of MDPI and/or the editor(s). MDPI and/or the editor(s) disclaim responsibility for any injury to people or property resulting from any ideas, methods, instructions or products referred to in the content.

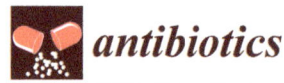

Review

Carbonic Anhydrase Inhibitors as Novel Antibacterials in the Era of Antibiotic Resistance: Where Are We Now?

Alessio Nocentini [1], Clemente Capasso [2],*, and Claudiu T. Supuran [1],*

1. NEUROFARBA Department, Section of Pharmaceutical and Nutraceutical Sciences, University of Florence, 50019 Firenze, Italy
2. Department of Biology, Agriculture and Food Sciences, Institute of Biosciences and Bioresources, CNR, 80131 Napoli, Italy
* Correspondence: clemente.capasso@ibbr.cnr.it (C.C.); claudiu.supuran@unifi.it (C.T.S.)

Abstract: Resistance to antibiotic treatment developed by bacteria in humans and animals occurs when the microorganisms resist treatment with clinically approved antibiotics. Actions must be implemented to stop the further development of antibiotic resistance and the subsequent emergence of superbugs. Medication repurposing/repositioning is one strategy that can help find new antibiotics, as it speeds up drug development phases. Among them, the Zn^{2+} ion binders, such as sulfonamides and their bioisosteres, are considered the most promising compounds to obtain novel antibacterials, thus avoiding antibiotic resistance. Sulfonamides and their bioisosteres have drug-like properties well-known for decades and are suitable lead compounds for developing new pharmacological agent families for inhibiting carbonic anhydrases (CAs). CAs are a superfamily of metalloenzymes catalyzing the reversible reaction of CO_2 hydration to HCO_3^- and H^+, being present in most bacteria in multiple genetic families (α-, β-, γ- and ι-classes). These enzymes, acting as CO_2 transducers, are promising drug targets because their activity influences microbe proliferation, biosynthetic pathways, and pathogen persistence in the host. In their natural or slightly modified scaffolds, sulfonamides/sulfamates/sulamides inhibit CAs in vitro and in vivo, in mouse models infected with antibiotic-resistant strains, confirming thus their role in contrasting bacterial antibiotic resistance.

Keywords: carbonic anhydrase; sulfonamides; inhibitors; antibiotic resistance; bacteria

1. Introduction

Antibiotic resistance is a worldwide emergency that kills more people than HIV/AIDS and malaria combined [1]. It kills around 30,000 people in Europe each year, with Italy accounting for one-third of them [2,3]. In addition, antibiotic-resistant illnesses have a significant effect on public health services [4]. Antibiotic resistance is the ability of bacteria to counteract the action of one or more of the commune FDA-approved antibiotics (Figure 1) [4,5]. The antibiotics reported in Figure 1 act as suppressors of cell wall synthesis, inhibitors of proteins or nucleic acids synthesis, membrane destroyers, antimetabolites, and competitive antagonists of substrates used in biosynthetic reactions [6]. It is essential to understand that humans and other animals do not acquire antibiotic resistance; instead, this phenomenon is developed by bacteria harbored in humans and animals [3]. When placed under selective pressure due to antibiotics, bacteria that have acquired a greater capacity for resistance (by DNA mutation or DNA genetic transfer) will have a greater chance of surviving and instead will occupy the environment vacated by bacteria that have been eliminated by therapy [7].

Thus, to treat infections caused by those resistant bacteria, one strategy is to administer other antibiotics to which they are sensitive. However, they might also acquire resistance to the new class of antibiotics (multi-resistant organisms), and so switching to a new type of antibiotic is required until we arrive at bacteria resistant to all antibiotics (pan-resistant microorganisms) [8]. The antibiotic resistance phenomenon is associated with the

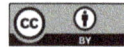

misuse and overprescribing of these drugs, as well as the inappropriate administration of antibiotics to companion animals and animals in the agriculture industry [9,10]. In livestock farms or aquacultures all over the world, antibiotics are routinely used not only to treat diseases, as is the case in human medicine but also to prevent diseases and as promoters of animal growth [11]. Furthermore, the rising discharge of antibiotics into waterways and soils poses a risk to all microorganisms in these habitats [11]. Thus, bacteria can become resistant and infect people who came in touch with the polluted environment, animals, or meat. Therefore, policies must be put in place to combat both the spread and future development of antibiotic resistance, as well as the oncoming wave of superbugs [12].

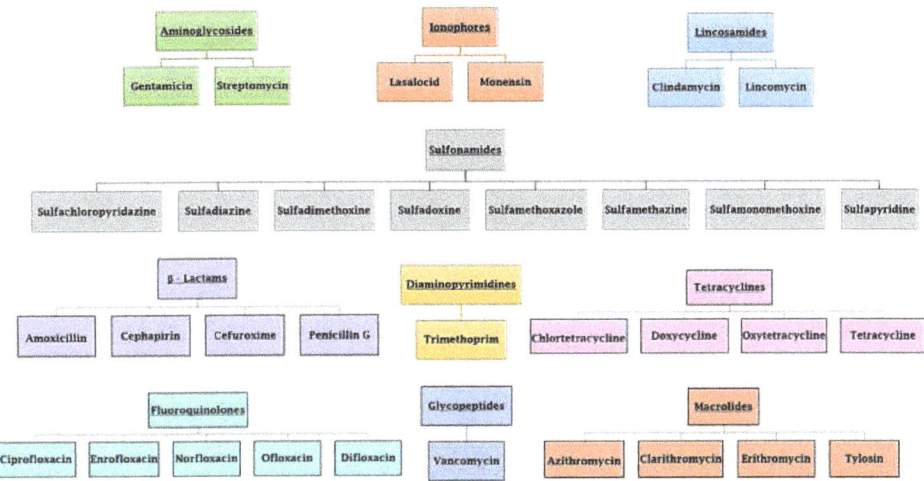

Figure 1. Various types of FDA-approved antibiotics. Class and antibiotic name are reported.

How do we intervene to stop antibiotic resistance? There is no shortage of strategies for dealing with the antibiotic resistance [13–16]. Among them, one may consider: (i) community- and healthcare-based approaches for infection control and prevention; (ii) vaccine preparation, which may have a good chance of preventing bacterial illnesses (up to date, only for *Streptococcus pneumoniae*, one of the six most hazardous antibiotic-resistant bacteria, exists such a vaccine); (iii) reduction of the use of antibiotics in non-human infection-treatment contexts, such as livestock farms; (iv) appropriate antibiotic use, as well as stopping their use for the management of viral infections; (v) maintenance of investments to make second-line antibiotics available, and the development of novel antibiotics and especially those with novel modes of action less susceptible to the onset of resistance, which can save lives [13–16]. This last strategy is fundamental, but new drug development takes a long time; most candidate compounds were in the research and development pipelines for over a decade before they made it to market [17]. Moreover, the most critical points are that the majority of the new antibiotics in development are variants of preexisting antibiotic classes, do not have a novel mechanism of action, and only a small number of them are expected to be effective against the **ESKAPE** pathogens (*Enterococcus faecium*, *Staphylococcus aureus*, *Klebsiella pneumoniae*, *Acinetobacter baumanii*, *Pseudomonas aeruginosa*, and *Enterobacter*). Finally, the future of antibiotics is shaky because of questions about their effectiveness and safety [18,19].

In this context, the drug repurposing or drug repositioning strategy offers the potential to "fast-track" the identification of novel antibiotics, since it speeds up the drug research process and reduces the time to market [20]. FDA-approved medications are considered the "existing drugs," and their repurposing reduces clinical development risk, making them attractive candidates [20].

2. A Superfamily of CO$_2$ Transducer Biomolecules: The Carbonic Anhydrase

2.1. Bacterial Carbonic Anhydrase

Carbon dioxide (CO$_2$) is a gas released into the atmosphere due to cellular respiration and oxidative metabolism, and all living creatures are responsible for its production [21]. In most cases, the process of transporting this waste gas out of cells is carried out by passive diffusion [22]. In many cases, the CO$_2$ channels, controlled by CO$_2$ levels inside the cell, make this transfer easier. However, CO$_2$ is not merely a waste product; it can also trigger various cellular signaling pathways to increase bacteria virulence and pathogenicity [23]. Bacteria can adapt to their environment by sensing and responding to CO$_2$, enhancing thus their chances of survival. This may be crucial because bacteria have to adapt to the relatively low CO$_2$ levels of the outer atmosphere for the higher CO$_2$ levels found inside most multicellular host organisms [23]. Bacteria, for example, may upregulate virulence factors at host physiologic CO$_2$ levels rather than ambient CO$_2$ levels to aid colonization or infection. Several such examples are *Vibrio cholerae*, which causes cholera, and produces enterotoxin as carbon dioxide levels rise, whereas bicarbonate produced by the CO$_2$ hydration is the first positive effector of the primary *V. cholerae* virulence gene transcription activator (ToxT), responsible for the cholera virulence cascade [24]. *Pseudomonas aeruginosa*, which can lead to infections in the blood, lungs (pneumonia), or other regions of the body following surgery, lives in vastly varying CO$_2$ settings depending on whether or not it is colonizing a host [25].

Biomolecules in microbes related to CO$_2$-sensitive pathways or acting as a CO$_2$ transducer have been proposed as appealing targets for medicines, since they control cell development and the subsequent synthesis of chemicals, enhancing the pathogen persistence in the host [26,27]. In this context, a crucial role is played by a superfamily of molecules known as carbonic anhydrases (CAs, EC 4.2.1.1). CAs can be thought as molecules that, rather than instantly detecting a change in CO$_2$, serve as CO$_2$ transducers, adjusting its levels [23,28]. With their activity, the CAs encoded by the bacterial genome of pathogenic and non-pathogenic bacteria provide the indispensable CO$_2$ and HCO$_3^-$/protons to microbial biosynthetic pathways, catalyzing the reversible reaction of CO$_2$ hydration to HCO$_3^-$ and H$^+$ (CO$_2$ + H$_2$O $\rightleftharpoons$ HCO$_3^-$ + H$^+$) [28]. Here, we stress the fact that the non-catalytic CO$_2$ hydration/dehydration reaction is too slow at physiological pH values to fulfill the organism's metabolic demands ($k_{cat\,(hydration)}$ = 0.15 s^{-1}; $k_{cat\,(dehydration)}$ = 50.0 s^{-1}) [29].

The classification system for CAs uses the Greek letters to represent the eight distinct families (or classes): α, β, γ, δ, ζ, η, θ, and ι [29–33]. The eight distinct CA-classes descend from the same ancestor, yet exhibit significant evolutionary diversity. The representative amino acid sequences of each CA-class show low sequence similarity, characteristic folds, and structures compared to the polypeptide chain of other CAs belonging to a different class [34–38]. In contrast, the mechanism involved in the reversible hydration of CO$_2$ is strictly conserved across all CA-classes, illustrating the CA superfamily's convergent evolution [34–38]. CAs are generally metalloenzymes with catalytic sites that contain a metal ion cofactor required for catalysis (Figure 2). The ion cofactor in many CAs is Zn^{2+}, which is coordinated by three amino acid residues from the protein backbone [29,30,39]. The fourth metal ion ligand is a water molecule/hydroxide ion that acts as the nucleophile in the enzyme's catalytic cycle. Metal ions other than Zn^{2+}, such as Co^{2+}, Cd^{2+}, Fe^{2+}, and Mn^{2+}, can be coordinated by several CA-classes [40–47]. Recently, it has been demonstrated that the newly discovered CA-class, the ι-CA, shows catalytic activity without the need for metal ions, as shown from the X-ray crystal structure of *Anabaena* sp. [48]. The CA-classes differ in the amino acid residues involved in metal coordination [49–52]. For example, the ion metal is coordinated by three His residues in the α, β, and γ-CAs and presumably θ-classes [42,45,53,54]; one His and two Cys residues in the β- and ζ-CAs [41]; and two His and one Gln residue in the η-class. α-CAs usually act as monomers or dimers; β-CAs only behave as dimers, tetramers, or octamers. To perform their catalytic activity, the γ-CAs must be trimers [55]. A tandemly repeated hexapeptide characterizes γ-CA monomers and is required for the left-hand fold of trimeric-helix structures. The X-ray structure of the θ-CAs was remarkably similar to that of some β-CAs [42,45,53,54]. The crystal structure of ζ-CA showed three slightly different active sites on the same polypeptide chain. Regarding the structural organization of δ- and η-CAs, no data are currently available, and a homology modelling of the η-CA was built [56]. Interestingly, only the α, η, θ, and ι -CAs have been shown to catalyze the esters/thioesters hydrolysis, while the other CA families lacked any detectable esterase activity [29,30,39,57–59]. Presently, four CA-classes (α, β, γ, and ι) have been demonstrated to exist in bacteria, and their distribution is noteworthy [34–38]. In many cases, the bacterial genome encodes for the three CA-classes (α, β, and γ) and rarely for the ι- class. However, it is common to find bacteria whose genomes encodes just one or two CAs, and very rarely none [27,29,33,49]. Moreover, the structural variations between bacterial and human α-CAs allow for the synthesis of inhibitors that target the bacterial enzyme but not the mammalian ones. Again, in some cases, the pathogenic bacterial genome encodes for CA-classes, which are absent in mammals, whose genome encodes only for α-CA, increasing the likelihood of success in treating the bacterial illness with compounds that act only on the bacterial CAs. Interestingly, for each CA-class has been obtained the X-ray crystallographic structures (Figure 3). It has been observed that α-CAs reside in the periplasmic region of bacteria cells and prevent CO_2 loss from bacteria by converting CO_2 into bicarbonate, which is then transported inside the cytoplasm by bicarbonate transporters [29–31,33]. On the other hand, cytoplasmic β- and γ -CA classes are responsible for carrying out intracellular functions such as maintaining CO_2 and HCO_3^- equilibrium and regulating pH. Recently, β, γ, and ι-CAs with signal peptide at N-terminus have been found, attributing them a putative periplasmic localization and a physiological role similar to those mentioned above for the α-CAs [31,32,39,57–59].

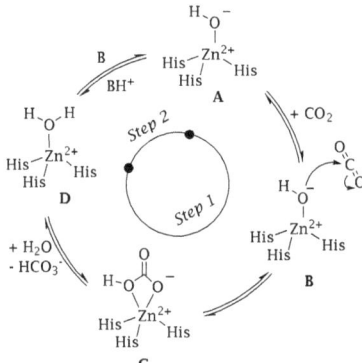

Figure 2. CA catalytic mechanism schematically represented for a α-class isoform.

2.2. CAs Help Bacteria to Survive

In the literature, many shreds of evidence support the opinion that the activity of CAs is connected to the survival of microbes because these enzymes are essential for supporting numerous physiological functions involving dissolved inorganic carbon, such as transport and supply of CO_2 or HCO_3^-, pH homeostasis, secretion of electrolytes/toxins, and biosynthetic processes [29,33,60]. For example, it has been proven in vivo that bacterial growth at ambient CO_2 concentrations is dependent on CA activity in bacteria such as *Ralstonia eutropha* (Gram-negative bacterium found in soil and water) and *Escherichia coli* (Gram-negative bacterium) [61–63]. In *E. coli*, the two β-CAs (CynT and CynT2) generate HCO_3^- to prevent bicarbonate depletion from cyanate breakdown and bacterial expansion at atmospheric CO_2 concentrations, respectively [62,63]. More intriguing is the in vivo evidence that CAs have a role in the proliferation of harmful bacteria such as *Mycobacterium tuberculosis* [64–68], *Helicobacter pylori* [69–71], *Vibrio cholerae* [72], *Brucella suis* [65–68], *Salmonella enterica* [73–75], and *Pseudomonas aeruginosa* [76]. CAs encoded by the genome of *H. pylori*, a Gram-negative, microaerophilic bacteria that colonizes the human stomach, are essential for the pathogen's acid acclimation and, consequently, survival in the severe environment typical of this organ, with pH values as low as 1.5–2.0 [69–71]. In addition to CAs, urease is the other enzymatic system used by the microbe for growing in this extreme environment. Under acidic conditions, urea goes into the cytoplasm through the urea channel. In the bacterial cytoplasm, $2NH_3$ and CO_2 are produced by the hydrolysis of urea [69–71]. The resulting CO_2 is then hydrated by β-CA, while the periplasmic α-CA hydrates the CO_2 diffused in the periplasm. The produced ions (H^+) by the CA-catalyzed reaction are used to form NH_4^+ by reacting with NH_3^+ in the periplasm and cytoplasm, which neutralizes the entering acid in the above environments [69–71]. In the case of the pathogenic bacterium *Vibrio cholerae*, a Gram-negative bacterium already mentioned above, CAs are involved in the production of sodium bicarbonate, which stimulates the development of cholera toxin [24]. It has been proposed that *V. cholerae* employs CAs to colonize the host [72]. Again, the brucellosis causal agent, *Brucella suis*, a non-motile Gram-negative coccobacillus, and *Mycobacterium tuberculosis*, a pathogenic bacterium that causes tuberculosis, were demonstrated to require functional CAs to proliferate [64–68]. Furthermore, through in vivo gene expression investigations on the bacterium *Salmonella enterica*, the MIG5 gene, which encodes for a CA that is significantly expressed during bacterial infection, has been found [73–75]. The deletion of the gene encoding this CA (psCA1) in the *Pseudomonas aeruginosa* reduced pathogenicity by decreasing calcium salt depositions [77].

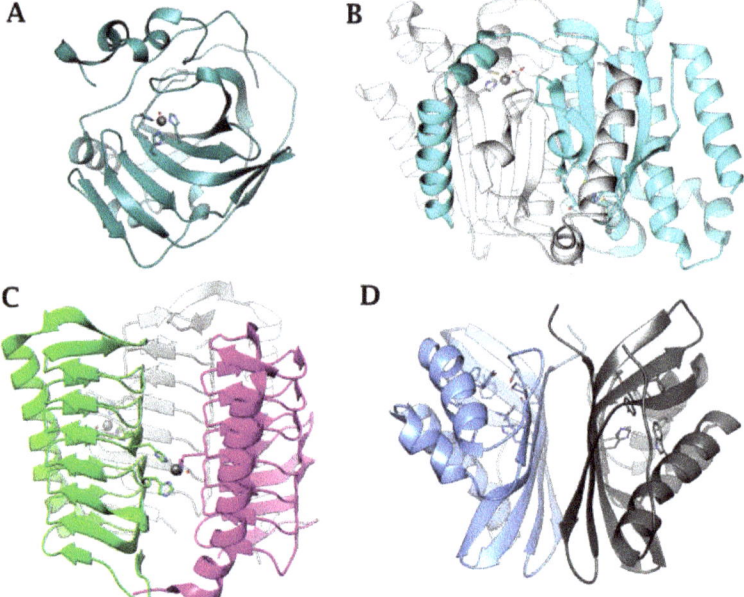

Figure 3. Ribbon view of (**A**) α-CA from *Neisseria gonorrhoeae* (PDB 1KOQ), (**B**) β-CA from *Escherichia coli* (PDB 1I6O), (**C**) γ-CA from *Burkholderia pseudomallei* (PDB 7ZW9), (**D**) ι-CA from *B. territorii* built by homology using PDB 3H51 as a template.

2.3. Carbonic Anhydrase Sulfonamide Inhibitors

Because the many biochemical processes mentioned above involve the activity of bacterial CAs, their inhibition may reduce the pathogen's survival and fitness. The good news is that CA inhibition suppresses bacterial growth differently from those demonstrated by traditional antibiotics, toward which the bacteria have developed or are developing antibiotic resistance. As reported in the scientific literature, many unique chemical classes of CA inhibitors (CAIs) exist [60]. The CAIs are classified into four distinct types based on how the inhibitors bind and inhibit the CA metalloenzymes. Four types of inhibitor-enzyme binding are currently known, based on whether the binding involves the catalytic metal ion or the metal coordinated-water molecule or how the active site is obstructed [78]. Therefore, there are metal ion binders (anion, sulfonamides and their bioisosteres, dithiocarbamates, xanthates, and so on); chemicals that bind to the zinc-coordinated water molecule/hydroxide ion (phenols, polyamines, thioxocoumarins, sulfocumarins); compounds that obstruct the active site entrance (coumarins and related isosteres); and compounds that bind out of the active site (carboxylate) [78].

Among these types, the Zn^{2+} ion binders, in particular, the sulfonamides and their bioisosteres, are considered the most promising compounds for the realization of novel antibacterials, avoiding antibiotic resistance [78–81]. Here, we emphasize that the sulfonamides/sulfamates/sulfamides able to inhibit the CA specifically are nonantibiotic inhibitors characterized by a primary sulfonamide moiety, having the following chemical formula: R-X-SO$_2$-NH$_2$, where R can be an aromatic, heterocyclic, aliphatic, or sugar scaffold, X = nothing, O or NH. Thus, sulfanilamide led to the discovery of the sulfa drugs and benzenesulfonamide CAIs of the type. They constitute an important class of drugs since they have drug-like properties well-known for decades and are suitable lead compounds for developing new pharmacological agent families for inhibiting CAs. Among them are the commercial derivatives 1–24 (Figure 4) and the clinically used agent **AAZ-EPA** (Figure 5). The series **AAZ-EPA** include acetazolamide (**AAZ**), methazolamide (**MZA**), ethoxzolamide (**EZA**), and dichlorophenamide (**DCP**) are classical, systemically working antiglaucoma CAIs. Dorzolamide (**DZA**) and brinzolamide (**BRZ**) are topically acting antiglaucoma agents. Benzolamide (**BZA**) is an orphan drug belonging to this class of pharmacological agents. Zonisamide (**ZNS**), sulthiame (**SLT**), and sulfamic acid ester topiramate (**TPM**) are widely used antiepileptic drugs. Sulpiride (**SLP**) and indisulam (**IND**) were also shown by our group to belong to this class of pharmacological agents, together with the COX2 selective inhibitors celecoxib (**CLX**) and valdecoxib (**VLX**). Saccharin (**SAC**) and the diuretic hydrochlorothiazide (**HCT**) are also known to act as CAIs. Famotidine (**FAM**) and epacadostat (**EPA**) are CAI sulfamide drugs clinically used respectively as a histamine H2 receptor antagonist and a selective indoleamine-2,3-dioxygenase 1 inhibitor. These inhibitors bind Zn (II) in a tetrahedral geometry, forming an extended network of hydrogen bonds with the enzyme amino acid residues, whereas the aromatic/heterocyclic portions of the inhibitor interact with the hydrophilic and hydrophobic residues found in the enzyme catalytic cavity, according to enzyme-inhibitor X-ray crystallographic data (Figure 6) [60].

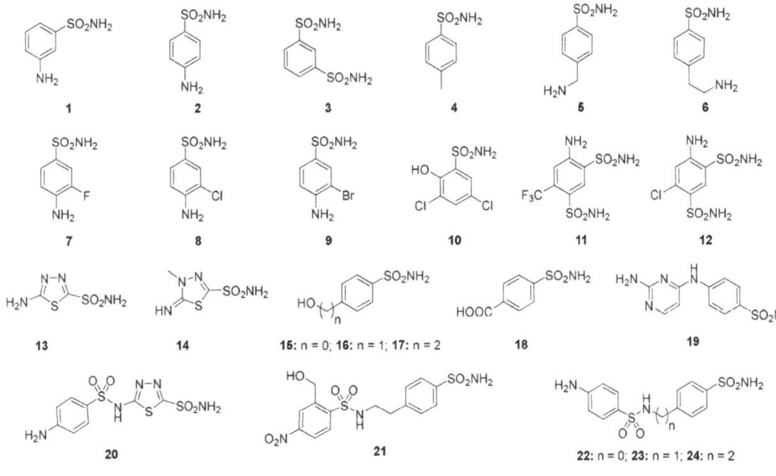

Figure 4. Structure of commercially available sulfonamide derivatives 1–24.

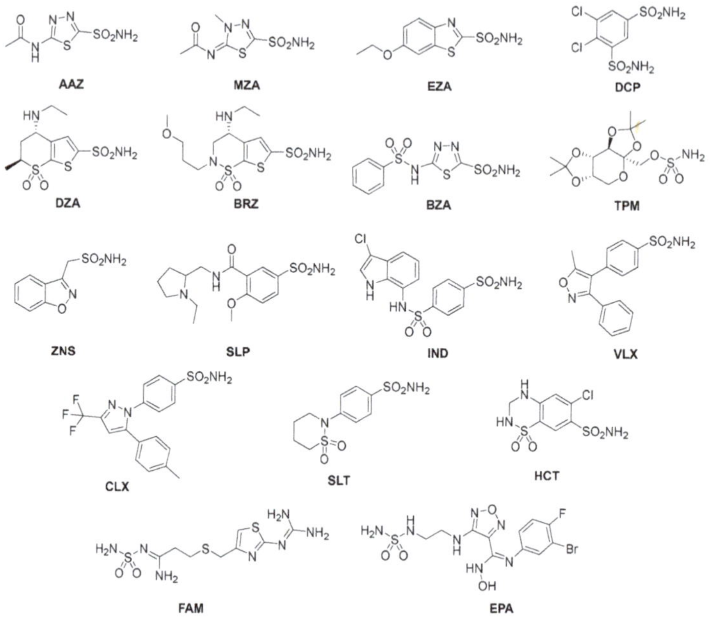

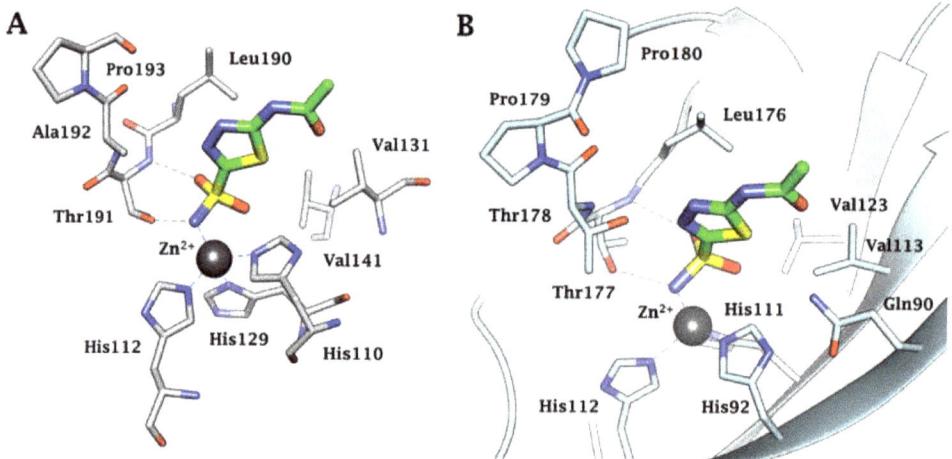

Figure 5. Structure of clinically used sulfonamide/sulfamate/sulfamide derivatives **AAZ-HCT**.

Figure 6. (**A**) Active site view of the α-CA of *Helicobacter pylori* in adduct with **AAZ** (4YGF). (**B**) Active site ribbon view of the α-CA of *N. gonorrhoeae* in adduct with **AAZ** (8DYQ). H-bonds are represented as black dashed lines.

3. Where Are We NOW with the Inhibition of the Bacterial CAs

In the last decade, several in vitro experiments were conducted employing the CAIs outlined in the preceding paragraph to inhibit the four bacterial CA classes (α, β, γ, and ι). Many of these studies were focused on bacterial CAs derived from pathogenic bacteria, such as *Mycobacterium tuberculosis*, *Vibrio cholerae*, *Francisella tularensis*, *Burkholderia pseudomallei*, *Porphyromonas gingivalis*, *Legionella pneumophila*, *Clostridium perfringens*, *Mammaliccosu sciuri*, etc. [36,82–85]. Most sulfonamide CAIs exert potent inhibition on most recombinant CAs belonging to the bacteria mentioned above [34,86–90]. The most interesting aspect was that, some of these CAIs, including acetazolamide and methazolamide, significantly limit the growth of bacteria in cell cultures [91]. In this context, some experimental shreds of evidence prove that the inhibition of bacteria CAs can be potentially used to combat the resistance of many pathogens to the existing antimicrobial drugs.

For example, ethoxzolamide (**EZA**), an authorized diuretic and carbonic anhydrase inhibitor, kills *Helicobacter pylori* in vitro, suggesting it could be turned into an anti-*H. pylori* medication [92].

The influence of the selective CA inhibitor **AAZ** on the bacterial lifecycle was tested by analyzing the growth of *E. coli* and its consumption of glucose, added as the only carbon source to the bacterial culture media [93]. Carbon sources are required for biosynthetic activities and metabolism is directly correlated with the rate at which carbon sources are used. The FDA-approved carbonic anhydrase **AAZ** was able to interfere with *E. coli* growth and glucose uptake at 31.2 µg/mL. Intriguingly, **AAZ** resulted in a good inhibitor of the two recombinant *E. coli* CAs, β-CA (CynT2) and γ-CA (EcoCAγ), with a K_I of 227 and 248 nM, respectively [94,95]. AAZ prevents sugar consumption due to its inhibitory action on bacterial CAs, which are directly engaged in providing CO_2/HCO_3^- required for the bacterial metabolic need [93].

It has been reproposed the FDA-approved carbonic anhydrase drug **AAZ** could be used to design potent antienterococcal agents. The authors, modifying the **AAZ** scaffold, arrived at two leads possessing improved potency against clinical vancomycin-resistant enterococci (VRE) strains [96]. The classical **AAZ** showed a MIC of 2 µg/mL, while the two leads had a MIC = 0.007 µg/mL and 1 µg/mL, respectively. **DZA**, another classical CAIs, resulted in MIC values of 1–8 µg/mL against a panel of clinical VRE isolates [97]. Based on the results of homology modeling and molecular dynamics simulations, the authors demonstrated that the α and γ CAs encoded by the Vancomycin-Resistant Enterococcus are the intracellular targets of the compounds [96,98]. In addition, **AAZ** fared better than linezolid (a standard drug for VRE infections) when tested in two in vivo VRE mouse models –murine colonization–reduction and VRE septicemia [99].

Finally, **AAZ** inhibited the growth of the Gram-negative bacterium *Neisseria gonorrhoeae* both in the in vitro as well as in vivo mouse model of a gonococcal genital tract infection [100,101]. Recently, Portela et al. [102] demonstrated that sulfonamide pretreatment has a positive outcome on the strength of dentin and the prevention of *Streptococcus mutans* colonization in teeth treated with two potent bacterial CA sulfonamide inhibitors [102].

It is also interesting to note that over the last few years, there has been a significant focus on developing non-classical CAIs for treating multiple diseases due to the prevalence of sulfonamide allergies among the general population as well as their use as potential new antibacterials [103]. The classes of non-classical inhibitors that show strong potential as lead compounds for isoform-specific drug design include phenols, polyamines, carboxylic acids, and coumarins and their derivatives. These compounds can anchor to the zinc-bound water/hydroxide ion or bind outside the active site to block substrate entry, exhibiting atypical binding mechanisms of the classical sulfonamide CAIs [103].

4. Conclusions

The well-known zinc-binding groups (ZBGs), such as the primary sulfonamide (-SO_2NH_2), primary sulfamate (-OSO_2NH_2), and sulfamide (-$NHSO_2NH_2$), which are present in the structure of several clinically-approved drugs and an increasing number of investigational medicines, have been proven to affect the inhibition of the CAs encoded by pathogenic bacteria [78–81]. Intriguingly, various types of these nonantibiotic sulfonamides, many of which offer pharmacologic applications as antiglaucoma, antiobesity, antitumor, or diuretic, resulted in potent inhibitors (k_I in the nanomolar range) of such CAs. These findings prompt scientists to consider the CAIs as a new approach to fight antibiotic resistance developed by bacteria versus the common FDA-approved antibiotics. Unlike common antibiotics, the CAIs impair the growth of pathogenic bacteria through a novel mechanism of action: perturbating/depleting the intracellular levels of CO_2 and HCO_3^-, which are necessary to microbial biosynthetic pathways. In addition, the antibacterial growth due to the CA inhibition is strongly supported by the fact that the slow non-catalytic CO_2 hydration/dehydration reaction is unable to restore these levels. These attractive facts led to the writing of fascinating manuscripts that discuss the repurposing of drugs such as ethoxzolamide (**EZA**), acetazolamide (**AZA**), and dorzolamide (**DZA**) as treatments for interfering with the life cycle of *E. coli, Helicobacter pylori, Neisseria gonorrhoeae*, and vancomycin-resistant enterococci.

In conclusion, the licensed sulfonamides/sulfamates/sulfamides acting as CAIs exhibit antibacterial properties in their native or slightly modified scaffolds [97], hypothesizing that the CAIs can be potentially employed either by themselves or in conjunction with an antibiotic or even as "antibiotic adjuvants" to increase the effectiveness of certain antibiotics.

Author Contributions: Supervision, C.T.S. and C.C.; Writing—original draft, C.C.; Writing—review and editing, A.N., C.T.S. and C.C. All authors have read and agreed to the published version of the manuscript.

Funding: This research was funded by the Italian Ministry of University and Research, project FISR2019_04819 BacCAD (to C.T.S. and C.C.).

Institutional Review Board Statement: Not applicable.

Informed Consent Statement: Not applicable.

Data Availability Statement: Not applicable.

Acknowledgments: We are grateful to Valentina Brasiello for her assistance.

Conflicts of Interest: The authors declare no conflict of interest.

References

1. Doolan, J.A.; Williams, G.T.; Hilton, K.L.F.; Chaudhari, R.; Fossey, J.S.; Goult, B.T.; Hiscock, J.R. Advancements in antimicrobial nanoscale materials and self-assembling systems. *Chem. Soc. Rev.* **2022**, *51*, 8696–8755. [CrossRef]
2. Wagenlehner, F.M.E.; Dittmar, F. Re: Global Burden of Bacterial Antimicrobial Resistance in 2019: A Systematic Analysis. *Eur. Urol.* **2022**, *82*, 658–670. [CrossRef]
3. European Food Safety Authority; European Centre for Disease Prevention and Control. The European Union Summary Report on Antimicrobial Resistance in zoonotic and indicator bacteria from humans, animals and food in 2019–2020. *EFSA J.* **2022**, *20*, e07209.
4. Reardon, S. Resistance to last-ditch antibiotic has spread farther than anticipated. *Nature* **2017**. [CrossRef]
5. Uruen, C.; Garcia, C.; Fraile, L.; Tommassen, J.; Arenas, J. How Streptococcus suis escapes antibiotic treatments. *Vet. Res.* **2022**, *53*, 91–123. [CrossRef]
6. Kapoor, G.; Saigal, S.; Elongavan, A. Action and resistance mechanisms of antibiotics: A guide for clinicians. *J. Anaesthesiol. Clin. Pharmacol.* **2017**, *33*, 300–305. [CrossRef]
7. Oz, T.; Guvenek, A.; Yildiz, S.; Karaboga, E.; Tamer, Y.T.; Mumcuyan, N.; Ozan, V.B.; Senturk, G.H.; Cokol, M.; Yeh, P.; et al. Strength of Selection Pressure Is an Important Parameter Contributing to the Complexity of Antibiotic Resistance Evolution. *Mol. Biol. Evol* **2014**, *31*, 2387–2401. [CrossRef]
8. Magiorakos, A.P.; Srinivasan, A.; Carey, R.B.; Carmeli, Y.; Falagas, M.E.; Giske, C.G.; Harbarth, S.; Hindler, J.F.; Kahlmeter, G.; Olsson-Liljequist, B.; et al. Multidrug-resistant, extensively drug-resistant and pandrug-resistant bacteria: An international expert proposal for interim standard definitions for acquired resistance. *Clin. Microbiol. Infect.* **2012**, *18*, 268–281. [CrossRef]
9. Sulis, G.; Pai, M.; Gandra, S. Comment on: Global consumption of antimicrobials: Impact of the WHO Global Action Plan on Antimicrobial Resistance and 2019 coronavirus pandemic (COVID-19). *J. Antimicrob. Chemother.* **2022**, *77*, 2891–2892. [CrossRef]
10. Iwu, C.D.; Patrick, S.M. An insight into the implementation of the global action plan on antimicrobial resistance in the WHO African region: A roadmap for action. *Int. J. Antimicrob. Agents* **2021**, *58*, 106411–106417. [CrossRef]
11. Cycon, M.; Mrozik, A.; Piotrowska-Seget, Z. Antibiotics in the Soil Environment-Degradation and Their Impact on Microbial Activity and Diversity. *Front. Microbiol.* **2019**, *10*, 338–382. [CrossRef]
12. Pusparajah, P.; Letchumanan, V.; Goh, B.H.; McGaw, L.J. Editorial: Novel Approaches to the Treatment of Multidrug-Resistant Bacteria. *Front. Pharmacol.* **2022**, *13*, 972935–972937. [CrossRef]
13. da Silva, T.H.; Hachigian, T.Z.; Lee, J.; King, M.D. Using computers to ESKAPE the antibiotic resistance crisis. *Drug Discov. Today* **2022**, *27*, 456–470. [CrossRef]

14. Nataraj, B.H.; Mallappa, R.H. Antibiotic Resistance Crisis: An Update on Antagonistic Interactions between Probiotics and Methicillin-Resistant *Staphylococcus aureus* (MRSA). *Curr. Microbiol.* **2021**, *78*, 2194–2211. [CrossRef]
15. Aslam, B.; Wang, W.; Arshad, M.I.; Khurshid, M.; Muzammil, S.; Rasool, M.H.; Nisar, M.A.; Alvi, R.F.; Aslam, M.A.; Qamar, M.U.; et al. Antibiotic resistance: A rundown of a global crisis. *Infect. Drug Resist.* **2018**, *11*, 1645–1658. [CrossRef]
16. Hansen, M.P.; Hoffmann, T.C.; McCullough, A.R.; van Driel, M.L.; Del Mar, C.B. Antibiotic Resistance: What are the Opportunities for Primary Care in Alleviating the Crisis? *Front. Public Health* **2015**, *3*, 35–41. [CrossRef]
17. Sun, D.X.; Gao, W.; Hu, H.X.; Zhou, S.M. Why 90% of clinical drug development fails and how to improve it? *Acta Pharm. Sin. B* **2022**, *12*, 3049–3062. [CrossRef]
18. Mancuso, G.; Midiri, A.; Gerace, E.; Biondo, C. Bacterial Antibiotic Resistance: The Most Critical Pathogens. *Pathogens* **2021**, *10*, 1310. [CrossRef]
19. Miethke, M.; Pieroni, M.; Weber, T.; Bronstrup, M.; Hammann, P.; Halby, L.; Arimondo, P.B.; Glaser, P.; Aigle, B.; Bode, H.B.; et al. Towards the sustainable discovery and development of new antibiotics. *Nat. Rev. Chem.* **2021**, *5*, 726–749. [CrossRef]
20. Krishnamurthy, N.; Grimshaw, A.A.; Axson, S.A.; Choe, S.H.; Miller, J.E. Drug repurposing: A systematic review on root causes, barriers and facilitators. *BMC Health Serv. Res.* **2022**, *22*, 970. [CrossRef]
21. Mitchell, A.P. Fungal CO_2 sensing: A breath of fresh air. *Curr. Biol.* **2005**, *15*, R934–R9366. [CrossRef]
22. Michenkova, M.; Taki, S.; Blosser, M.C.; Hwang, H.J.; Kowatz, T.; Moss, F.J.; Occhipinti, R.; Qin, X.; Sen, S.; Shinn, E.; et al. Carbon dioxide transport across membranes. *Interface Focus* **2021**, *11*, 20200090–20200107. [CrossRef]
23. Cummins, E.P.; Selfridge, A.C.; Sporn, P.H.; Sznajder, J.I.; Taylor, C.T. Carbon dioxide-sensing in organisms and its implications for human disease. *Cell Mol. Life Sci.* **2014**, *71*, 831–845. [CrossRef]
24. Shimamura, T.; Watanabe, S.; Sasaki, S. Enhancement of enterotoxin production by carbon dioxide in Vibrio cholerae. *Infect. Immun.* **1985**, *49*, 455–456. [CrossRef]
25. Lotlikar, S.R.; Hnatusko, S.; Dickenson, N.E.; Choudhari, S.P.; Picking, W.L.; Patrauchan, M.A. Three functional beta-carbonic anhydrases in *Pseudomonas aeruginosa* PAO1: Role in survival in ambient air. *Microbiology* **2013**, *159 Pt 8*, 1748–1759. [CrossRef]
26. Supuran, C.T.; Capasso, C. A Highlight on the Inhibition of Fungal Carbonic Anhydrases as Drug Targets for the Antifungal Armamentarium. *Int. J. Mol. Sci.* **2021**, *22*, 4324. [CrossRef]
27. Capasso, C.; Supuran, C.T. Bacterial, fungal and protozoan carbonic anhydrases as drug targets. *Expert Opin. Ther. Targets* **2015**, *19*, 1689–1704. [CrossRef]
28. Campestre, C.; De Luca, V.; Carradori, S.; Grande, R.; Carginale, V.; Scaloni, A.; Supuran, C.T.; Capasso, C. Carbonic Anhydrases: New Perspectives on Protein Functional Role and Inhibition in *Helicobacter pylori*. *Front. Microbiol.* **2021**, *12*, 629163–629174. [CrossRef]
29. Supuran, C.T.; Capasso, C. An Overview of the Bacterial Carbonic Anhydrases. *Metabolites* **2017**, *7*, 56. [CrossRef]
30. Capasso, C.; Supuran, C.T. An overview of the alpha-, beta- and gamma-carbonic anhydrases from Bacteria: Can bacterial carbonic anhydrases shed new light on evolution of bacteria? *J. Enzym. Inhib. Med. Chem.* **2015**, *30*, 325–332. [CrossRef]
31. Nocentini, A.; Supuran, C.T.; Capasso, C. An overview on the recently discovered iota-carbonic anhydrases. *J. Enzym. Inhib. Med. Chem.* **2021**, *36*, 1988–1995. [CrossRef]
32. Supuran, C.T.; Capasso, C. New light on bacterial carbonic anhydrases phylogeny based on the analysis of signal peptide sequences. *J. Enzym. Inhib. Med. Chem.* **2016**, *31*, 1254–1260. [CrossRef]
33. Supuran, C.T.; Capasso, C. Biomedical applications of prokaryotic carbonic anhydrases. *Expert Opin. Ther. Pat.* **2018**, *28*, 745–754. [CrossRef]
34. Annunziato, G.; Angeli, A.; D'Alba, F.; Bruno, A.; Pieroni, M.; Vullo, D.; De Luca, V.; Capasso, C.; Supuran, C.T.; Costantino, G. Discovery of New Potential Anti-Infective Compounds Based on Carbonic Anhydrase Inhibitors by Rational Target-Focused Repurposing Approaches. *ChemMedChem* **2016**, *11*, 1904–1914. [CrossRef]
35. Ozensoy Guler, O.; Capasso, C.; Supuran, C.T. A magnificent enzyme superfamily: Carbonic anhydrases, their purification and characterization. *J. Enzym. Inhib. Med. Chem.* **2016**, *31*, 689–694. [CrossRef]
36. Del Prete, S.; Vullo, D.; De Luca, V.; Carginale, V.; Ferraroni, M.; Osman, S.M.; AlOthman, Z.; Supuran, C.T.; Capasso, C. Sulfonamide inhibition studies of the beta-carbonic anhydrase from the pathogenic bacterium *Vibrio cholerae*. *Bioorganic Med. Chem.* **2016**, *24*, 1115–1120. [CrossRef]
37. Del Prete, S.; De Luca, V.; De Simone, G.; Supuran, C.T.; Capasso, C. Cloning, expression and purification of the complete domain of the eta-carbonic anhydrase from *Plasmodium falciparum*. *J. Enzym. Inhib. Med. Chem.* **2016**, *31*, 54–59. [CrossRef]
38. Capasso, C.; Supuran, C.T. An Overview of the Carbonic Anhydrases from Two Pathogens of the Oral Cavity: *Streptococcus mutans* and *Porphyromonas gingivalis*. *Curr. Top. Med. Chem.* **2016**, *16*, 2359–2368. [CrossRef]
39. Del Prete, S.; Nocentini, A.; Supuran, C.T.; Capasso, C. Bacterial iota-carbonic anhydrase: A new active class of carbonic anhydrase identified in the genome of the Gram-negative bacterium *Burkholderia territorii*. *J. Enzym. Inhib. Med. Chem.* **2020**, *35*, 1060–1068. [CrossRef]
40. Pinard, M.A.; Lotlikar, S.R.; Boone, C.D.; Vullo, D.; Supuran, C.T.; Patrauchan, M.A.; McKenna, R. Structure and inhibition studies of a type II beta-carbonic anhydrase psCA3 from *Pseudomonas aeruginosa*. *Bioorganic Med. Chem.* **2015**, *23*, 4831–4838. [CrossRef]
41. Ferraroni, M.; Del Prete, S.; Vullo, D.; Capasso, C.; Supuran, C.T. Crystal structure and kinetic studies of a tetrameric type II beta-carbonic anhydrase from the pathogenic bacterium *Vibrio cholerae*. *Acta Crystallogr. Sect. D Biol. Crystallogr.* **2015**, *71 Pt 12*, 2449–2456. [CrossRef]

42. De Simone, G.; Monti, S.M.; Alterio, V.; Buonanno, M.; De Luca, V.; Rossi, M.; Carginale, V.; Supuran, C.T.; Capasso, C.; Di Fiore, A. Crystal structure of the most catalytically effective carbonic anhydrase enzyme known, SazCA from the thermophilic bacterium *Sulfurihydrogenibium azorense*. *Bioorganic Med. Chem. Lett.* **2015**, *25*, 2002–2006. [CrossRef]
43. Zolnowska, B.; Slawinski, J.; Pogorzelska, A.; Chojnacki, J.; Vullo, D.; Supuran, C.T. Carbonic anhydrase inhibitors. Synthesis, and molecular structure of novel series N-substituted N′-(2-arylmethylthio-4-chloro-5-methylbenzenesulfonyl)guanidines and their inhibition of human cytosolic isozymes I and II and the transmembrane tumor-associated isozymes IX and XII. *Eur. J. Med. Chem.* **2014**, *71*, 135–147.
44. De Luca, L.; Ferro, S.; Damiano, F.M.; Supuran, C.T.; Vullo, D.; Chimirri, A.; Gitto, R. Structure-based screening for the discovery of new carbonic anhydrase VII inhibitors. *Eur. J. Med. Chem.* **2014**, *71*, 105–111. [CrossRef]
45. Di Fiore, A.; Capasso, C.; De Luca, V.; Monti, S.M.; Carginale, V.; Supuran, C.T.; Scozzafava, A.; Pedone, C.; Rossi, M.; De Simone, G. X-ray structure of the first 'extremo-alpha-carbonic anhydrase', a dimeric enzyme from the thermophilic bacterium Sulfurihydrogenibium yellowstonense YO3AOP1. *Acta Crystallogr. Sect. D Biol. Crystallogr.* **2013**, *69 Pt 6*, 1150–1159. [CrossRef]
46. Supuran, C.T. Structure-based drug discovery of carbonic anhydrase inhibitors. *J. Enzym. Inhib. Med. Chem.* **2012**, *27*, 759–772. [CrossRef]
47. Supuran, C.T. Carbonic anhydrases—An overview. *Curr. Pharm. Des.* **2008**, *14*, 603–614. [CrossRef]
48. Hirakawa, Y.; Senda, M.; Fukuda, K.; Yu, H.Y.; Ishida, M.; Taira, M.; Kinbara, K.; Senda, T. Characterization of a novel type of carbonic anhydrase that acts without metal cofactors. *BMC Biol.* **2021**, *19*, 105. [CrossRef]
49. Supuran, C.T.; Capasso, C. Carbonic Anhydrase from Porphyromonas Gingivalis as a Drug Target. *Pathogens* **2017**, *6*, 30. [CrossRef]
50. Capasso, C.; Supuran, C.T. An Overview of the Selectivity and Efficiency of the Bacterial Carbonic Anhydrase Inhibitors. *Curr. Med. Chem.* **2015**, *22*, 2130–2139. [CrossRef]
51. Capasso, C.; Supuran, C.T. Sulfa and trimethoprim-like drugs—Antimetabolites acting as carbonic anhydrase, dihydropteroate synthase and dihydrofolate reductase inhibitors. *J. Enzym. Inhib. Med. Chem.* **2014**, *29*, 379–387. [CrossRef]
52. Capasso, C.; Supuran, C.T. Anti-infective carbonic anhydrase inhibitors: A patent and literature review. *Expert Opin. Ther. Pat.* **2013**, *23*, 693–704. [CrossRef] [PubMed]
53. James, P.; Isupov, M.N.; Sayer, C.; Saneei, V.; Berg, S.; Lioliou, M.; Kotlar, H.K.; Littlechild, J.A. The structure of a tetrameric alpha-carbonic anhydrase from *Thermovibrio ammonificans* reveals a core formed around intermolecular disulfides that contribute to its thermostability. *Acta Crystallogr. Sect. D Biol. Crystallogr.* **2014**, *70 Pt 10*, 2607–2618. [CrossRef]
54. Huang, S.; Xue, Y.; Sauer-Eriksson, E.; Chirica, L.; Lindskog, S.; Jonsson, B.H. Crystal structure of carbonic anhydrase from *Neisseria gonorrhoeae* and its complex with the inhibitor acetazolamide. *J. Mol. Biol.* **1998**, *283*, 301–310. [CrossRef] [PubMed]
55. Kisker, C.; Schindelin, H.; Alber, B.E.; Ferry, J.G.; Rees, D.C. A left-hand beta-helix revealed by the crystal structure of a carbonic anhydrase from the archaeon *Methanosarcina thermophila*. *EMBO J.* **1996**, *15*, 2323–2330. [CrossRef] [PubMed]
56. De Simone, G.; Di Fiore, A.; Capasso, C.; Supuran, C.T. The zinc coordination pattern in the eta-carbonic anhydrase from *Plasmodium falciparum* is different from all other carbonic anhydrase genetic families. *Bioorganic Med. Chem. Lett.* **2015**, *25*, 1385–1389. [CrossRef] [PubMed]
57. De Luca, V.; Petreni, A.; Carginale, V.; Scaloni, A.; Supuran, C.T.; Capasso, C. Effect of amino acids and amines on the activity of the recombinant iota-carbonic anhydrase from the Gram-negative bacterium *Burkholderia territorii*. *J. Enzym. Inhib. Med. Chem.* **2021**, *36*, 1000–1006. [CrossRef] [PubMed]
58. De Luca, V.; Petreni, A.; Nocentini, A.; Scaloni, A.; Supuran, C.T.; Capasso, C. Effect of Sulfonamides and Their Structurally Related Derivatives on the Activity of iota-Carbonic Anhydrase from *Burkholderia territorii*. *Int. J. Mol. Sci.* **2021**, *22*, 571. [CrossRef]
59. Petreni, A.; De Luca, V.; Scaloni, A.; Nocentini, A.; Capasso, C.; Supuran, C.T. Anion inhibition studies of the Zn(II)-bound iota-carbonic anhydrase from the Gram-negative bacterium *Burkholderia territorii*. *J. Enzym. Inhib. Med. Chem.* **2021**, *36*, 372–376. [CrossRef]
60. Supuran, C.T.; Capasso, C. Antibacterial carbonic anhydrase inhibitors: An update on the recent literature. *Expert Opin. Ther. Pat.* **2020**, *30*, 963–982. [CrossRef]
61. Kusian, B.; Sultemeyer, D.; Bowien, B. Carbonic anhydrase is essential for growth of *Ralstonia eutropha* at ambient CO_2 concentrations. *J. Bacteriol.* **2002**, *184*, 5018–5026. [CrossRef] [PubMed]
62. Cronk, J.D.; Endrizzi, J.A.; Cronk, M.R.; O'Neill, J.W.; Zhang, K.Y. Crystal structure of *E. coli* beta-carbonic anhydrase, an enzyme with an unusual pH-dependent activity. *Protein Sci.* **2001**, *10*, 911–922. [CrossRef] [PubMed]
63. Merlin, C.; Masters, M.; McAteer, S.; Coulson, A. Why is carbonic anhydrase essential to *Escherichia coli*? *J. Bacteriol.* **2003**, *185*, 6415–6424. [CrossRef] [PubMed]
64. Nishimori, I.; Minakuchi, T.; Maresca, A.; Carta, F.; Scozzafava, A.; Supuran, C.T. The beta-carbonic anhydrases from *Mycobacterium tuberculosis* as drug targets. *Curr. Pharm. Des.* **2010**, *16*, 3300–3309. [CrossRef] [PubMed]
65. Kohler, S.; Ouahrani-Bettache, S.; Winum, J.Y. Brucella suis carbonic anhydrases and their inhibitors: Towards alternative antibiotics? *J. Enzym. Inhib. Med. Chem.* **2017**, *32*, 683–687. [CrossRef] [PubMed]
66. Singh, S.; Supuran, C.T. 3D-QSAR CoMFA studies on sulfonamide inhibitors of the Rv3588c beta-carbonic anhydrase from *Mycobacterium tuberculosis* and design of not yet synthesized new molecules. *J. Enzym. Inhib. Med. Chem.* **2014**, *29*, 449–455. [CrossRef]

67. Ceruso, M.; Vullo, D.; Scozzafava, A.; Supuran, C.T. Sulfonamides incorporating fluorine and 1,3,5-triazine moieties are effective inhibitors of three beta-class carbonic anhydrases from *Mycobacterium tuberculosis*. *J. Enzym. Inhib. Med. Chem.* **2014**, *29*, 686–689. [CrossRef]
68. Carta, F.; Maresca, A.; Covarrubias, A.S.; Mowbray, S.L.; Jones, T.A.; Supuran, C.T. Carbonic anhydrase inhibitors. Characterization and inhibition studies of the most active beta-carbonic anhydrase from *Mycobacterium tuberculosis*, Rv3588c. *Bioorganic Med. Chem. Lett.* **2009**, *19*, 6649–6654. [CrossRef]
69. Modak, J.K.; Tikhomirova, A.; Gorrell, R.J.; Rahman, M.M.; Kotsanas, D.; Korman, T.M.; Garcia-Bustos, J.; Kwok, T.; Ferrero, R.L.; Supuran, C.T.; et al. Anti-Helicobacter pylori activity of ethoxzolamide. *J. Enzym. Inhib. Med. Chem.* **2019**, *34*, 1660–1667. [CrossRef]
70. Ronci, M.; Del Prete, S.; Puca, V.; Carradori, S.; Carginale, V.; Muraro, R.; Mincione, G.; Aceto, A.; Sisto, F.; Supuran, C.T.; et al. Identification and characterization of the alpha-CA in the outer membrane vesicles produced by *Helicobacter pylori*. *J. Enzym. Inhib. Med. Chem.* **2019**, *34*, 189–195. [CrossRef]
71. Buzas, G.M. Helicobacter pylori—2010. *Orv. Hetil.* **2010**, *151*, 2003–2010. [CrossRef] [PubMed]
72. Abuaita, B.H.; Withey, J.H. Bicarbonate Induces *Vibrio cholerae* virulence gene expression by enhancing ToxT activity. *Infect. Immun.* **2009**, *77*, 4111–4120. [CrossRef] [PubMed]
73. Rollenhagen, C.; Bumann, D. Salmonella enterica highly expressed genes are disease specific. *Infect. Immun.* **2006**, *74*, 1649–1660. [CrossRef]
74. Nishimori, I.; Minakuchi, T.; Vullo, D.; Scozzafava, A.; Supuran, C.T. Inhibition studies of the beta-carbonic anhydrases from the bacterial pathogen *Salmonella enterica* serovar Typhimurium with sulfonamides and sulfamates. *Bioorganic Med. Chem.* **2011**, *19*, 5023–5030. [CrossRef]
75. Vullo, D.; Nishimori, I.; Minakuchi, T.; Scozzafava, A.; Supuran, C.T. Inhibition studies with anions and small molecules of two novel beta-carbonic anhydrases from the bacterial pathogen *Salmonella enterica* serovar Typhimurium. *Bioorganic Med. Chem. Lett.* **2011**, *21*, 3591–3595. [CrossRef]
76. Lotlikar, S.R.; Kayastha, B.B.; Vullo, D.; Khanam, S.S.; Braga Reygan, E.; Murray, A.B.; McKenna, R.; Supuran, C.T.; Patrauchan, M.A. *Pseudomonas aeruginosa* β-carbonic anhydrase, psCA1, is required for calcium deposition and contributes to virulence. *Cell Calcium.* **2019**, *84*, 102080–102095. [CrossRef] [PubMed]
77. Guragain, M.; King, M.M.; Williamson, K.S.; Pérez-Osorio, A.C.; Akiyama, T.; Khanam, S.; Patrauchan, M.A.; Franklin, M.J. The *Pseudomonas aeruginosa* PAO1 Two-Component Regulator CarSR Regulates Calcium Homeostasis and Calcium-Induced Virulence Factor Production through Its Regulatory Targets CarO and CarP. *J. Bacteriol.* **2016**, *198*, 951–963. [CrossRef] [PubMed]
78. Supuran, C.T. Advances in structure-based drug discovery of carbonic anhydrase inhibitors. *Expert Opin. Drug Discov.* **2017**, *12*, 61–88. [CrossRef]
79. Supuran, C.T. Structure and function of carbonic anhydrases. *Biochem. J.* **2016**, *473*, 2023–2032. [CrossRef]
80. Supuran, C.T. Carbonic anhydrase inhibition and the management of neuropathic pain. *Expert Rev. Neurother* **2016**, *16*, 961–968. [CrossRef]
81. Supuran, C.T. Drug interaction considerations in the therapeutic use of carbonic anhydrase inhibitors. *Expert Opin. Drug Metab. Toxicol.* **2016**, *12*, 423–431. [CrossRef] [PubMed]
82. Del Prete, S.; Vullo, D.; Osman, S.M.; AlOthman, Z.; Supuran, C.T.; Capasso, C. Sulfonamide inhibition profiles of the beta-carbonic anhydrase from the pathogenic bacterium *Francisella tularensis* responsible of the febrile illness tularemia. *Bioorganic Med. Chem.* **2017**, *25*, 3555–3561. [CrossRef] [PubMed]
83. Vullo, D.; Del Prete, S.; Di Fonzo, P.; Carginale, V.; Donald, W.A.; Supuran, C.T.; Capasso, C. Comparison of the Sulfonamide Inhibition Profiles of the beta- and gamma-Carbonic Anhydrases from the Pathogenic Bacterium *Burkholderia pseudomallei*. *Molecules* **2017**, *22*, 421. [CrossRef] [PubMed]
84. Del Prete, S.; Vullo, D.; De Luca, V.; Carginale, V.; Osman, S.M.; AlOthman, Z.; Supuran, C.T.; Capasso, C. Comparison of the sulfonamide inhibition profiles of the alpha-, beta- and gamma-carbonic anhydrases from the pathogenic bacterium *Vibrio cholerae*. *Bioorganic Med. Chem. Lett.* **2016**, *26*, 1941–1946. [CrossRef]
85. Dedeoglu, N.; DeLuca, V.; Isik, S.; Yildirim, H.; Kockar, F.; Capasso, C.; Supuran, C.T. Sulfonamide inhibition study of the beta-class carbonic anhydrase from the caries producing pathogen *Streptococcus mutans*. *Bioorganic Med. Chem. Lett.* **2015**, *25*, 2291–2297. [CrossRef]
86. Cau, Y.; Mori, M.; Supuran, C.T.; Botta, M. Mycobacterial carbonic anhydrase inhibition with phenolic acids and esters: Kinetic and computational investigations. *Org. Biomol. Chem.* **2016**, *14*, 8322–8330. [CrossRef]
87. Modak, J.K.; Liu, Y.C.; Supuran, C.T.; Roujeinikova, A. Structure-Activity Relationship for Sulfonamide Inhibition of *Helicobacter pylori* alpha-Carbonic Anhydrase. *J. Med. Cheml* **2016**, *59*, 11098–11109. [CrossRef]
88. Supuran, C.T. Bortezomib inhibits bacterial and fungal beta-carbonic anhydrases. *Bioorganic Med. Chem* **2016**, *24*, 4406–4409. [CrossRef]
89. Supuran, C.T. Legionella pneumophila Carbonic Anhydrases: Underexplored Antibacterial Drug Targets. *Pathogens* **2016**, *5*, 44. [CrossRef]
90. Vullo, D.; Kumar, R.S.S.; Scozzafava, A.; Ferry, J.G.; Supuran, C.T. Sulphonamide inhibition studies of the beta-carbonic anhydrase from the bacterial pathogen *Clostridium perfringens*. *J. Enzym. Inhib. Med. Chem.* **2018**, *33*, 31–36. [CrossRef]

91. Shahidzadeh, R.; Opekun, A.; Shiotani, A.; Graham, D.Y. Effect of the carbonic anhydrase inhibitor, acetazolamide, on *Helicobacter pylori* infection in vivo: A pilot study. *Helicobacter* **2005**, *10*, 136–138. [CrossRef] [PubMed]
92. Buzas, G.M. *Helicobacter pylori*—2021. *Orv. Hetil.* **2021**, *162*, 1275–1282. [CrossRef] [PubMed]
93. De Luca, V.; Carginale, V.; Supuran, C.T.; Capasso, C. The gram-negative bacterium Escherichia coli as a model for testing the effect of carbonic anhydrase inhibition on bacterial growth. *J. Enzym. Inhib. Med. Chem.* **2022**, *37*, 2092–2098. [CrossRef] [PubMed]
94. Del Prete, S.; Bua, S.; Supuran, C.T.; Capasso, C. Escherichia coli gamma-carbonic anhydrase: Characterisation and effects of simple aromatic/heterocyclic sulphonamide inhibitors. *J. Enzym. Inhib. Med. Chem.* **2020**, *35*, 1545–1554. [CrossRef]
95. Del Prete, S.; De Luca, V.; Bua, S.; Nocentini, A.; Carginale, V.; Supuran, C.T.; Capasso, C. The Effect of Substituted Benzene-Sulfonamides and Clinically Licensed Drugs on the Catalytic Activity of CynT2, a Carbonic Anhydrase Crucial for *Escherichia coli* Life Cycle. *Int. J. Mol. Sci.* **2020**, *21*, 4175. [CrossRef]
96. Kaur, J.; Cao, X.; Abutaleb, N.S.; Elkashif, A.; Graboski, A.L.; Krabill, A.D.; AbdelKhalek, A.H.; An, W.; Bhardwaj, A.; Seleem, M.N.; et al. Optimization of Acetazolamide-Based Scaffold as Potent Inhibitors of Vancomycin-Resistant Enterococcus. *J. Med. Chem.* **2020**, *63*, 9540–9562. [CrossRef]
97. Abutaleb, N.S.; Elhassanny, A.E.M.; Flaherty, D.P.; Seleem, M.N. In vitro and in vivo activities of the carbonic anhydrase inhibitor, dorzolamide, against vancomycin-resistant enterococci. *Peerj* **2021**, *9*, e11059. [CrossRef]
98. An, W.W.; Holly, K.J.; Nocentini, A.; Imhoff, R.D.; Hewitt, C.S.; Abutaleb, N.S.; Cao, X.F.; Seleem, M.N.; Supuran, C.T.; Flaherty, D.P. Structure-activity relationship studies for inhibitors for vancomycin-resistant Enterococcus and human carbonic anhydrases. *J. Enzym. Inhib. Med. Chem.* **2022**, *37*, 1838–1844. [CrossRef]
99. Abutaleb, N.S.; Elkashif, A.; Flaherty, D.P.; Seleem, M.N. In Vivo Antibacterial Activity of Acetazolamide. *Antimicrob. Agents Chemother.* **2021**, *65*, 65–70. [CrossRef]
100. Abutaleb, N.S.; Elhassanny, A.E.M.; Seleem, M.N. In vivo efficacy of acetazolamide in a mouse model of *Neisseria gonorrhoeae* infection. *Microb. Pathog.* **2022**, *164*, 105454–105458. [CrossRef]
101. Hewitt, C.S.; Abutaleb, N.S.; Elhassanny, A.E.M.; Nocentini, A.; Cao, X.F.; Amos, D.P.; Youse, M.S.; Holly, K.J.; Marapaka, A.K.; An, W.W.; et al. Structure-Activity Relationship Studies of Acetazolamide-Based Carbonic Anhydrase Inhibitors with Activity against *Neisseria gonorrhoeae*. *ACS Infect. Dis.* **2021**, *7*, 1969–1984. [CrossRef] [PubMed]
102. Portela, M.B.; Barboza, C.M.; da Silva, E.M.; de Moraes, D.C.; Simão, R.A.; de Souza, C.R.; Cardoso, V.D.S.; Ferreira-Pereira, A.; Vermelho, A.B.; Supuran, C.T. Dentine biomodification by sulphonamides pre-treatment: Bond strength, proteolytic inhibition, and antimicrobial activity. *J. Enzym. Inhib. Med. Chem.* **2023**, *38*, 319–329. [CrossRef] [PubMed]
103. Lomelino, C.L.; Supuran, C.T.; McKenna, R. Non-Classical Inhibition of Carbonic Anhydrase. *Int. J. Mol. Sci.* **2016**, *17*, 1150. [CrossRef] [PubMed]

Disclaimer/Publisher's Note: The statements, opinions and data contained in all publications are solely those of the individual author(s) and contributor(s) and not of MDPI and/or the editor(s). MDPI and/or the editor(s) disclaim responsibility for any injury to people or property resulting from any ideas, methods, instructions or products referred to in the content.

MDPI AG
Grosspeteranlage 5
4052 Basel
Switzerland
Tel.: +41 61 683 77 34
www.mdpi.com

Antibiotics Editorial Office
E-mail: antibiotics@mdpi.com
www.mdpi.com/journal/antibiotics

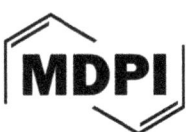

Disclaimer/Publisher's Note: The statements, opinions and data contained in all publications are solely those of the individual author(s) and contributor(s) and not of MDPI and/or the editor(s). MDPI and/or the editor(s) disclaim responsibility for any injury to people or property resulting from any ideas, methods, instructions or products referred to in the content.

www.ingramcontent.com/pod-product-compliance
Lightning Source LLC
LaVergne TN
LVHW070408100526
838202LV00014B/1412